Oxford Medical Publications

Cancer in children:
clinical management

Cancer in children:
clinical management

Fourth Edition

Edited by
P.A. Voûte
Department of Paediatric Oncology, Emma Kinderziekenhuis, Academic Medical Center, University of Amsterdam, The Netherlands

C. Kalifa
Department of Paediatric Oncology, Institut Gustave Roussy, Villejuif, France

and

A. Barrett
Department of Radiation Oncology, Beatson Oncology Centre, Western Infirmary, Glasgow, U.K.

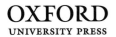
OXFORD
UNIVERSITY PRESS

OXFORD
UNIVERSITY PRESS

Great Clarendon Street, Oxford OX2 6DP

Oxford University Press is a department of the University of Oxford.
It furthers the University's objective of excellence in research, scholarship,
and education by publishing worldwide in

Oxford New York

Athens Auckland Bangkok Bogotá Beunos Aires Calcutta
Cape Town Chennai Dar es Salaam Delhi Florence Hong Kong Istanbul
Karachi Kuala Lumpur Madrid Melbourne Mexico City Mumbai
Nairobi Paris São Paulo Singapore Taipei Tokyo Toronto Warsaw
with associated companies in Berlin Ibadan

Oxford is a registered trade mark of Oxford University Press
in the UK and in certain other countries

Published in the United States
by Oxford University Press Inc., New York

© P. A. Voûte, C. Kalifa, A. Barrett and the contributors listed on p. xi, 1998

The moral rights of the author have been asserted

Database right Oxford University Press (maker)

First edition published 1975
Second edition published 1986
Third edition published 1992
Fourth edition published 1998
Reprinted 1999, 2001

A catalogue record for this book is available from the British Library

Library of Congress Cataloging in Publication Data
Cancer in children : clinical management / edited by P. A. Voûte, C. Kalifa,
and A. Barrett.—4th ed.
(Oxford medical publications)
Incluces bibliographical references and index.
1. Tumours in children. I. Voûte, P. A. (Paul Antoine), 1906–
II. Kalifa, C. (Chantal) III. Barrett, Ann. IV. Series.
[DNLM: 1. Neoplasms–in infancy & childhood. 2. Neoplasms—
therapy. QZ275 C2146 1998]
RC281.C4C37 1998
618.92′994–dc21
DNLM/DLC
for Library of Congress 97–34660 CIP

ISBN 0 19 262897 6

Printed in Great Britain by Biddles Ltd, *www.biddles.co.uk*

Preface

Since the last edition of this book, published in 1992, advances in molecular biology have taught us much about the mechanisms of development of malignant disease in children. Progress in the treatment of these diseases has continued—not with the spectacular improvements which were seen in the 1970s, but with continuing refinement of treatment approaches to maintain excellent cure rates for many tumours and to minimize the acute and long-term sequelae which cause us, our patients, and their families so much concern. We hope this fourth edition will serve as a useful introduction to this fascinating, fruitful, and frustrating branch of medicine.

We should like to thank all who have helped with the preparation of this book, but especially Tres Stafford for her invaluable assistance, and Annette Thain for her patience in obtaining and checking literature references.

A. Barrett   Glasgow, U.K.
C. Kalifa   Villejuif, France
P.A. Voûte   Amsterdam, The Netherlands
February 1998

Contents

Introduction

The progress which has been achieved in the treatment of childhood cancer is in many ways a remarkable success story. From being an almost lethal disease 20 – 30 years ago, more than 70% of children with cancer can now be offered treatment with cure as the most likely outcome. This progress is the result of basic research and the testing of new knowledge through multi-institutional and multi-national clinical trials.

However, this progress has its dark side. For any family, the diagnosis of cancer in one of its children turns its life upside down. The diagnostic process is complicated, the therapy very demanding or even life-threatening, and the possibility of relapse a constant threat to the child and family. The problems of long-term sequelae are a matter for continuing concern. Furthermore, it remains a sad fact that in spite of all the progress made, childhood cancer is still the leading cause of death from disease in children above 1 year of age in industrialized countries. The remaining third that we are still unable to cure with present strategies remains a tremendous challenge.

In fact it can be said that we have three important challenges: first we need to find effective therapy for the third whom we cannot cure with current strategies; secondly we want to get rid of long-term sequelae in the patients we are able to cure today; and thirdly we would like to spread the knowledge of effective treatment of childhood cancer to areas and countries where no such service is available. To meet these challenges, we need to recruit more people and more countries into the battle. An up-to-date, comprehensive, but not overwhelmingly complex textbook is a necessary prerequisite for such recruitment, and for people already active in the field to continuously update themselves.

Cancer in Children has for many of us represented the introduction into this exciting field and is already a 'classic'. We should be grateful to the editors who have taken on the work of editing this fourth edition. I hope that this up-to-date review will attract more scientists and clinicians to our field, will help to spread current knowledge in this area to new groups and countries, and will provide an update for the elderly amongst us.

The International Society of Paediatric Oncology (SIOP), of which I have the honour of being the current President, is happy to endorse this book and to recommend it for use alongside the teaching courses in Paediatric Oncology organized by SIOP and the European School of Oncology.

Sverre Lie
President of the
International Society
of Paediatric Oncology

1998
Oslo, Norway

Abbreviations

AFP	alpha-fetoprotein
AIDS	Acquired Immune Deficiency Syndrome
BFM	Berlin Frankfurt Münster Group
BMT	Bone Marrow Transplantation
BWTSG	Brazilian Wilms' Tumour Study Group
CCG	Children's Cancer Group
CESS	Co-operative Ewing's Sarcoma Study
CHOP	Children's Hospital of Philadelphia
CMV	Cytomegalovirus
EBV	Epstein-Barr Virus
EFS	Event-free survival
ENSG	European Neuroblastoma Study Group
FAB	French American British classification of leukaemias
G-CSF	Granulocyte-Colony Stimulating Factor
GPOH	German Paediatric Oncology Haematology Group
HCG	Human choriogonadotrophin
HSV	Herpes Simplex Virus
IARC	International Agency for Research on Cancer
IESS	Intergroup Ewing's Sarcoma Study
LESG	Late Effects Study Group
LNESG	Localized Neuroblastoma European Study Group
NOHPO	Nordic Organization of Haematology and Paediatric Oncology
NWTS	National Wilms' Tumour Study
OS	Overall survival
POG	Paediatric Oncology Group
SIOP	International Society of Paediatric Oncology
SMN	Second malignant neoplasm
UKCCSG	United Kingdom Children's Cancer Study Group
VZV	Varicella-Zoster Virus
WBC	white blood cell count
WT	Wilms' Tumour

Contributors

F Aubier Department of Pediatric Oncology, Institut Gustave-Roussy, Paris, France

A Barrett Beatson Oncology Centre, Western Infirmary, Glasgow, UK

H Budka Department of Neuropathology, University Hospital, Vienna, Austria

M Büyükpamukçu Department of Paediatric Oncology, Hacettepe University, Ankara, Turkey

B de Camargo Department of Paediatric Oncology, A C Camargo Hospital, Sao Paulo, Brazil

H Caron Department of Paediatric Oncology, Emma Kinderziekenhuis, Academic Medical Center, University of Amsterdam, Netherlands

G Chantada Hemato-oncology Unit, Hospital de Pediatria, Buenos Aires, Argentina

A W Craft University of Newcastle upon Tyne, Newcastle, UK

Th. Czech Department of Neurosurgery, University Hospital, Vienna, Austria

K Dieckmann Department of Radiology and Radiobiology, University Hospital, Vienna

B Dockhorn- Dworniczak Department of Pathology, University Hospital, Münster, Germany

G J Draper Childhood Cancer Research Group, University of Oxford, UK

H Gadner Department of Paediatric Haematology, St Anna Children's Hospital, Vienna

M Gaze The Meyerstein Institute of Oncology, Middlesex Hospital, UK

N Grois Department of Paediatric Haematology, St Anna Children's Hospital, Vienna

G Gustafsson Department of Paediatrics, Karolinska Sjukhuset, Stockholm, Sweden

H Ikeda Department of Surgery, Gunma Children's Medical Centre, Japan

H Jürgens Department of Paediatric Haematology/Oncology, University of Münster, Germany

A Lasorella Division of Paediatric Oncology, Catholic University, Rome, Italy

J Lemerle Department of Paediatric Oncology, Institut Gustave-Roussy, Paris, France

S O Lie   Department of Paediatrics, Rikshospitalet, The National Hospital, Oslo, Norway

R Mastrangelo   Division of Paediatric Oncology, Catholic University, Rome, Italy

O Oberlin   Department of Paediatric Oncology, Institut Gustave-Roussy, Paris, France

A Pearson   Department of Child Health, Royal Victoria Infirmary, Newcastle upon Tyne, UK

F Pein   Department of Paediatric Oncology, Institut Gustave-Roussy, Paris, France

R Pötter   Department of Radiology and Radiobiology, University Hospital, Vienna, Austria

R Riccardi   Division of Paediatric Oncology, Catholic University, Rome, Italy

E Schvartzman   Hemato-oncology Unit, Hospital de Pediatria, Buenos Aires, Argentina

M Schwab   German Cancer Research Center, Cytogenetics Division, Germany

I Slavc   Department of Paediatrics, University Hospital, Vienna, Austria

L A Smets   Department of Experimental Therapy, Netherlands Cancer Institute, Amsterdam, The Netherlands

M C G Stevens   Department of Oncology, Birmingham Children's Hospital, Birmingham, UK

C A Stiller   Childhood Cancer Research Group, University of Oxford, UK

Y Tsuchida   Department of Surgery, Gunma Children's Medical Center, Japan

F de Vathaire   Department of Statistics and Epidemiology, Institut Gustave-Roussy, Paris, France

P A Voûte   Department of Paediatric Oncology, Emma Kinderziekenhuis, Academic Medical Center, University of Amsterdam, Netherlands

S Weitzman   Division of Haematology/Oncology, Hospital for Sick Children, Ontario, Canada

D Wimberger-Prayer   Department of Radiodiagnosis, University Hospital, Vienna, Austria

W Winkelmann   Department of Orthopaedics, University Hospital, Münster, Germany

M Yule   Department of Oncology, Royal Hospital for Sick Children, Glasgow, UK

1 The epidemiology of cancer in children

C.A. Stiller and G.J. Draper

Introduction

Although childhood cancer is rare, accounting for under 1% of all cancer in industrialized countries, it is of great scientific interest for a number of reasons. Several types of cancer are virtually unique to childhood, whereas the carcinomas most frequently seen in adults—those of lung, female breast, stomach, large bowel, and prostate—are extremely rare among children. Some of the most striking progress in cancer treatment has been made in paediatric oncology. Investigation of childhood tumours has led to major advances in the understanding of the genetic aetiology of cancer. In this chapter we consider the classification of childhood cancer, the principles of cancer registration, incidence and survival rates, and aetiology.

Classification

The great majority of malignant neoplasms occurring in adults are carcinomas, and so the International Classification of Diseases, by which cancers other than leukaemias, lymphomas, and melanomas are classified purely by site of origin, is reasonably satisfactory for the presentation of their incidence rates. In contrast, childhood cancers exhibit great histological diversity, and some types of tumour can arise in many different primary sites. It is therefore more appropriate for childhood cancers to be classified according to histology. A special classification was accordingly devised (Birch and Marsden 1987), with groups defined by the codes for morphology in addition to topography in the International Classification of Diseases for Oncology (ICD-O). This was used for the monograph *International Incidence of Childhood Cancer* (Parkin *et al.* 1988) and became the standard classification for reports on the descriptive epidemiology of childhood cancer. A modified version has recently been published as the *International Classification of Childhood Cancer* (Kramarova *et al.* 1996), with groups defined according to the codes in the second edition of ICD-O. This is now recommended for the presentation of incidence rates, and will be used for a forthcoming second volume of *International Incidence of Childhood Cancer*. The classification contains 12 main diagnostic groups, most of which are in turn divided into subgroups. The main groups are: I leukaemia; II lymphoma and reticuloendothelial neoplasms; III central nervous system and miscellaneous intracranial and intraspinal neoplasms; IV sympathetic nervous system tumours; V retinoblastoma; VI renal tumours; VII hepatic tumours; VIII malignant bone tumours; IX soft-tissue sarcomas; X germ-cell, trophoblastic, and other gonadal neoplasms; XI carcinoma and other malignant epithelial neoplasms; XII other and unspecified malignant neoplasms. Most of these groups are limited to malignant neoplasms, but there are two exceptions. Benign and unspecified intracranial and intraspinal tumours, including choroid plexus papilloma, ganglioglioma, non-malignant gliomas, craniopharyngioma, pituitary adenoma, pinealoma, meningioma, and tumours of unspecified type are included in group III because they are ascertained by many cancer registries. For the same reason, non-malignant intracranial and intraspinal germ-cell tumours are also included (in group X).

Childhood cancer registration

The aim of a cancer registry is to collect information on all cases of cancer occurring within a geographically defined population. Sometimes there are insufficient resources to maintain a population-based registry, but it may nevertheless be possible to collect similar data on all cases seen in one or more hospitals or pathology departments. In the absence of population-based data, these series can still yield much useful information, and several population-based cancer registries trace their origins to hospital or pathology series. The amount of data collected on each case varies enormously between registries, but the minimum consists of the patient's name, sex, date of diagnosis and age at diagnosis, and sufficient information on the primary site and histological type of the neoplasm for it to be coded according to whatever system is used, preferably ICD-O. Most registries collect the patient's date of birth where known, as this is particularly useful for linking data on the same patient from different sources, and for detecting duplicates. The basis of diagnosis is also usually recorded, at least to the extent of whether there was histological verification. There can be many different sources of information, of which the most frequently used are clinical records, pathology records, death certificates, and other cancer registries. The registration data should be checked for internal consistency. Computer programs which do this for age, sex, primary site, and histological type are included in the IARC Technical Report, *International Classification of Childhood Cancer* (Kramarova *et al.* 1996). The IARC monograph, *Cancer Registration: Principles and Methods* (Jensen *et al.* 1991), gives detailed information on many aspects of setting up and maintaining a cancer registry. The operating methods of many individual registries are described in *International Incidence of Childhood Cancer* (Parkin *et al.* 1988).

Population-based cancer registries now cover the whole or part of more than 50 countries. As childhood cancer accounts for a very small proportion of all cancer, registries which restrict their coverage to children are able to collect more detailed information on each case. There are population-based national childhood cancer registries in Great Britain, Germany, Hungary, and Australia, and a national childhood leukaemia registry in the Netherlands. Regional childhood cancer registries operate in the Greater Delaware Valley in the USA, in several regions of Great Britain and France, and in the provinces of Torino in Italy and Valencia in Spain. In many countries, including those such as the USA, Japan, and Spain, where there is no national population-based cancer registration, registers of patients are maintained by national organizations of paediatric oncologists or by clinical trial groups. The registry in Germany is operated in particularly close collaboration with clinical trials, using a common follow-up system.

Incidence

Incidence in Great Britain

Table 1.1 gives numbers of cases and incidence rates for the 12 main groups and principal sub-groups of the International Classification of Childhood Cancer in England and Wales during 1981–90. The pattern of incidence is typical of that found among the mainly White populations of industrialized countries in Europe, North America, and Oceania, though some of the rates are towards the lower end of the usual range for these populations. The total age-standardized annual incidence was 122 per million children, giving a cumulative risk of 1 in 564 of developing cancer during the first 15 years of life. About a third of all childhood cancers are leukaemias, predominantly acute lymphoblastic leukaemia (ALL). Brain and spinal tumours are the second most common diagnostic group, accounting for 20–25% of registrations, astrocytomas being the most frequent histological type. Lymphomas account for 10% of registrations, and non-Hodgkin lymphoma (NHL) has a somewhat higher incidence than Hodgkin's disease. Neuroblastoma and Wilms' tumour, the two most frequent embryonal tumours of childhood, each account for 6–7% of registrations, as do soft-tissue sarcomas, while retinoblastoma accounts for 3%. Nearly all of the remaining cases are bone sarcomas, germ-cell tumours, and epithelial tumours. Of this last group, malignant melanoma, skin carcinoma, and thyroid carcinoma are the most frequent, but none of them accounts for more than 1% of all childhood cancer.

Within childhood, the total incidence of cancer is highest, over 150 per million, in the first 5 years of life, compared with 90–100 at age 5–14. The age-incidence distribution varies considerably between diagnostic groups. There is a marked peak in the incidence of ALL at age 2–3 years. Early age peaks are also found for all of the distinctive embryonal tumours. The highest incidence of neuroblastoma, retinoblastoma, and hepatoblastoma is in the first year of life, but for Wilms' tumour the peak occurs slightly later. In contrast, Hodgkin's disease and bone sarcomas are virtually never seen before the age of two, and their incidence increases steeply throughout childhood and adolescence. Among boys, the incidence of testicular germ-cell tumours is highest in early childhood, and the start of the sharp increase in incidence during adolescence and early adulthood is barely noticeable before the age of 15; among girls, ovarian germ-cell tumours are rare until the postpubertal increase, which begins at an earlier age than it does among boys.

International variations

There is considerable systematic variation in the many types of childhood cancer between different regions of the world and between ethnic groups in the same country (Parkin *et al.* 1988; Stiller and Parkin 1996).

Leukaemia

In the USA, Blacks have a substantially lower incidence of ALL and the early childhood peak is very much attenuated. By contrast, there is little evidence of ethnic variations in the incidence of childhood leukaemia in the UK; in particular the pattern of occurrence of ALL among both Blacks and children of South Asian ethnic origin is very similar to that among Whites, with a marked peak in early childhood. In the former socialist countries of central and eastern Europe,

Table 1.1 Registration rates for childhood cancers in England and Wales, 1981–90

Diagnostic group	Total registrations	Annual rates per million for age groups			Age-standardized	Cumulative	Sex ratio M/F
		0–4	5–9	10–14			
All cancers	11 355	166.5	93.1	95.3	122.2	1774	1.2
I Leukaemia	3705	62.7	31.1	22.5	40.8	581	1.2
Lymphoid	2959	51.5	25.7	15.7	32.8	464	1.2
Acute non-lymphocytic	596	8.4	4.3	5.8	6.3	92	0.9
Chronic myeloid	88	1.4	0.7	0.6	1.0	13	1.9
Other specified	8	0.1	0.1	0.1	0.1	1	–
Unspecified	54	1.1	0.2	0.3	0.6	8	0.8
II Lymphoma	1134	6.1	11.3	17.7	11.2	175	2.2
Hodgkin's disease	489	1.1	4.1	9.8	4.6	75	2.1
Non-Hodgkin	559	4.2	6.4	6.9	5.7	87	2.3
Burkitt's	46	0.4	0.6	0.4	0.5	7	3.5
Other reticuloendothelial	17	0.2	0.1	0.2	0.2	2	–
Unspecified	23	0.2	0.2	0.3	0.2	3	–
III Brain and spinal	2549	29.6	28.0	22.3	27.0	399	1.1
Ependymoma	275	4.7	1.9	1.9	3.0	43	1.3
Astrocytoma	977	10.7	10.8	9.1	10.3	153	1.0
Primitive neuroectodermal	540	7.1	6.5	3.4	5.8	85	1.6
Other glioma	388	3.7	5.2	3.4	4.1	60	1.0
Miscellaneous	219	1.3	2.2	3.3	2.2	33	1.1
Unspecified	150	2.1	1.3	1.3	1.6	23	0.9
IV Sympathetic nervous system	797	21.2	3.2	0.6	9.4	125	1.0
Neuroblastoma	781	20.9	3.2	0.4	9.3	122	1.0
Other	16	0.3	–	0.2	0.2	2	–
V Retinoblastoma	310	9.2	0.5	–	3.7	48	1.1
VI Renal	655	16.1	3.9	0.6	7.7	103	0.9
Wilms' tumour	645	16.0	3.9	0.4	7.6	101	0.9
Renal carcinoma	10	0.1	0.1	0.2	0.1	1	–
VII Hepatic	101	2.2	0.5	0.5	1.1	15	1.3
Hepatoblastoma	75	2.1	0.2	0.1	0.9	11	1.4
Hepatic carcinoma	26	0.1	0.3	0.4	0.3	4	1.3
VIII Malignant bone	546	0.8	4.3	11.7	5.1	83	0.9
Osteosarcoma	284	0.2	1.7	6.8	2.6	43	0.9
Chondrosarcoma	10	–	0.0	0.3	0.1	1	–

Table 1.1 *Continued*

Diagnostic group	Total registrations	Annual rates per million for age groups			Age-standardized	Cumulative	Sex ratio M/F
		0–4	5–9	10–14			
Ewing's sarcoma	235	0.5	2.3	4.4	2.2	36	0.9
Other specified	11	0.0	0.1	0.2	0.1	1	–
Unspecified	6	0.1	0.1	0.1	0.1	0	–
IX Soft-tissue sarcoma	774	11.1	6.2	6.9	8.3	120	1.1
Rhabdomyosarcoma	488	7.9	4.4	3.1	5.3	76	1.2
Fibrosarcoma	105	1.2	0.8	1.2	1.1	16	1.0
Kaposi's	1	–	–	0.0	0.0	0	–
Other specified	123	1.2	0.7	1.9	1.2	18	1.1
Unspecified	57	0.8	0.3	0.7	0.6	8	1.3
X Germ-cell and gonadal	397	6.1	1.6	4.5	4.2	61	0.9
Intracranial and intraspinal germ-cell	100	0.9	0.8	1.4	1.0	15	1.5
Other non-gonadal germ-cell	94	2.4	0.2	0.3	1.1	14	0.3
Gonadal germ-cell	181	2.8	0.6	2.2	1.9	27	1.2
Gonadal carcinoma	14	–	0.1	0.4	0.1	2	–
Other and unspecified	8	0.0	0.0	0.2	0.1	1	–
XI Carcinoma and epithelial	343	1.0	2.1	7.4	3.2	52	0.8
Adrenocortical carcinoma	14	0.2	0.1	0.1	0.2	2	–
Thyroid carcinoma	54	–	0.2	1.4	0.5	8	0.5
Nasopharyngeal carcinoma	31	0.0	0.1	0.8	0.3	4	1.7
Melanoma	110	0.6	0.9	1.8	1.1	16	0.9
Skin carcinoma	61	–	0.3	1.6	0.5	9	0.8
Other and unspecified	73	0.1	0.5	1.6	0.7	11	0.8
XII Other and unspecified	44	0.5	0.4	0.5	0.5	6	1.4
Other specified	6	0.1	0.0	0.1	0.1	0	–
Other unspecified	38	0.4	0.3	0.5	0.4	5	1.4

Source: National Registry of Childhood Tumours.

the early childhood peak is also less marked and the total incidence is again lower (Parkin *et al.* 1996). A similar pattern is found in many developing countries of Asia and Latin America. There is little international variation in the incidence of ANLL.

Lymphomas

Childhood Hodgkin's disease has a relatively high incidence, particularly among younger children, in developing countries of Latin America and the Middle East. Lymphomas, both Hodgkin's disease and NHL, are more common among South Asian children in Britain than among Whites, and the excess of Hodgkin's disease is again greatest among younger children. The highest incidence of Burkitt's lymphoma, sometimes as large as 80 per million, is found in a broad geographic band of tropical Africa where malaria is endemic, and the incidence is also high in Papua New Guinea; in both of these regions, Burkitt's lymphoma is the most common childhood cancer. Elsewhere it is harder to identify patterns of incidence for Burkitt's lymphoma since many cases may have been registered simply as NHL. The incidence of all NHL, including Burkitt's, is relatively high in Mediterranean countries and the Middle East and in some Latin American countries.

Brain and spinal tumours

In the USA, the incidence of brain and spinal tumours is lower among Black children than among Whites, while in Britain, children of South Asian, and perhaps especially Indian, ethnic origin also have a lower incidence. In developing countries the recorded incidence of brain and spinal tumours is often low, sometimes as little as 5 per million. It is unclear to what extent this reflects underascertainment, particularly in areas without neurological services, rather than a reduced underlying risk.

Neuroblastoma

The recorded incidence of neuroblastoma in several countries is much higher than in Britain, particularly in the first year of life, possibly because of increased detection of otherwise silent tumours during routine health checks. In the USA, neuroblastoma has a lower incidence among Blacks than Whites in infancy, but the rates are similar for the two ethnic groups at the age of 1 year and above. Recorded incidence in developing countries is often very low, but in some African registries it is similar to that among US Blacks. Thus it seems likely that there is little variation in underlying risk, and that recorded incidence reflects the proportions of tumours that are diagnosed and registered.

Retinoblastoma

Retinoblastoma occurs in two distinct forms, heritable and non-heritable. Heritable retinoblastoma includes all cases of bilateral retinoblastoma and a few children with unilateral tumours, and the incidence is apparently constant throughout the world. Non-heritable retinoblastoma is always unilateral, and there are large variations in incidence. In the USA, Blacks have a higher incidence than Whites, and the incidence is substantially higher in many developing countries, particularly in sub-Saharan Africa.

Wilms' tumour

Variations in the incidence of Wilms' tumour depend largely on ethnic group rather than geographical area. Black children in the USA, the UK, and Africa have a higher incidence than Whites, though their age distributions are similar. Children of East Asian ethnic origin in the USA and Asia have a lower incidence than White children, and the deficit is more marked after the first year of life.

Liver tumours

Hepatoblastoma has apparently constant incidence throughout the world. The incidence of hepatic carcinoma in children is highest in regions of the world where the disease is also common among adults, namely East and South-East Asia, Melanesia, and sub-Saharan Africa. Nearly all childhood cases in these high-risk regions occur in chronic carriers of hepatitis B.

Sarcomas

Of the two principal types of childhood bone sarcoma, osteosarcoma appears to have a similar incidence in most populations, though it may be lower in Asia. Black children in the United States, but apparently not Black populations in Africa, have a somewhat higher incidence than Whites. In contrast, there are striking variations in the incidence of Ewing's sarcoma. This tumour has very low incidence in East and South-East Asia, and among Black populations in Africa, the USA, and Britain. Ewing's sarcoma appears to be rather more common in Australia than in other regions of the world.

Rhabdomyosarcoma is the most common soft-tissue sarcoma of childhood in most populations. In South and East Asia, and also among Asian children in Britain, its incidence is around half that in White children. In the USA, Black children have a lower incidence of rhabdomyosarcoma than Whites, but fibrosarcoma is somewhat more common. Kaposi's sarcoma is extremely rare in children in most regions of the world, but in East and Central Africa, where it is endemic among adults, the incidence among children was about 2 per million around 1970. Since then, there have been very large increases, and around 1990, rates of 10–14 per million were recorded. The great majority of the increase is clearly related to the AIDS epidemic, which has been particularly severe in the region.

Other cancers

There is little evidence for variations in the incidence of germ-cell tumours. Gonadal germ-cell tumours seem to be somewhat more common in East Asia and also among South Asian children in Britain, though incidence rates in India are unremarkable.

By far the highest incidence of childhood thyroid carcinoma, around 80 per million, has been recorded in areas of Belarus contaminated by radiation from the Chernobyl nuclear reactor explosion. The existence of the excess is not in doubt, both because the rates are 50 times as great as those seen elsewhere and because of the aggressive histological type in many cases. The true size of the excess risk is hard to determine, however, as some cases may have been detected particularly early by intensive screening and it is well known that thyroid cancer in other populations can be undetected for many years after onset.

The highest incidence of nasopharyngeal carcinoma among children is in North Africa, a region of intermediate risk for adults, where it accounts for around 10% of all childhood cancers. In East Asian countries, where incidence is highest among adults, children have only a moderately elevated incidence, up to 0.8 per million, while in the USA the incidence among Black children is about 1 per million, nine times that among Whites in the same country. The highest relative frequency of oral carcinoma in childhood, 3% of all childhood cancers, has been found in Bangladesh, and this may be related to betel nut chewing.

There is an exceptionally high incidence of skin carcinoma, both squamous cell and basal cell, among children in Tunisia, where the great majority of cases are associated with xeroderma pigmentosum. Malignant melanoma has a very high incidence in Australia and New Zealand, where it is also a very common cancer among adults, resulting from high levels of sun exposure.

Trends in incidence

The most striking increases in incidence of any childhood cancers, those relating to Kaposi's sarcoma in East and Central Africa and to thyroid carcinoma in Belarus, have been described above. Otherwise, any changes have been much more modest (Draper *et al.* 1994). (The very large increases in recorded incidence of neuroblastoma in Japan and some other areas with population screening of course represent increased detection rather than a change in underlying risk.) The best documented trend concerns ALL, the commonest childhood cancer in all developed countries. The early childhood peak started to emerge in mortality data in England and Wales in the 1920s, and it was certainly well established among White children in the USA by the early 1940s. A further modest rise, particularly in early childhood, took place in some Western countries until the late 1970s. Meanwhile, increasing incidence in early childhood among US Blacks led to the emergence of a moderate peak in the age-incidence curve for this ethnic group. Small increases have also been observed in some Western populations for a number of other childhood cancers, notably brain tumours, neuroblastoma, and soft-tissue sarcomas. It is not yet clear, however, how much any of these increases is attributable to changes in diagnostic practice rather than in underlying risk.

Clusters

A cluster of cases of a disease may be defined as the occurrence of a substantially larger number of cases than expected in a small geographically defined population, usually during a short period of time. There have been many reports of clusters of childhood leukaemia and other cancers. Among the most well known are those in the vicinity of the British nuclear sites at Sellafield and Dounreay, though it is now generally accepted that they are unlikely to result from radiation exposure. Reported clusters need to be investigated carefully, the first stage being to check that the details of diagnosis, dates, and location are correct and the incidence rate is indeed high. Cluster investigations may yield clues to the aetiology of the particular cases or of the disease in general, though they are usually disappointing in this respect. It is also important to address the concerns of the local population, often with respect to the role of possible environmental pollution. In order to systematize the investigation of clusters, guidelines have been published in the USA, and a handbook is in preparation in Britain.

Survival rates

In contrast to the very small improvements in prognosis that have occurred for many of the common cancers of adults, the past 30 years have seen dramatic increases in the survival rates of most types of childhood cancer. Figures 1.1–1.3 show the five-year survival rates for children in Britain diagnosed in successive quinquennia between 1962 and 1991 separately for the principal diagnostic groups. During this period, survival improved substantially for virtually all diagnostic groups, though the main advances for different types of cancer have occurred at different times. In the 1960s, there were particularly marked improvements in the prognosis for children with Hodgkin's disease and Wilms' tumour. The 1970s saw large improvements for a wide range of diagnoses, most notably ALL and NHL. In the 1980s, survival rates increased for children with ANLL, bone sarcomas, and germ-cell tumours. There has, however, been disappointingly little improvement in survival from brain tumours or neuroblastoma. Detailed comparisons of survival rates between countries are subject to a number of methodological problems, principally concerned with the precise definition of cases eligible for analysis and with the methods used to obtain follow-up information. In general, however, comparisons with population-based data from other countries, including the USA (Miller *et al.* 1995), Germany (Kaatsch *et al.* 1995), and Australia (Giles *et al.* 1995), indicate that the survival rates achieved most recently in Britain are typical of those for industrialized countries.

The spectacular increases in survival rates described here are undoubtedly largely due to advances in treatment and supportive care. At the same time as these developments in therapy, however, there was also a substantial movement towards concentration of treatment at relatively few specialist centres, at some of which very large numbers of children are treated. Also, whereas at one time there were national clinical trials only for acute leukaemia and a handful of other diagnostic groups, in many countries there are now national or international trials and studies open for entry of children with all but the rarest types of cancer, and the proportions of eligible children that are entered in these trials have also increased. For several diagnostic groups, survival rates have been found to be higher among children who were treated at specialist centres, or who were entered in clinical trials regardless of the treatment arm (Stiller 1994).

Follow-up

As survival rates have improved for nearly all childhood cancers, the number of long-term survivors has greatly increased and these survivors already include a substantial number of adults. Several large studies of survivors from childhood cancer are now in progress, addressing such topics as the criteria for cure, quality of life, risk of second primary neoplasms, fertility, and the health of the survivors' offspring. Late effects and long-term follow-up are discussed from a clinical point of view in Chapter 7. We summarize here the epidemiological data. Although late relapses can occur, the great majority of five-year survivors may be regarded as cured, only one tenth of them dying of recurrent tumour or a treatment-related cause during the ensuing 10 years. Among five-year survivors diagnosed in Britain during 1971–85, 9% had died by 1990; 73% of the deaths were due to recurrent tumour, 7% to a second primary neoplasm, and 15% to other treatment-related effects (Robertson *et al.* 1994). In two large population-based studies, the risk

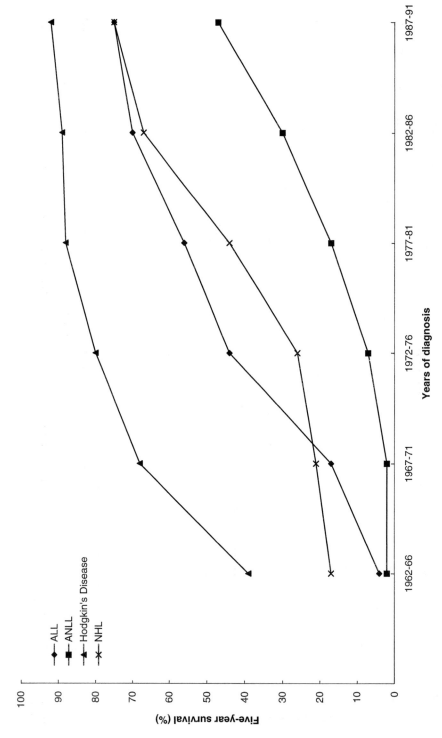

Fig. 1.1 Actuarial five-year survival rates (per cent) for children diagnosed in Britain during 1962–91 with ALL, ANLL, Hodgkin's disease, and NHL (including Burkitt's). (National Registry of Childhood Tumours.)

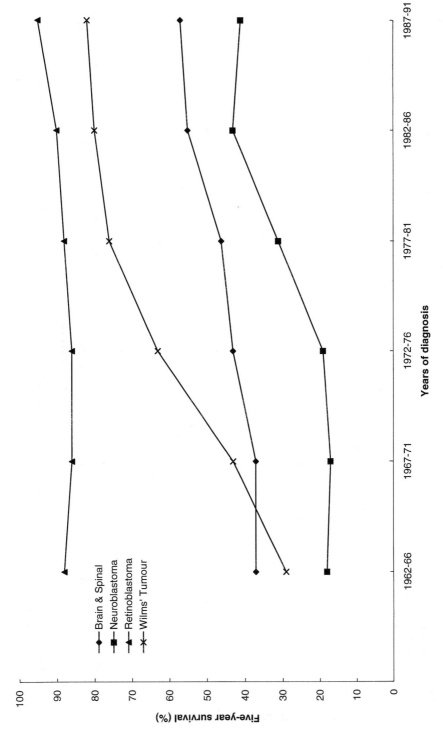

Fig. 1.2 Actuarial five-year survival rates (per cent) for children diagnosed in Britain during 1962–91 with brain and spinal tumours, neuroblastoma, retinoblastoma, and Wilms' tumours. (National Registry of Childhood Tumours.)

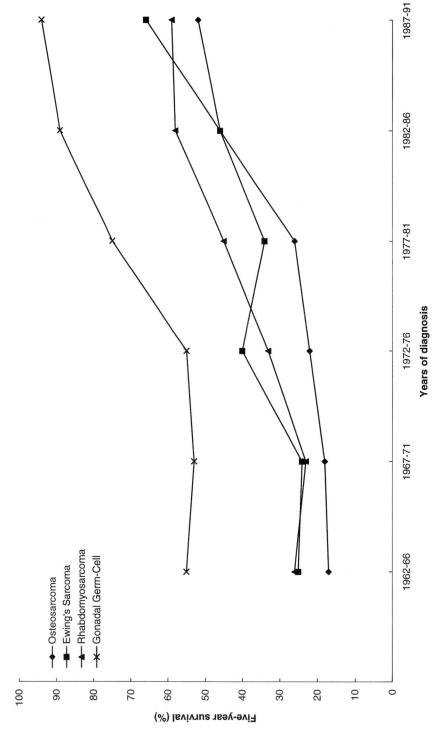

Fig. 1.3 Actuarial five-year survival rates (per cent) for children diagnosed in Britain during 1962–91 with osteosarcoma, Ewing's sarcoma, rhabdomyosarcoma, and malignant gonadal germ-cell tumours. (National Registry of Childhood Tumours.)

of developing a second primary neoplasm within 25 years of diagnosis of childhood cancer was 4%, four to six times the risk in the general population (Hawkins and Stevens 1996). The risks vary considerably, however, between different types of childhood cancer, being especially high among survivors of heritable retinoblastoma. It should also be stressed that these risk estimates, at least for longer intervals following diagnosis, are based on survivors who were treated before the era of intensive chemotherapy, though many did of course receive radiotherapy. Also, virtually nothing is yet known of the risks to survivors beyond the age of about 40, when the population incidence of several common cancers begins to rise markedly.

Some forms of treatment for cancer cause infertility, but many survivors go on to have children of their own. Most children of survivors are still very young. It is particularly important to follow up the offspring of survivors of cancer in childhood for two reasons. Some childhood cancers are known to have a predominantly genetic aetiology and the risk of transmission to future generations needs to be assessed. The question of whether treatment-related germ-cell mutagenesis causes cancer, congenital malformations, or other genetic disease in the offspring of survivors also needs to be studied, and the risks, if any, estimated. Estimates of the risks to offspring of survivors are discussed in the section on genetic epidemiology below.

The aetiology of childhood cancer

Little is known about the causes of childhood cancer. International comparisons of the type described above, together with case-control and cohort studies, have suggested a variety of possible aetiological factors, but these have seldom been convincing or replicated in further studies. On the other hand, studies of the genetics of childhood cancer have been much more rewarding both in their practical application to problems of childhood cancer and in terms of basic science.

Environmental factors

Possible causes of childhood cancer, both generally and for specific diagnostic groups, have been investigated in a large number of studies, particularly in Britain and the United States. The two factors that have attracted most attention are radiation, both ionizing and non-ionizing, and the role of infections—in the child, in the mother, and in the community. The other factors studied include parental characteristics, environmental exposures of both child and parents, particularly *in utero* exposures, and occupational exposures of both parents. Concern about possible environmental causes of genetic damage has led to studies of preconception exposures of the parents.

Ionizing radiation

Probably the first, and still the largest, case-control study of childhood cancer was that carried out by Dr Alice Stewart and her colleagues. An early report from this study claimed that antenatal radiography, used mainly in the third trimester of pregnancy for obstetric reasons, significantly increased the probability of the subsequent child developing cancer. Although this result was initially greeted with considerable scepticism, it is now widely accepted as correct; the most useful presentation of the results is that by Bithell and Stewart (1975). For children born between about 1945 and 1965 there was a 40–50% increase in the risk of childhood cancer if the mother was given about two or three abdominal X-rays during pregnancy. It should be emphasized that antenatal radiography probably caused at most about 5% of childhood cancers even when it was more widely used and doses were higher than they are now. Both the number of pregnant women X-rayed and the doses of radiation have greatly decreased since the time of Stewart's work; indeed, radiography has been largely replaced by the use of ultrasound. (There is no evidence that ultrasound causes childhood cancer.)

Other childhood exposures to radiation, e.g. that used in treating tinea capitis in early childhood or, particularly, the large doses given during radiotherapy, are also carcinogenic. The possibility that some childhood cancers are caused by natural radiation (gamma, radon) has been suggested but is unproven. Clearly, on the usual assumption of a linear dose-response relationship for the carcinogenic effects of radiation, one would expect some cases to be caused by background gamma radiation.

The report that has caused both the most public concern and scientific interest in this area was probably that by Gardner *et al.* (1990) which stated that preconception exposure of the father could lead to childhood leukaemia and NHL. Because of the relatively small doses involved (from employment in the nuclear industry), doubts were raised about the validity of this finding, although the study appeared to be epidemiologically sound. Subsequent studies have failed to confirm the association reported by Gardner.

Non-ionizing radiation

In recent years concern has been expressed over the possible carcinogenic effects of non-ionizing radiation both in adults and in children. Ultraviolet radiation from sunlight is known to cause melanoma and other skin cancers. Concern has been expressed about exposure arising from electric power transmission and use—both from power lines and from domestic exposure. In spite of a very large research effort, however, the question of whether such exposures do have carcinogenic effects is unresolved. Electric and magnetic fields do not appear to damage DNA and it has been suggested that their mode of action, if any, is as a promoter. Research on this topic has been reviewed on several occasions, most recently by a committee of the National Research Council in the United States (National Research Council 1996). Its report concluded that 'the current body of evidence does not show that exposure to these [power frequency electric and magnetic] fields presents a human-health hazard. Specifically no conclusive and consistent evidence shows that exposures to residential electric and magnetic fields produce cancer ...'. The committee paid particular attention to studies of residential exposure to magnetic fields as measured by 'wire codes' (a means of assessing electric and magnetic field exposures on the basis of electric wiring configurations) in relation to childhood leukaemia, but concluded that while there was evidence for an association this did not amount to evidence for causation.

Parental occupation and socioeconomic status

Any association observed between childhood disease and parental occupations may reflect either specific exposures or lifestyle factors associated with particular occupations. Furthermore, a parent may well be in the same occupation before the conception of the child, during pregnancy, and subsequently; thus it may be difficult to determine whether any observed association is attributable to exposure occurring before conception, *in utero*, or postnatally.

A large number of papers have been published analysing occupation in general or specific occupations, and using a variety of study designs. It is inevitable that in a large series of studies, some of which include analyses of many different occupations, a number of statistically significant results will be reported. In such circumstances it is necessary to determine whether there is consistency between different studies and whether there is any evidence of a 'dose-response' effect, i.e. in this instance, whether the risk is higher for children of parents who have been more heavily exposed to the suspected occupational mutagen or who have worked longer in the occupation. As judged by these criteria, there appears to be no parental occupation for which there is sufficient evidence that it is causally associated with childhood cancer. For a review, see O'Leary *et al.* (1991).

Occupational category is of course closely related to socioeconomic status. Thus, if there is an effect on childhood cancer of lifestyle or standards of living, this could appear as an effect of an occupation which happens to be in the high-risk group as defined by socioeconomic status. The possibility of such an association with socioeconomic status has been investigated both in case-control studies and in 'ecological' studies, i.e. by comparing incidence rates for areas classified according to socioeconomic status of their resident populations. For childhood leukaemia there is good evidence that incidence increases with increasing socioeconomic status. The reasons for this are unknown, though one explanation is suggested below.

Infections

The possible role of infections, specially viruses, in the aetiology of childhood cancer has been studied in a number of ways. Viruses are known to be implicated in some human cancers, and these may occur in children, e.g. Burkitt's lymphoma (Epstein-Barr virus) and liver carcinoma (hepatitis B). Case-control studies have included analyses of exposures to infectious illnesses both for the children themselves and for their mothers while pregnant. Positive findings have been reported but there is no conclusive evidence from these studies. Perhaps the most persuasive evidence for the involvement of an infectious agent in childhood leukaemia comes from studies of clustering and of incidence rates in different types of geographical area (Alexander 1993; Kinlen 1995).

The latter author, in a remarkable series of studies, has shown that childhood leukaemia rates increase as a result of 'population mixing', i.e. when people from several different areas come together. This observation has been repeated in a variety of different situations in which such population mixing occurs. Kinlen's explanation is that such situations are conducive to the spread of an infectious agent or agents among a previously unexposed, and therefore susceptible, group, and that childhood leukaemia may represent an unusual response to such agents. It is not suggested that leukaemia is itself an infectious disease. Stiller and Boyle (1996) studied migration patterns within England and Wales and found that higher childhood leukaemia rates occurred where migration was higher. Their findings are in agreement with Kinlen's, and the authors suggest that they may also account for the differences in rates for different socioeconomic groups already referred to.

Other possible aetiological factors

A wide variety of other possible factors has been studied; Stiller (1997) should be consulted for a recent extended review and references. The cell types involved in childhood cancers and the shape of the age distribution, with a peak for the typical cancers of childhood at a very early age, have led many investigators to concentrate on events occurring during pregnancy, or even before conception.

Preconception factors

The fact that some childhood cancers are attributable to germ-cell mutations has led many investigators to study parental exposure to possible mutagens. Such studies have included various types of exposure to ionizing radiation (including the occupational exposures mentioned above) and to chemicals. Again, no consensus has emerged; in a recent paper Sorahan *et al.* (1997) have presented evidence that smoking by fathers before the time of conception possibly increases the chance of cancer in the child.

In utero exposures

The effects of *in utero* ionizing radiation have already been referred to. It is well known that diethylstilboestrol given to pregnant women to avert a threatened miscarriage can cause vaginal adenocarcinoma in their daughters—though these occur mainly in young women rather than children. This finding, together with studies of transplacental carcinogenesis in laboratory animals, has suggested that other drugs given to women during pregnancy may cause childhood cancer. A number of positive findings have been published but no firm causal associations have been established. Similarly, smoking in pregnancy has been widely studied but is not established as a risk factor for childhood cancer.

Postnatal exposures

Ionizing radiation and infections have already been discussed. Many other environmental factors have been studied but once again there is no consensus. Some support has been found for the suggestion by Preston-Martin *et al.* (1982) that childhood brain tumours may be caused by *N*-nitroso compounds. The suggestion that intramuscular vitamin K, given to neonates to prevent vitamin K deficiency bleeding, doubles the risk of childhood cancer has led to a series of further studies. It seems clear that the original findings will not be confirmed. However, it remains possible that vitamin K itself or some other constituent of the particular formulation that has been most widely studied, Konakion, is carcinogenic, though with a smaller risk than originally suggested.

Other drugs have occasionally been reported as risk factors and, of course, cytotoxic drugs given in the course of treatment for cancer are known causes of further cancers, but there is no evidence to suggest that any substantial numbers of childhood cancers are attributable to these or other drugs.

Genetic epidemiology

A detailed discussion of the genetic aspects of childhood cancer is given in Chapter 2 of this volume. In the present chapter we concentrate on genetic epidemiology, i.e. the estimation of risks of childhood cancer for family members of affected children and for individuals who have genetic conditions known to predispose to childhood cancer.

The most obvious example of a genetically determined cancer is retinoblastoma. About 40% of cases have the heritable form of this disease. The pattern of inheritance is that of a dominant autosomal gene with about 90% penetrance, but the gene is in fact the first example of a tumour suppressor gene, Rb1: about 90% of individuals who inherit the mutated form of this gene from a parent subsequently suffer a mutation of the wild type, or normal, allele leading to loss of heterozygosity and the development of retinoblastoma. A variety of other cancers is also now known to occur in these individuals.

There is an obvious genetic element in some other childhood cancers, notably Wilms' tumour, but the pattern of inheritance in Wilms' tumour is a great deal more complicated and the proportion of clearly hereditary cases much smaller.

Some familial aggregations arise through the association of childhood and adult tumours with known genetic disease such as neurofibromatosis, tuberous sclerosis, Fanconi's anaemia, ataxia telangiectasia, xeroderma pigmentosum, and Bloom's syndrome, though the actual number of cases of childhood cancer in which these conditions occur is rather small. There are also well-documented associations with congenital abnormalities; the strongest association with such a condition is Down syndrome, which occurs in a small percentage of cases of childhood leukaemia.

Relatives of affected children

Various authors have studied the siblings, twins, offspring, and, to a lesser extent, the parents of children with cancer.

Siblings and twins

There are many case-reports on the incidence of cancer among siblings and twins of affected cases but few systematic studies of the magnitude of the risk.

The largest population studies of childhood cancer among siblings are those carried out by Miller (1971) in the United States and Draper *et al.* (1977, 1996) in Britain. From the first two British studies the authors concluded that if one child in a family has malignant disease then, in the absence of any further information about the existence of genetic disease in that family, and excluding twins and retinoblastoma, the siblings of that child have approximately double the risk of the general population, i.e. a risk of approximately 1 in 300 as compared with the average risk of about 1 in 600. A similar conclusion can be drawn from Miller's paper when due allowance is made for his method of ascertaining cases. Unfortunately, risk estimates have not yet been made for the more recent data. It seems probable that as more becomes known about the genetic element in childhood cancer, the risk estimates will increase for families where familial syndromes have been identified, while those for the remaining families will decrease. One would, of course, expect there to be occasional families with two affected siblings purely by chance. A doubling of the risks for siblings as compared with the general population implies that half of the families so affected are in fact due to chance. (Incidentally, this implies that laboratory studies of these families will be expected to find nothing of interest at least 50% of the time.) We emphasize that the 1 in 300 risk quoted above is for a sibling of an affected child as calculated at birth; the calculated risk is less for siblings who are a few years old when the affected child is diagnosed. The estimated risk is also lower if there are other, unaffected children in the family.

The risks are higher if there are two affected children in the family and where there is known genetic disease of a type associated with cancer. The special case of retinoblastoma is dealt with by Draper *et al.* (1992); the risk for a subsequent sibling following an apparently sporadic case of retinoblastoma, i.e. where there is no previous family history, appears to be about 2% if the affected sibling has bilateral disease, and 1% if it is unilateral. This is lower than has previously been suggested, and is lower still if there are other, unaffected siblings.

The risk that the co-twin of a twin with cancer will also be affected is of particular concern, and more so if the twins are monozygous. In general, both twins and childhood cancer are too rare for any quantitative estimates of risk to be made. It seems likely that the risk for a dizygotic co-twin of an affected case will be at least as high as that for ordinary siblings, but no data are available. Nearly all the published cases of childhood cancer in twins are like-sexed pairs and are known or assumed to be monozygous. The fact that in case-reports of affected twin pairs the two children almost invariably have the same diagnosis and tend to be diagnosed at the same age is an indication that such cases may be genetic in origin. One would expect there to be an increased risk for the monozygous co-twins of affected cases, but in general there are insufficient data to estimate such risks; the fact that the co-twins of the great majority of cases do not develop cancer (Draper *et al.* 1996) implies that the risk to co-twins is, in general, not very high. The exception to this is childhood leukaemia, where perhaps 25% of co-twins of monozygotic cases also develop the disease. However, as first pointed out by Chaganti *et al.* (1979), it appears likely that many of these cases are due to *in utero* transfer of leukaemia cells rather than being genetically determined.

Risks to offspring

The risks to offspring of childhood cancer survivors (Hawkins and Stevens 1996) correspond well with those from the studies of siblings. In general they are low, the main exception being for retinoblastoma, though even here, as for siblings, the risks in cases of sporadic retinoblastoma appear to be lower than previously suggested: for a child of a unilateral case, and where it is not known whether the disease is of the hereditary type, the estimated risk is 1% (Draper *et al.* 1996). Similarly, a few offspring of survivors of Wilms' tumour develop the same disease, but in a study of 382 offspring of survivors of childhood leukaemia and non-Hodgkin lymphoma followed up for a median period of 5.8 years, no cases of these diseases developed (Hawkins *et al.* 1995).

Other family members

Studies of the families of children with cancer are discussed by Birch (1994). Perhaps the most striking finding to emerge from these studies is the extent of the occurrence in some of the families of the Li-Fraumeni syndrome (Li and Fraumeni 1969) in which a variety of childhood cancers and some adult types, notably breast cancer in young women, are observed. Some of these families are now known to be associated with mutations of the p53 tumour suppressor gene.

Acknowledgements

We are grateful to Betty Roberts and Sue Medhurst for secretarial assistance and to Pat Brownbill for the production of survival curves. This work was undertaken by the Childhood Cancer

Research Group which receives support from the Department of Health; the views expressed in this publication are those of the authors and not necessarily those of the Department of Health.

References

Alexander, F.E. (1993). Viruses, clusters and clustering of childhood leukaemia: a new perspective? *European Journal of Cancer*, 29A, 1424–1443.

Birch, J.M. (1994). Family cancer syndromes and clusters. *British Medical Bulletin*, 50, 624–639.

Birch, J.M., and Marsden, H.B. (1987). A classification scheme for childhood cancer. *International Journal of Cancer*, 40, 620–624.

Bithell, J.F., and Stewart, A. (1975). Pre-natal irradiation and childhood malignancy. A review of British data from the Oxford survey. *British Journal of Cancer*, 31, 271–287.

Chaganti, R.S.K., Miller, D.R., Meyers, P.A., and German, J. (1979). Cytogenetic evidence of the intrauterine origin of acute leukaemia in monozygotic twins. *New England Journal of Medicine*, 300, 1032–1034.

Draper, G.J., Heaf, M.M., and Kinnier Wilson, L.M. (1977). Occurrence of childhood cancers among sibs and estimation of familial risks. *Journal of Medical Genetics*, 14, 81–90.

Draper, G.J., Sanders, B.M., Brownbill, P.A., and Hawkins, M.M. (1992). Patterns of risk of hereditary retinoblastoma and applications to genetic counselling. *British Journal of Cancer*, 66, 211–219.

Draper, G.J., Kroll, M.E., and Stiller, C.A. (1994). Childhood cancer. In *Cancer Surveys*, Vol. 19/20: *Trends in Cancer Incidence and Mortality*. (ed. R. Doll, J.F. Fraumeni and C.S. Muir), pp. 493–517, Cold Spring Harbor Laboratory Press, Plainview, New York.

Draper, G.J., Sanders, B.M., Lennox, E.L., and Brownhill, P.A. (1996). Patterns of childhood cancer among siblings. *British Journal of Cancer*, 74, 152–158.

Gardner, M.J., Snee, M.P., Hall, A.J., Powell, C.A., Downes, S., and Terrell, J.D. (1990). Results of case-control study of leukaemia and lymphoma among young people near Sellafield nuclear plant in West Cumbria. *British Medical Journal*, 300, 423–429.

Giles G., Waters, K., Thursfield, V., and Farrugia, H. (1995). Childhood cancer in Victoria, Australia, 1970–1989. *International Journal of Cancer*, 63, 794–797.

Hawkins, M.M., and Stevens, M.C.G. (1996). The long term survivors. *British Medical Bulletin*, 52, 898–923.

Hawkins, M.M., Draper, G.J., and Winter, D.L. (1995). Cancer in the offspring of the survivors of childhood leukaemia and non-Hodgkin lymphomas. *British Journal of Cancer*, 71, 1335–1339.

Jensen, O.M., Parkin, D.M., MacLennan, R., Muir, C.S., and Skeet, R.G. (ed.) (1991). *Cancer Registration: Principles and Methods*. IARC Scientific Publications, No. 95. International Agency for Research on Cancer, Lyon.

Kaatsch, P., Haaf, G., and Michaelis, J. (1995). Childhood malignancies in Germany—methods and results of a nationwide registry. *European Journal of Cancer*, 31A, 993–999.

Kinlen, L.J. (1995). Epidemiological evidence for an infective basis in childhood leukaemia. *British Journal of Cancer*, 71, 1–5.

Kramarova, E., Stiller, C.A., Ferlay, J., Parkin, D.M., Draper, G.J., Michaelis, J., *et al.* (ed.) (1996). *International Classification of Childhood Cancer*. IARC Technical Report No. 29. International Agency for Research on Cancer, Lyon.

Li, F.P., and Fraumeni, J.F. (1969). Rhabdomyosarcoma in children: epidemiologic study and identification of a familial cancer syndrome. *Journal of the National Cancer Institute*, 43, 1365–1373.

Miller, R.W. (1971). Deaths from childhood leukaemia and solid tumours among twins and other sibs in the United States, 1960–67. *Journal of the National Cancer Institute*, 46, 203–209.

Miller, R.W., Young, J.L., and Novakovic, B. (1995). Childhood cancer. *Cancer*, 75, 395–405.

National Research Council (1996). Possible health effects of exposure to residential electric and magnetic fields. National Academy Press, Washington DC.

O'Leary, L.M., Hicks, A.M., Peters, J.M., and London, S. (1991). Parental occupational exposures and risk of childhood cancer: a review. *American Journal of Industrial Medicine*, 20, 17–35.

Parkin, D.M., Stiller, C.A., Draper, G.J., Bieber, C.A., Terracini, B., and Young, J.L. (ed.) (1988). *International Incidence of Childhood Cancer*. IARC Scientific Publications, No. 87 International Agency for Research on Cancer, Lyon.

Parkin, D.M., Clayton, D., Black, R.J., Masuyer, E., Friedl, H.P., Ivanov, E., *et al.* (1996). Childhood leukaemia in Europe after Chernobyl: 5 year follow-up. *British Journal of Cancer*, 73, 1006–1012.

Preston-Martin, S., Yu, M.C., Benton, B., and Henderson, B.E. (1982). *N*-Nitroso compounds and childhood brain tumours: A case-control study. *Cancer Research*, 42, 5240–5245.

Robertson, C.M., Hawkins, M.M., and Kingston, J.E. (1994). Late deaths and survival after childhood cancer: implications for cure. *British Medical Journal*, 309, 162–166.

Sorahan, T., Lancashire, R.J., Hulten, M.A., Peck, I., and Stewart, A.M. (1997). Childhood cancer and parental use of tobacco: deaths from 1953 to 1955. *British Journal of Cancer*, 75, 134–138.

Stiller, C.A. (1994). Centralized treatment, entry to trials, and survival. *British Journal of Cancer*, 70, 352–362.

Stiller, C.A. (1997). Aetiology and epidemiology. In *Paediatric Oncology. Clinical practice and controversies*. (ed. C.R. Pinkerton and P.N. Plowman) pp. 3–26. Chapman and Hall Medical, London.

Stiller, C.A., and Boyle, P.J. (1996). Effect of population mixing and socioeconomic status in England and Wales, 1979–85, on lymphoblastic leukaemia in children. *British Medical Journal*, 313, 1297–1300.

Stiller, C.A., and Parkin, D.M. (1996). Geographic and ethnic variations in the incidence of childhood cancer. *British Medical Bulletin*, 52, 682–703.

2 Genetic elements of childhood cancer

M. Schwab

Introduction

Genetic alterations have a fundamental role in the development of cancer, both in children and adults. The simplified concept is that specific genes normally involved in central regulatory processes, like cell division, differentiation, or signal transduction, can be structurally damaged or eliminated from the cellular genome by exogenous or endogenous causes. The alteration or deletion of normal gene function can initiate tumourogenesis or can provide a selective growth advantage to a benign tumour cell. Cancer in children, although rare compared with cancer in adults, has provided basic insights into genetic mechanisms of tumourogenesis. This chapter will present major concepts of the role of genetic alterations in tumourogenesis and will discuss their clinical potential.

Oncogenes *versus* tumour-suppressor genes

Genetic damage underlying tumourogenesis may affect two classes of genes which either alone or in combination with each other contribute to neoplastic growth: oncogenes and tumour-suppressor genes.

Oncogenes act positively and are often referred to as 'dominant' modulators of cellular growth. They result from normal cellular genes through three major molecular pathways: point mutation, with the consequence of a small but significant change in protein function; translocation, by which two different chromosomes exchange genomic material and thereby can disrupt the normal gene structure; and amplification, which results in the acquisition of multiple copies of a normally single copy gene. In contrast, tumour-suppressor genes contribute to tumourogenesis by their functional impairment or inactivation, which can result from point mutation or complete gene deletion (Fig. 2.1). Their normal activity results in tumour suppression. Tumour-suppressor genes act 'recessively' at the cellular level. Because every cell has two copies of each gene, the functional inactivation or deletion of one copy of the tumour-suppressor gene normally remains without consequence, due to the activity of the normal remaining copy. The tumour-suppressing activity is lost once both copies have become inactivated.

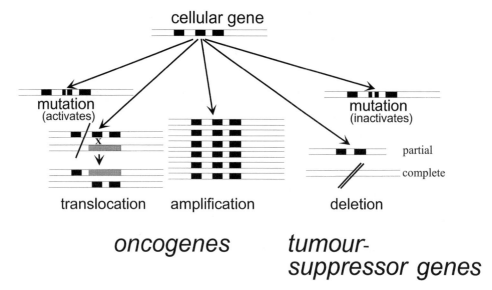

Fig. 2.1 Molecular pathways for the activation of oncogenes and inactivation of tumour-suppressor genes.

Somatic *versus* germ-line changes

Genetic damage can occur at two levels of the human genome. Tumourogenesis is restricted to the individual when the genome of a somatic cell is affected. In contrast, damage in a germ cell will be inherited by the progeny and represents the starting point for a family afflicted with cancer. Germ-line damage causes high susceptibility to cancer, and generally the targets of damage are tumour-suppressor genes. Because the second copy of the tumour-suppressor gene usually remains normal and active, tumourogenesis is suppressed and the development of the embryo is normal, due to the 'recessive' character of the alteration. The activity of an oncogene, due to its 'dominant' character, would deregulate cellular growth at an early stage of development and therefore not allow embryonic growth. An exception may be multiple endocrine neoplasia type 2A and 2B, in which a dominantly acting oncogene called *RET* is transmitted through the germ line in the hereditary form of the disease (Santoro *et al.* 1995).

Although the germ-line loss of a tumour-suppressor gene usually allows normal growth, the developing embryo or the young child does have an enhanced tumour susceptibility. This is due to the fact that, in general terms, every gene has a statistical likelihood of undergoing mutational change. A simple calculation may illustrate this connection between enhanced tumour susceptibility and mutation rate. A gene with a mutation rate of 10^{-7} will mutate statistically once in 10^7 cells. If the two gene copies are intact, both alleles will be inactivated at a cell number of 10^{14}, which is roughly the total number of cells in an adult. A child who has inherited only one normal copy of a gene will suffer from a mutation of this gene once 10^7 cells have been reached. Because most tumour-suppressor genes contribute to tumourogenesis with a tissue-specific restriction, the cell number of the particular tissue type or organ is the critical determinant for tumour onset. This has been best demonstrated for hereditary cases of retinoblastoma, which usually develops in young children (Fig. 2.2). The calculation shows that the likelihood of the

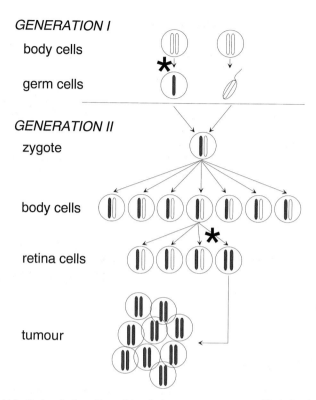

Fig. 2.2 Two-hit model for the inactivation of two alleles of a tumour-suppressor gene. The hallmark of this model is that the first mutation occurs in a germ-line cell with the consequence of a susceptible second generation that has only one intact allele. This allele can be inactivated in a somatic cell.

second normal gene copy mutating in the young children is high (90–95%) because the number of cells in the retina of the young child easily amounts to 10^7. As a consequence, the vast majority of children carrying one damaged allele and developing normally during early childhood will still develop cancer, due to mutational inactivation of the second allele. These children have inherited a high susceptibility to cancer.

Even though the ability of environmental factors to damage the human genome both at the somatic and germ-line level is widely discussed, we have to get used to the idea that a proportion of cancer-associated genomic changes result from endogeneous processes. Candidate mechanisms are failure of DNA-repair systems during the replication of DNA (Modrich 1991; Karran 1996) or errors of DNA recombination enzymes that are normally responsible for the developmental recombination of DNA sequences, for instance the rearrangement of immunoglobulin or T cell receptor loci (Rabbitts 1991).

Cellular functions of oncogenes and tumour-suppressor genes

The proteins encoded by oncogenes and tumour-suppressor genes operate throughout the cell and affect various regulatory processes (Bishop 1991). Many proteins are members of signal transduction pathways and include growth factors (like epidermal growth factor, EGF, and platelet derived growth factor, PDGF), their receptors, G proteins (like RAS), cytoplasmic proteins (e.g. APC) of as yet unidentified function) and nuclear proteins, presumably involved in the regulation of gene transcription (retinoblastoma protein; Wilms' tumour protein; von Hippel-Lindau protein). This diversity of protein functions in different types of tumours has challenged the early contention that a solution to the cancer problem might be at hand quickly.

Over the past years we have come closer to describing some of the activities of oncoproteins. Yet, in most instances, we are completely ignorant about which of these activities are eventually related to tumourogenesis. This situation is aggravated by the fact that oncoproteins usually do not have specific biological functions of their own, like simple metabolic enzymatic reactions. Instead, they can have multiple functions, i.e. they act in a pleiotropic way, in different cell types during different phases of the cell cycle or different stages of cellular differentiation. Their functions are usually modified by physical interactions with various other proteins. It is very clear that the genetics of tumourogenesis has far outpaced the understanding of the biochemistry and cellular biology of oncoprotein products. In no case is the biochemical contribution to tumourogenesis of any protein encoded by an oncogene or a tumour-suppressor gene completely clear. We can only describe some of the activities and guess about their relationship to tumourogenesis. This situation is exemplified by types of childhood tumours for which the genetic changes initiating tumourogenesis appear known.

Retinoblastoma

Historically, the retinoblastoma gene (*RB*) was the first human tumour-suppressor gene to be isolated. The study of the genetics of familial retinoblastoma led the way to describing inheritance patterns and to postulate the development of this tumour as the result of two independent mutations which inactivate the two alleles of the same gene found on chromosome 13q14 (Knudson 1971; Knudson and Strong 1972; Weinberg 1992). This paradigmatic setting would seem to rapidly lead to understanding of this type of cancer. Intensive work over the past years has taught us otherwise—the more we have learned about the functions of the RB protein, the less we seem to understand about how its functional loss relates to retinoblastoma.

One possibly important clue to pRB activity has been thought to come from the observation that the protein undergoes changes in phosphorylation during the cell cycle: hypophosphorylated protein during G_1-phase bound to a nuclear structure contrasts with hyperphosphorylated pRB in S-, G_2-, and M-phase residing in the cytoplasm (Weinberg 1992). This suggests that the nuclear association of pRB with an as yet unidentified binding partner might be related to pRB function. But this possibility becomes even more complex with the observation that at least 10 additional, distinct polypeptides of as yet unidentified function can bind to pRB. One of the working hypotheses is now that pRB might suppress the growth-modulating activity of one of these binding partners by sequestration.

The specificity with which *RB* inactivation elicits retinoblastoma, although second tumours like osteosarcomas can develop, remains a mystery. The *RB* gene is expressed in virtually all cell types, and loss of both alleles in children with hereditary forms of retinoblastoma therefore results in loss of function in all cell types. On the somatic level, *RB* alleles have been found deleted in common cancers in adults, such as prostate carcinomas, a third of bladder and

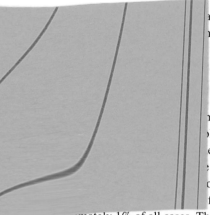

ally all small-cell lung cancers. These tumours have not been
...ce in patients with inherited *RB* inactivation had been cured of

...na, develops at high incidence (~10%) as bilateral cancers. By
...lastoma, it has been hypothesized that bilateral tumours occur
...etic lesion. This model requires that susceptible individuals
...e germ line; the other would be inactivated in the somatic cell
...ong 1972). In contrast to the relatively high frequency of famil-
...familial transmission of Wilms' tumour is documented in only
approximately 1% of all cases. This would suggest that new germ-line mutations are responsible
for the development of most familial Wilms' tumours (Haber and Housman 1992).

The Wilms' tumour gene (referred to as *WT1*) was isolated from chromosome 11p13 (Haber and
Housman 1992). In contrast to the ubiquitously expressed *RB* gene, *WT1* is expressed in a very
restricted number of tissues, with a strong developmental regulation in the kidney. *WT1* appears to
encode a transcription factor potentially regulating the expression of other genes. Understanding
the biological functions of *WT1* will critically depend on the identification of the corresponding
target genes regulated by *WT1*. *WT1* mutations have exclusively been found in Wilms' tumours,
and patients with germ-line inactivation of *WT1* do not have an increased incidence of other types
of cancer. The inactivation patterns include rare gross deletions or rearrangements, but small internal deletions are most common. Individuals with bilateral tumours are heterozygous for *WT1*
mutation in their germ line (as analysed from normal tissue) and have functional loss of the second
allele in both tumours, in perfect agreement with the Knudson two-hit model.

In contrast to retinoblastoma, which is associated exclusively with *RB* inactivation, Wilms'
tumour is genetically heterogeneous, and it appears that at least two additional loci may be
involved in tumourogenesis. Some Wilms' tumours appear to result from genomic changes in
band 11p15, rather than 11p13 to which *WT1* maps. A third, as yet unidentified locus, has been
implicated in inherited predisposition to Wilms' tumour. Linkage analyses have excluded 11p13
and 11p15 from transmission of disease susceptibility.

Neuroblastoma

In spite of some reports of familial neuroblastoma, this tumour should be regarded as developing
sporadically in at least the vast majority of cases. It is not known if any specific genomic alteration initiates neuroblastoma, but there are two types of genetic damage that appear centrally
involved in tumour development. A high proportion of tumours has alteration (deletion or
translocation) of distal chromosome 1p (Schwab *et al.* 1996), and it has been postulated that this
genomic region harbours a neuroblastoma suppressor locus. Attempts to isolate this alleged locus
have so far been unsuccessful, mainly because the genomic damage has been insufficiently
defined and because the genetic information in distal 1p has remained largely unexplored.

The second type of genetic damage involves amplification of the gene *MYCN* (Schwab *et al.*
1995). The tumour cells often carry hundreds of copies of the gene in addition to the two alleles

that are normally present. Amplification of *MYCN* occurs with high specificity in neuronal tumours and in addition to neuroblastoma rarely in brain tumours, retinoblastomas, and small cell lung cancers. A reasonable understanding of the mechanism by which *MYCN* becomes amplified in neuroblastomas has been developed, but the molecular challenges that initiate the amplification process have remained largely unknown. The *MYCN* gene encodes a nuclear protein that has properties of a transcription factor. The gene belongs to the *MYC*-family, with other members being *MYCC* and *MYCL*. The best characterized *MYC* and *MYCN* genes appear to have very similar activities when subjected to a variety of functional tests. Yet, the ubiquitous expression of *MYC* contrasts with the neuropreferential expression of *MYCN*, and neuroblastomas amplify only *MYCN* but never *MYC*. An understanding of *MYCN* function during normal development and in tumourogenesis might come from determining the identity of targets of transcriptional regulation. More recent developments also suggest that the MYCN protein is one member of a multiprotein complex. This situation, which presumably holds for all oncoproteins, presents an enormous challenge for finding out what is the contribution of *MYCN* to neuroblastoma.

Ewing's tumour

Ewing's tumour belongs to a group of small round cell, peripheral, primitive, neuroectodermal tumours (pPNET), which also includes peripheral neuroepithelioma and Askin tumour. When undifferentiated, these tumours are difficult to distinguish from each other as well as from rhabdomyosarcoma and neuroblastoma. Roughly 85% of pPNETs have been found to carry a t (11;22)(q29;12). This translocation fuses a gene *EWS* on chromosome 22 in frame with a member of the *ETS* family of transcription factors *FLI1* on chromosome 11. The expressed chimaeric protein has both DNA-binding and transactivation properties. Most of the remaining 15% of pPNETs have a variant t(21;22)(q22;q12) which results in a fusion of *EWS* with another member of the *ETS* family, *ERG*, which is very closely related to *FLI1*. A corresponding EWS/ERG fusion protein is expressed (Sorensen and Triche 1996).

The situation in which chromosome-specific translocations result in fusion proteins that have functional domains of both protein partners is highly reminiscent of the translocations in leukaemias, particularly CML, in which domains of the *ABL* and *BCR* genes are fused. While a misguided recombinase system normally responsible for immunoglobulin or T-cell receptor gene rearrangements may be involved in specific translocations in leukaemias (Rabbitts 1991), the molecular mechanism dictating gene-specific translocations in Ewing's sarcoma is unknown. It is not at all clear how the chimeric fusion proteins might contribute to tumourogenesis, although some speculations have been raised (Sorensen and Triche 1996).

Clinical potential of genomic alterations

Although an understanding of the biochemical contribution that genomic alterations make to tumourogenesis is far away, the specificity of genomic damage offers a clinically useful potential for different types of tumours (Sheer and Squire 1996). Direct benefits can be expected from two areas, diagnosis and prognosis, while foundations for therapeutic interventions on the basis of genomic alterations of oncogenes and tumour-suppressor genes have yet to be developed.

Identification of high-risk individuals in cancer famili

A major area for diagnostic potential lies in the identification
cancer families. The knowledge of specific genetic damage i
hood cancers, particularly retinoblastoma and Wilms' tumou
all family members for genetic damage in their germ line (J
cancers with a hereditary background, such as familial aden
forms of breast cancer, von Hippel-Lindau disease, and ot'
risk of cancer development can be evaluated in individual
retinoblastoma) as well as in individuals with new germ-l'
simple blood test. Somatic mutations are restricted to the tu...
tumours cannot be determined from normal cells of the individual.

Diagnosis and monitoring of therapeutic effect

Malignancies that have suffered a reciprocal translocation, particularly leukaemias (Rabbitts
1991), can be detected by molecular approaches with great precision, and the diagnosis of different types of leukaemias is possible when they might otherwise be confused with one another.
Using the polymerase chain reaction (PCR), it is now possible to detect the presence of one
leukaemic cell among one million normal cells (Crescenzi *et al.* 1988). This approach allows the
extremely sensitive detection of residual leukaemic cells in patients after therapy, or in bone
marrow that is being evaluated for autologous transplantation.

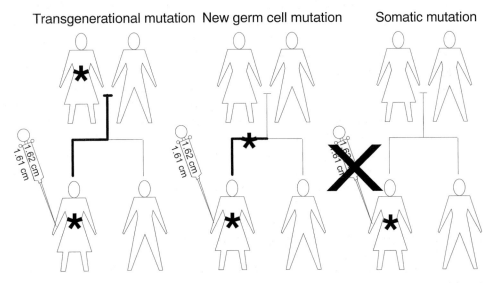

Fig. 2.3 Identification of high-risk patients in cancer families. If the corresponding mutation is stably transmitted through
the germ line (transgenerational mutation), high- and low-risk family members can be readily identified by determining the
gene status in normal peripheral blood lymphocytes. New germ-cell mutations, which are the starting point for a cancer
family, can be identified similarly. A somatic mutation is confined to the tumour cells and cannot be identified by analysing
normal cells.

Prognosis

Genomic lesions are obviously important determinants of tumour cell growth. Consequently, efforts have been undertaken to determine whether particular genomic alterations offer the possibility of evaluating the future course a tumour might take. The clinical debut of oncogenes is represented by the amplification of *MYCN* in neuroblastomas. The amplified *MYCN* is a strong, independent indicator of future aggressive tumour growth and of poor patient outcome (Schwab and Amler 1990). Determining the status of *MYCN* has become routine clinically in designing therapeutic regimens. More recent studies suggest that patients with low stage tumours without *MYCN* amplification do not benefit from chemotherapy.

Virtually all types of genetic lesions found in tumours have been or are being evaluated for prognostic usefulness. Although statistically significant correlations between individual parameters and prognosis have emerged in many settings, most have not been sufficiently reliable in decision making when it comes to therapy-design for the individual patient.

Genetic therapies

The application of established therapeutic approaches has done little over the past years to improve the survival rates of patients with most types of tumours, although there are positive exceptions. The rapid pace at which disease-associated genes have been identified over the past years has promoted the idea that an ideal approach to the cure of patients with cancers would be to reverse the adverse effect of genomic damage by genetic means. In a simplified form, this genetic therapy would, for instance, involve the introduction of a normal copy of a tumour-suppressor gene into tumour cells that have suffered damage of this gene. The expectation would be that the normal gene copy would be expressed and supply the tumour cell with the normal gene function and eventually abrogate the tumour phenotype.

Although this approach appears simple, and has been shown to work in tissue culture systems, a multitude of obstacles prohibits any clinical application at this time. The most serious problem is targeting and introducing the corresponding genes into the tumour cell. Even in tissue culture systems, in which diluted cellular monolayers can be exposed to saturating doses of exogenous gene copies, only a fraction of the cells actually take up the genes and assume a less aggressively growing phenotype. Cells of a solid tumour mass are difficult to challenge with exogenous gene copies. The problem of tumour-cell-specific targeting and of efficient introduction of exogenous gene copies remains unsolved.

Clonal variation of tumour cells is another serious problem. The cells of an advanced tumour have usually suffered damage at multiple genetic loci, and populations of genetically different cells exist within the tumour. Even if the problems of efficient targeting and introduction of exogenous gene copies into tumour cells might be solved, the genetic tumour cell heterogeneity will remain a serious obstacle. After all, tumour cells are genetically unstable and can evolve into new populations that acquire resistance against strong, selective forces. It is conceptually unclear at present how genetic therapies that have failed so far to correct relatively simple monogenic metabolic diseases can be employed to reverse a genetically extremely complex cancer disease.

Conclusions

Over past years, the identification of genetic elements in human cancer, both in children and adults, has progressed rapidly. Unfortunately, this has not lead to clear definition of the biochemical mechanisms involved in the metamorphosis of the normal cell to malignancy. The initial naive idea that learning about a particular oncogene or suppressor gene function means understanding cancer development has been replaced by a feeling that every single question answered entails more complicated problems to solve. This is in part due to the pleiotropic activity of the proteins encoded by oncogenes and tumour-suppressor genes. They can assume different functions depending on their status of post-transcriptional modification and dependent on the physical interaction with a multiplicity of other protein partners. While isolated activities can be described, it remains to be seen if we ever proceed to a full understanding of the role such polypeptide complexes have during normal development and tumourogenesis.

For the near future, the greatest promise, and benefit for the patient, lies in the application of genomic alterations as diagnostic and prognostic tools. In recognition of this potential, the corresponding technologies are rapidly entering clinical practice. In the long run, the further search for genetic damage in cancer cells and the identification of biochemical functions of oncogenes and tumour-suppressor genes is the best we can do to understand tumourogenesis and to design approaches for causal intervention.

Acknowledgements

Work in the author's lab is supported by the Dr. Mildred Scheel Foundation, Deutsche Forschungsgemeinschaft, Heidelberg-Mannheim Comprehensive Cancer Center, DKFZ-Israel Cooperation, and General Funds from the DKFZ.

References

Bishop, J.M. (1991) Molecular themes in oncogenesis. *Cell*, 64, 235–248.

Crescenzi, M., Seto, G., Herzig, G.P., Weiss, P.D., Griffith, R.C., and Korsmeyer, S.J. (1988) Thermostable DNA polymerase chain amplification of t(14;18) chromosome breakpoints and detection of minmal residual disease. *Procedures of the National Academy of Sciences (USA)*, 85, 4869–4873.

Haber, D.A. and Housman, D.E. (1992) Role of the *WT1* gene in Wilms' tumour. *Cancer Surveys* 12, 105–117.

Karran, P. (1996) Microsatellite instability and DNA mismatch repair in human cancer. *Seminars in Cancer Biology*, 7, 15–24.

Knudson, A.G. (1971) Mutation and cancer: a statistical study. *Procedures of the National Academy of Sciences (USA)*, 68, 820–823.

Knudson, A.G. and Strong, L.C. (1972) Mutation and cancer: a model for Wilms' tumour of the kidney. *Journal of the National Cancer Institute*, 48, 313–324.

Modrich, P. (1991) Mechanisms and biological effects of mismatch repair. *Annual Review of Genetics*, 25, 229–253.

Rabbitts, T.H. (1991) Translocations, master genes, and differences between the origins of acute and chronic leukaemias. *Cell*, 67, 641–644.

Santoro, M., Carlomagno, F., Romano, A., Bottaro, D.P., Dathan, N.A., Grieco, M., *et al.* (1995) Activation of RET as a dominant transforming gene by germline mutations of MEN2A and MEN2B. *Science*, 267, 381–383.

Schwab, M. and Amler, L.C. (1990) Amplification of cellular oncogenes: A predictor of clinical outcome in human cancer. *Genes Chromosomes and Cancer*, 1, 181–193.

Schwab, M., Corvi, R., and Amler, L.C. (1995) N-*MYC* oncogene amplification: A consequence of genomic instability in human neuroblastoma. *Neuroscientist*, 1, 277–285

Schwab, M., Praml, C., and Amler, L.C. (1996) Genomic instability in 1p and human malignancies. *Genes Chromosomes and Cancer*, 16, 211–229.

Sheer, D. and Squire, J. (1996) Clinical applications of genetic rearrangements in cancer. *Cancer Biology*, 7, 25–32.

Sorensen, P.H.B. and Triche, T.J. (1996) Gene fusions encoding chimaeric transcription factors in solid tumours. *Cancer Biology*, 7, 3–14.

Weinberg, R.A. (1992) The retinoblastoma gene and gene product. *Cancer Surveys*, 12, 43–57.

3 Molecular basis of childhood cancer

L.A. Smets

Introduction

The past decades have witnessed spectacular advances in understanding the molecular biology of cancer. Central to this progress is the notion that cancer is a genetic disease, resulting from somatic and germ-line mutations. The human genome comprises about 10^5 genes that are edited by an estimated number of 10^3 regulatory genes. Regulatory genes encode hormones, hormone receptors, signal-transduction proteins, transcription factors, molecules involved in cell-cell interactions, and proteins that function in the surveillance of cell proliferation and genomic integrity. It is estimated that about 10^2 regulatory genes are potential oncogenes (proto-oncogenes) or tumour-suppressor genes, giving rise to cancer if mutated (Bishop 1991). The progress in detecting (combinations of) oncogenes in specific types of cancer has significantly improved our understanding of the aetiology of this disease (Vogelstein and Kinzler 1993). This knowledge, in conjunction with sophisticated analytical techniques, provides tools for more accurate diagnosis, allows more reliable genetic counselling and risk-classification, and offers a possibility of specific, defect-oriented therapies.

Important progress has also been made in the molecular biology of cellular factors that mediate the response to cytostatic treatment. These include the mechanisms by which cells can extrude foreign compounds—paramount to the development of multidrug resistance—and the gene systems that recognize and repair genomic damage after chemo- and radiotherapy. Finally, there is growing insight that cells frequently die by a genetically controlled process of active suicide or apoptosis, hinting at entirely novel therapeutic strategies.

The discovery of oncogenes and tumour-suppressor genes

Oncogenes

Cancer is traditionally used as a collective noun for a spectrum of widely different diseases, characterized by uncontrolled proliferation and metastatic spread. A genetic causation was suggested early by several observations: the genetic predisposition for some—mostly paediatric—tumours, the frequent observation of chromosomal aberrations in cancer cells, and the carcinogenic potential of mutagens. Moreover, dose-effect studies in animals had suggested that between 2–7 genetic events or hits are required for tumour induction with mutagenic/carcinogenic compounds. In parallel, tissue culture studies revealed the existence of discrete and permanent phenotypic changes in cancer cells: immortalization, low growth factor requirement, loss of control of growth and motility by cell-cell contact, and even the capacity to invade and destroy normal tissues.

The apparent link between genetic changes and stable phenotypic properties was confirmed by analysis of the genetic content of RNA containing retroviruses, long known as an aetiological factor in many types of cancer in rodents, poultry, and cattle. Retroviruses all contain genetic information for three virus-specific proteins (env, gag, pol). Tumourogenic viruses harbour an extra gene, called viral oncogene (v-*onc*), responsible for the malignant transformation of infected cells. Molecular probes against v-*oncs* and antibodies against their predicted protein structures revealed that v-*onc*-like genes were present in nearly all normal cells as potential cellular oncogenes (c-*onc* genes), and that the corresponding proteins were (over) expressed in some tumours. Thus, viral oncogenes are cellular genes, 'stolen' and activated during infectious cycles. Subsequently, slowly transforming viruses that do not contain v-*onc* genes were found randomly integrated into the DNA of normal tissues. In tumours, these viruses are non-randomly integrated in or near cellular oncogenes or tumour-suppressor genes, resulting in dysregulation of their expression.

The genetic origin of tumours without a viral aetiology was subsequently established in studies in which DNA, isolated from human tumour cells, was used to transform normal mouse cells by transfection. The human DNA sequence responsible for transformation was identified as a cellular oncogene, e.g. the mutated *ras* gene of bladder cancer cells (Fig. 3.1).

Tumour-suppressor genes

Studies involving viral infections or DNA transfection can detect dominant or gain-of-function oncogenes, i.e. genes that impose a transformed phenotype on normal cells. A novel class of recessive, loss-of-function oncogenes was indicated in fusions between normal and malignant

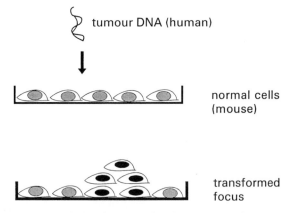

tumour DNA (human)

normal cells
(mouse)

transformed
focus

Fig. 3.1 Detection of human oncogenes by transfecting DNA from human cancer cells into a monolayer of normal mouse cells. A transformed mouse cell gives rise to a multilayered focus in the monolayer which can be propagated to isolate a (dominant) human oncogene.

cells. These somatic cell hybrids initially display a normal phenotype but become transformed after the loss of a specific chromosome that belongs to the normal fusion partner. This chromosome contains a gene that suppresses the malignant phenotype: a tumour-suppressor gene.

Activation of oncogenes

Oncogenes and tumour-suppressor genes are by origin normal genes involved in the regulation of cellular behaviour. In order to cause cancer, the normal gene or proto-oncogene must be 'activated', whereas both alleles of tumour-suppressor genes have to be eliminated by deletions or inactivating mutations. In the absence of overt chromosomal changes, deletion of tumour-suppressor genes is detected as loss of heterozygosity (LOH), i.e. the disappearance of polymorphic differences between two suspected allelic loci. Activation or deregulated gene expression includes overexpression of the oncoprotein, e.g. Bcl-2 in follicular lymphoma, or unscheduled expression when during normal development the gene should be silent, e.g. c-*myc* in mature T- or B-lymphoma cells. Activation of proto-oncogenes is caused by alterations that include gene amplification, chromosomal translocations and inversions, or by gene mutations.

Amplification

Amplification increases the gene copy number, leading to a proportional increase in (onco)protein production. The cytogenetic correlate of chromosomal amplification is tri- or tetrasomy, i.e. the presence of three or four copies of a particular chromosome. In such cases, it is very difficult to pinpoint the relevant oncogene among thousands of co-amplified normal genes. Moreover, concomitant amplification of tumour-suppressor genes may obscure the effect of oncogene amplification. Amplification may be limited to a small set of adjacent genes such as the cyclin *D1* gene in breast cancer or the *MDR1* gene in some types of multidrug resistance. These amplifications are detected by blotting techniques or by characteristic alterations in chromosomal banding pattern, called homogeneously staining regions (HSR). The classic example is the HSR in methotrexate-resistant cells, containing multiple copies of the gene encoding for dihydrofolate reductase. Amplified genes may be present in extrachromosomal elements or mini-chromosomes: double minutes (DMs). Overexpression of N-*myc* in neuroblastoma is frequently associated with many extranuclear DMs.

Translocation and inversion

During normal cell development, lineage-specific genes are assembled and activated by rearrangement. Rearranging genes are fragile at the joining ends and prone to breakage. These breaks may rejoin, in error, with breaks in other rearranging or actively transcribing genes to form non-random chromosomal translocations and inversions (Rabbitts 1994). The principal consequence of translocation and inversion is activation of a proto-oncogene, or the creation of a fusion gene encoding a chimaeric protein. Translocations involving chromosomes 2, 14, or 22, carrying the genes for Ig heavy and light chains, are a frequent finding in B-lineage lymphoma. Preferred partners in these translocations are c-*myc* on chromosome 8 and *bcl*-2 on chromosome

18, being deregulated if placed in juxtaposition with the Ig genes. Likewise, rearrangements of T cell receptor genes can lead to oncogene-activating translocations in T cell leukaemia and lymphoma. Most of the translocation partners are highly conserved transcription factors for differentiation, normally not expressed in T cells. An example is the *HOX11* gene on chromosome 10, which is activated by translocations 10;14 or 7;10.

In most cases, and notably so in solid tumours, the repercussion of translocations and inversions is gene fusion, resulting in the synthesis of chimaeric proteins. Increased tyrosine kinase activity of the BCR-ABL fusion protein is the consequence of translocation 9;22, the Philadelphia chromosome. In fact, most fusion proteins appear to be protein kinases or DNA-binding transcription factors, involved in the control of proliferation and differentiation.

Mutations

Mutations are a frequent cause of the inactivation of tumour-suppressor genes, but can also activate proto-oncogenes. Mutations in specific codons of *ras* genes have established an intriguing association between the chemical properties of a carcinogen, the nucleotide sequence of specific codons, and the sensitivity of particular tissues to a specific mutation. This is exemplified by the preferred mutation of codon 12 in Ki-*ras* in lung adenocarcinoma of smokers. Mutations can activate proto-oncogenes by interrupting downregulating activities. Thus, mutations can eliminate the intrinsic GTPase activity of *ras*-encoded G proteins, required for interrupting their activation after binding of GTP (see also section on functions of oncogenes and tumour-suppressor genes) or they can increase the production of mRNA and protein in case of mutations in c-*myc*. The tumour suppressor gene *p53* encodes a transcription factor and is mutated in 50% of human cancers. Mutated p53 protein is frequently more stable and the accumulated protein can block the function of the product of the normal allele in a dominant-negative way.

Multistep nature of cancer in adults and children

Although cancer is in essence a genetic disease, it differs from congenital abnormalities in several aspects (Vogelstein and Kinzler 1993). Cancer is, for the most part, caused by somatic mutations, and only rarely by germ-line mutations, mainly in paediatric tumours. Moreover, tumours do not arise from a single mutation, but clonally from several mutations that accumulate in a single progenitor cell. Because the probability of this accumulation is low, most cancers occur in older people. The accumulation is not entirely random, and certain mutations clearly precede others, e.g. in colorectal tumourogenesis. The non-random sequence of multiple genetic hits, driving the multi step process of tumour progression, is facilitated by genomic instability. For instance, mutations in *p53* inhibit DNA repair and promote survival of variant cells by blocking apoptosis.

Aetiology

Paediatric tumours arise early because there are mostly only two rate-limiting mutations involved, e.g. in retinoblastoma and Wilms' tumour (Grundy and Coppes 1996), and because one of these mutations can be inherited. In the latter case, the second, post-natal mutation is the inactivation of the other allele of a tumour-suppressor gene. Moreover, the number of hits required for the induction of a blastoma, the most frequent type of cancer in children, may be lower in their precursor cells than in those of other tissues. Finally, mutations in embryonic tissues affect expanding populations instead of steady-state renewal tissues in adults, putting more cells at risk for acquiring a second mutation.

Because paediatric cancers arise early, environmental factors play a minor role in their aetiology which is, instead, dominated by genetic inheritance and familial predisposition. Thyroid cancer from radiation exposures may be the exception to this rule. Apart from the rate of appearance, the spectrum of genetic changes in cancer of children also differs somewhat from that in adults. Thus, c-*myc*, which is highly expressed in embryonic tissues, is frequently involved in paediatric cancer, whereas *ras* genes are rarely so. Activation of *ras* occurs exclusively by mutation due to exposure to carcinogens. The low frequency of *ras* mutations in paediatric cancer therefore affirms the minor importance of environmental carcinogens. Virally-induced cancer accounts for 15% of all cancers, but rarely for paediatric tumours because of the long latency of induction, suggesting an indirect contribution to cancer development.

Although most genetic alterations in paediatric malignancies are shared with those in adult disease, there is a remarkable difference in the sequence of events. Thus, deletion/mutation of the tumour-suppressor genes *Rb* and *WTI* are primordial in retinoblastoma and Wilms' tumour, respectively, and frequently associated with hereditary predispositions. In adult tumours, changes in 'paediatric' tumour-suppressor genes occur in the course of tumour progression, e.g. the Ewing's sarcoma (*EWS*) gene in the *EWS-ATF-1* fusion gene involved in melanoma or *Rb* mutations in several adult tumours (lung, oesophagus).

A characteristic difference between paediatric and adult cancer is the role of chromosome amplification (aneuploidy). Aneuploidy is a frequent occurrence in adult tumours and invariably associated with poor prognosis. In contrast, aneuploidy in most solid tumours of children (rhabdomyosarcoma, retinoblastoma, neuroblastoma) is associated with a more favourable prognosis. In B-lineage ALL, a special form of aneuploidy, called hyperdiploidy and involving chromosomes 4, 6, 10, and 21, is considered the most important predictor of good response (Smets *et al.* 1995). The mechanisms by which aneuploidy affects prognosis are not known, but they have been associated with the metabolism of antimetabolite drugs in hyperdiploid ALL.

A more detailed description of oncogenic alterations in paediatric malignancies and in the predisposing syndromes can be found in Chapter 2 and in the chapters dealing with specific malignancies.

Functions of oncogenes and tumour-suppressor genes

Comparison of structural motifs in proteins encoded by (proto) oncogenes with those of known proteins can reveal their function. Antibodies raised against characteristic peptide sequences provide information on their expression and subcellular distribution in normal and malignant cells. Transfection of oncogenes and tumour-suppressor genes in suitable viral vectors and studies with transgenic animals in which specific genes are either overexpressed or deleted, are also potent investigational tools. The assembled information from these studies has yielded a quite coherent picture of how the most important oncogenes transform a normal cell. In a multi-cellular organism, the social behaviour of individual cells (proliferation, differentiation, migration) is governed by endocrine and paracrine signals (hormones, growth/differentiation factors) and by signals generated by cell-cell contact. The extracellular signals, perceived at the cell surface, are transduced to the nucleus to promote or repress gene transcription. Signal transduction pathways for growth/differentiation are characteristically composed of the following elements: an extracellular cell surface receptor, intracellular translating/amplifying receptor domains, and various second messengers (Ca²⁺ ions, lipid messengers, cyclic AMP, protein kinases) that act on nuclear transcription factors. For instance, the proto-oncogenes *jun* and *fos* are the targets of growth-factor-stimulated protein kinases STAT and MAPK in normal cells, but cause uncontrolled, factor-independent growth if constitutively activated.

The majority of oncoproteins are inappropriately acting elements of these signalling cascades. Fig. 3.2 illustrates how the expression of the oncogene *sis*, encoding the alpha chain of the platelet-derived growth factor, causes autocrine stimulation of cells which harbour the cognate receptor. Cells in which the intracellular domain of the EGF receptor—a tyrosine kinase encoded by *erbB*—is inappropriately expressed, can proliferate autonomously in the absence of the growth hormone or of an extracellular EGF receptor domain. The products of *ras* genes belong to a class of G proteins that amplify and transduce extracellular signals. Specific mutations in this gene prolong or intensify growth-stimulating signals leading to unscheduled responses. Other oncoproteins are chimaeric nuclear transcription factors that stimulate proliferation.

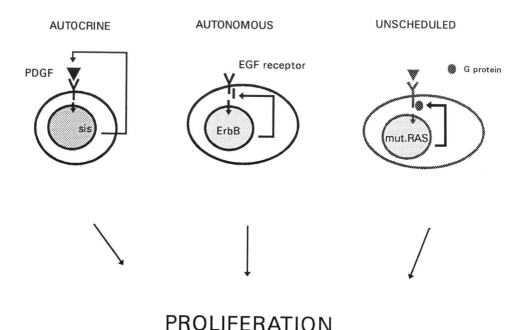

Fig. 3.2 Activation of proto-oncogenes stimulates proliferation. Activation of *sis* results in the release of the platelet-derived growth factor (PDGF) and autocrine growth (left). The protein encoded by *erbB* is a signal-transducing element of the EGF receptor and deregulation of its expression leads to autonomous growth in the absence of the growth factor (middle). Mutated *ras* encodes a constitutively activated G protein, involved in signal transduction (right).

Tumour-suppressor genes, on the other hand, are considered to belong to signalling pathways for differentiation. Most identified tumour-suppressor genes are nuclear factors that control transcription of differentiation factors. Loss of tumour-suppressor genes or incapacitating mutations relieve cells from restraints on proliferation. For instance, the *WT1* gene involved in Wilms' tumour promotes differentiation by suppressing a gene that encodes for the growth factor IGF-2. Deletion of both alleles of the *WT1* gene allows the expression of this growth factor, resulting in stimulated, neoplastic growth.

Genes that regulate cell survival

More recently, a class of oncogenes has been discovered which, unlike classical oncogenes and tumour-suppressor genes, regulates survival rather than proliferation. The target of survival-regulating genes is programmed cell death or apoptosis, that is, the controlled removal of redundant or unwanted cells during embryogenesis and tissue homeostasis. Apoptosis is under control by genes whose expression is frequently altered in cancer cells. In non-Hodgkin's lymphoma, translocation 14;18 deregulates the *bcl-2* gene, and the overexpressed 26 kDa Bcl-2 protein protects the cell against several triggers for apoptosis. Bcl-2 and related proteins such as Bcl-X$_1$ are counteracted by the products of death-promoting genes *bax*, *bad*, *bak*, and family members with which they can form heterodimers. The ratio of promoting and inhibiting proteins, e.g. Bcl-2/Bax, is therefore considered to act as a rheostat that determines the probability of survival after several types of cellular insult (Fig. 3.3). Induction of apoptosis is, in many but not all instances, associated with deregulated cell cycle control. Genes involved in cell cycle progression such as *p53* and c-*myc*, are therefore key players in many forms of apoptosis. The anti-apoptotic mechanism of Bcl-2 is not known, but there is upcoming evidence that the protein may prevent excessive cell cycle deregulation.

Cytostatic drugs and radiation often induce the final stages of apoptosis that include characteristic DNA degradation and the formation of apoptotic bodies. It has been postulated that *p53* status and the Bcl-2/Bax ratio determine the intrinsic sensitivity to cytostatic treatment of tumours by modulation of apoptosis. This may not be generally true because blocked apoptosis,

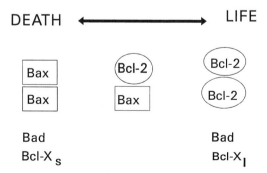

Fig. 3.3 Proteins that regulate apoptosis. Bax and related proteins promote apoptosis and can heterodimerize with apoptosis-inhibiting Bcl-2 and related proteins. The ratio of Bcl-2 to Bax is considered to act as a rheostat that controls the survival probability after cytotoxic insult.

e.g. in *p53*$^{-/-}$ cells exposed to radiation, may not prevent cell death from other causes such as mitotic failure or the loss of clonogenic capacity. Clinical studies have not established a clear relationship between *p53* status and apoptotic index with the initial response to treatment. Moreover, high Bcl-2 levels are sometimes associated with good prognosis. For instance, in ALL of childhood, highest levels of Bcl-2 are found in the most favourable prognostic group of patients with B-lineage disease and low WBC. The discrepancy between clinical and laboratory findings can be explained by the fact that the role of apoptosis-regulating genes may be context-dependent, i.e. by affecting tumour factors such as growth fraction, vascularization, and repopulation capacity. These factors, which are of minor importance or irrelevant in simple tissue culture systems, have a known impact on the response to chemo- and radiotherapy of tumour tissues. Moreover, delayed or blocked apoptosis may conceivably interfere with clinical outcome by promoting the survival of ectopic, metastasizing tumour cells or by allowing time for repair of critically damaged cells. The balance of all these factors may mitigate, if not outweigh, the putative antagonistic role of blocked apoptosis on the sensitivity of a specific tumour to a specific type of anticancer therapy (discussed in Cote *et al.* 1997).

Despite these controversies, induction of apoptosis is a stimulating strategic concept for novel types of cancer treatment. Ionizing radiation and various stress factors can kill some cell types by increasing the levels of ceramide, leading to apoptosis. Cytostatic drugs have been reported to kill T cells by activation of Fas/APO I -mediated apoptotic pathways. Such observations strongly challenge conventional concepts regarding cytotoxic mechanisms in chemo- and radiotherapy and the factors that determine the differential sensitivity of normal and malignant tissues to cytostatic treatment.

Genes that control the cell cycle

Because malignant transformation leads to neoplastic growth, the cell cycle is the stage for most actors in this tragedy: oncogenes and tumour-suppressor genes. These genes, when normal, have been assigned important functions in the maintenance of controlled proliferation and the surveillance of genomic integrity. Conversely, genes initially detected as regulators of the cell cycle are now increasingly found to be potential (proto) oncogenes. Genetic control of cell proliferation is thus highly integrated with control of cell survival and repair of genomic damage (Fig. 3.4). In the context of this chapter, only a brief summary of the most important aspects can be given.

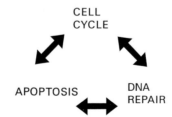

Fig. 3.4 Genetic controls on cell-cycle progression, repair of DNA damage, and apoptosis form a highly integrated system. Defects in any of these components are (co-)carcinogenic or responsible for tumour progression.

The cell cycle is composed of several distinct subcycles, such as the cell division cycle and the DNA replication cycle. These subcycles are driven and coordinated by the sequential expression of cyclins that are only expressed in specific phases of the cell cycle. Cyclins 'mix and match' with various cell-cycle-dependent kinases, CDKs, leading to activation of the intrinsic kinase activity of the CDK (Morgan 1995). The targets of activated cyclin/CDK complexes are the genes and proteins that function in cell-cycle checkpoints. Important cell-cycle checkpoints are: 'commitment to G_0–G_1 transition', 'progression through G_1–S', and 'chromatin integrity' during transition from G_2 to M phase. The activity of cyclin/CDK complexes is inhibited by various CDK-inhibiting proteins, CDKIs, such as p16, p21, and p27. The assembly of all these elements is a tightly controlled and integrated system of cell-cycle initiation and progression (Jacks and Weinberg 1996).

The cell-cycle checkpoint 'progression' has been studied in great detail. Central is the tumour-suppressor gene *Rb*, which is phosphorylated by the active cyclinD/CDK4 complex. Phosphorylated Rb protein releases the associated transcription activator E2F which is integral to G_1–S transition and the onset of DNA synthesis. DNA damage upregulates *p53* which in turn enhances the transcription of the CDKI protein p21, an inhibitor of cyclinD/CDK4. The effect of sensed DNA damage is cell-cycle arrest by inhibited Rb phosphorylation, allowing time for repair or stimulation of apoptosis, if repair fails. Consequently, overexpression of cyclins and CDKs on the one hand and inactivation of CDKIs and tumour-suppressor genes *p53* and *Rb* on the other, are documented cell-cycle deregulating, and thus potentially carcinogenic, events.

Loss of cell-cycle control is not only a prominent cause of cancer, it may also affect the sensitivity to cytostatic treatment. Many anticancer agents act on specific points in the cell cycle (DNA antimetabolites, mitotic spindle poisons) or require progression through cell-cycle subphases for cytotoxicity, e.g. of S-phase in the action of topoisomerase I and II inhibitors. Alterations in the control of cell-cycle progression can therefore increase or decrease the sensitivity to such agents (Waldman *et al.* 1996).

Because cell-cycle integrity is essential in normal development, nature tolerates only minor deviations from it. Cells that become deficient in cell-cycle control are therefore eliminated by apoptosis. This is convincingly demonstrated by the observation that overexpression of the pro-liferation-stimulating gene c-*myc* induces apoptosis in normal cells. In cancer cells, activation of c-*myc* must be accompanied by mutations that attenuate an apoptotic response or block its induction.

Genes that control the response to treatment

Cytostatic drugs kill their target cells in a balanced sequence of events: drug uptake/export through the plasma membrane, drug activation/inactivation in the cytoplasm, induction/repair of DNA damage, and death/survival at a given level of damage (Fig. 3.5). Because of their intrinsic genomic instability, resistance can emerge in tumours at any of these steps. The molecular biology of drug export, DNA repair, and cell survival is at the centre of today's research.

Multidrug resistance

A clinically important group of drugs consists of natural products (vincristine, anthracyclines, antibiotics, epidophyllotoxins). Despite widely different cytotoxic mechanisms, these drugs share

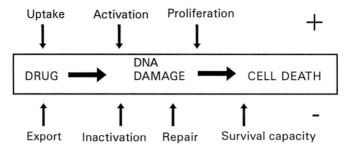

Fig. 3.5   The intrinsic sensitivity of tumour cells to cytostatic treatment is determined by a complex balance between promoting (+) and inhibiting (–) factors. Multidrug resistance by enhanced drug export and increased survival probability by blocked apoptosis are at the centre of today's research.

the structural property of being lipophilic, organic cations that accumulate in cells by facilitated diffusion, driven by an electrochemical gradient. Most natural products are foreign to our body and potentially toxic. A superfamily of highly conserved genes encodes for proteins that extrude organic cations, called the (ABC) transporter family because of a common structural motif that consists of an ATP-binding cassette. Overexpression of (ABC) transporter genes is the cause of primary or acquired multidrug resistance (MDR), an important cause of failed/ineffective chemotherapy in cancer of adults and children (Chan *et al.* 1996).

The best known drug exporter is the P-glycoprotein (P-gp) encoded by the *MDR1* gene (Borst 1991). P-gp is a 170-kDa membrane glycoprotein, constitutively expressed in organs with excretory or secretory functions (stomach, gut, pancreas, kidney). The presence of P-gp in the epithelia of these organs indicates its function in preventing exposure to xenobiotic compounds, and explains the intrinsic insensitivity of tumours of these organs to chemotherapy. P-gp is frequently upregulated during treatment of solid tumours and leukaemia by mutation or amplification of the *MDR1* gene or by post-translational modification. P-gp consists of membrane-spanning domains that form a pore in the plasma membrane. The cytoplasmic drug-binding domain is flanked by two nucleotide-binding sites that provide the energy for drug export by hydrolysis of ATP. The structure has considerable homology with exporter proteins in bacteria. P-gp-mediated multidrug resistance can be antagonized by reversal agents such as verapamil and cyclosporin A, that compete with drugs for binding to the exporter. The clinical effectiveness of these agents is disappointing, however, because of severe toxicity. More specific and less toxic second-generation reversal agents are under investigation.

In several MDR cell lines, natural products can be exported by a 190-kDa, MDR-related protein (MRP). The primary structure of MRP is only distantly related to that of P-gp, and its spectrum of exported drugs is somewhat different. For instance, the drug taxol is exported by P-gp but not by MRP. MRP has high affinity for glutathione-S-conjugated compounds, suggesting a function in detoxification by eliminating drug conjugates. The *MRP* gene is expressed in several normal tissues and tumours. Its role in primary and acquired drug resistance is under investigation. In neuroblastoma, expression of *MRP* correlates well with N-*myc* amplification and poor outcome of treatment (Norris et al. 1996). The alkaloid genestein is an experimental reversal agent for MRP.

In multidrug-resistant lung cancer cells that express neither P-gp nor MRP, a 110-kDa protein is overexpressed. The protein is called LRP, lung-cancer-related resistance protein, and has strong homology with the vault proteins. These proteins control transport between cytosolic and nucleosolic compartments. LRP does not require ATP, and it is uncertain whether LRP belongs to the (ABC) transporter family. Overexpression of LRP is associated with poor response to chemotherapy in AML and ovarian cancer.

DNA repair

Exposure to ionizing radiation and to most chemotherapeutic drugs culminates in the induction of DNA damage. The capacity to repair this damage is potentially important for sensitivity to chemo- and radiotherapy. The extreme sensitivity of cells and tissues from individuals with inherited repair-deficient syndromes (xeroderma pigmentosum, ataxia telangiectasia) attests to this view. DNA damage repair includes base and nucleotide excision repair, mismatch repair of spontaneous or adduct-induced replication errors, and repair of double strand breaks generated by radiation or by drugs such as topoisomerase I and II inhibitors. Over 40 human genes, involved in DNA repair and metabolism, have been cloned to date.

Nucleotidyl transferases remove methylated or alkylated DNA bases in cells exposed to nitrosureas and related compounds. Radiation-induced single base lesions are removed by DNA glycosylases, followed by repair of the apurinic/apyrimidinic site by endonucleases, DNA polymerase β, and ligases. Several genes encode proteins involved in the repair of mismatched base pairs. These genes are characteristically deficient in hereditary syndromes that predispose to cancer, e.g. the Lynch syndrome or hereditary nonpolyposis colon cancer (HNPPC). Cells affected by these mutations have increased genomic instability, reflected in microsatellite instability associated with the replication error positive (RER$^+$) phenotype (Loeb 1994). Double strand breaks are repaired in a complex sequence of recognition and binding of a heterodimer of Ku70 and Ku80 gene products, complexing with a DNA-dependent protein kinase, whose activity allows subsequent recruitment of other repair factors (Gottlieb and Jackson 1994).

In addition to dysfunctional DNA repair enzymes, cells can be deficient in signalling responses elicited by DNA damage and in the regulation of the cell cycle. The *p53* and *ATM* (mutated in ataxia telangectasia) genes, with germ-line mutations in the Li-Fraumeni and ataxia telangiectasia syndromes, respectively, are typically involved in the signalling of DNA damage and cell cycle control. Cell-cycle arrest by *p53* allows time for repair and induction of apoptosis, if repair fails. The gene is therefore considered a guardian of the genome. Whether induction of apoptosis is an alternative role of *p53* or the consequence of *p53*-mediated excessive cell-cycle deregulation is unknown.

DNA repair and sensitivity to treatment

Compared to the obvious importance of repair deficiencies in so-called mutator phenotypes to the induction of cancers, their impact on the intrinsic sensitivity to cytostatic treatment is less clear. Increased levels of DNA adduct-repairing transferases confer resistance to alkylating agents and platinum-containing drugs, but mismatch repair-deficient cells can tolerate increased levels of drug-induced DNA damage. Likewise, the role of p53 is complex. Functional p53 can conceivably increase resistance by allowing time for repair of damage, but also render cells more sensitive by induction of apoptosis. In irradiated cells, G_2 delay at the cell-cycle checkpoint for the repair of chromatin damage cells has been associated with both decreased and increased sensitivity.

Genetic control of DNA repair occurs not only in cancers but also in normal tissues. Accordingly, interpatient variation in the tolerance to radiotherapy might conceivably be traced back to a different expression of repair enzymes. Although screening for such differences would be valuable for treatment planning, it is obvious that this task is formidable in view of the many genes involved.

Apoptosis

Because cytostatic treatment often induces in the exposed cells the late manifestations of apoptosis, it has been postulated that blocked apoptosis by dysfunctional p53 or overexpressed Bcl-2 can be considered as a special form of multidrug resistance. As discussed (on pp. 37–8), this conclusion may not be generally true because of apparent discrepancies between clinical and laboratory findings.

Oncogenes at the bedside

The recent discoveries in the molecular biology of cancer have almost autocatalytically expanded our knowledge of this disease. It is a reasonable assumption that blueprints of all genetic changes in individual tumours will be available within 1–2 decades.

Many of these achievements are gradually filtering into clinical practice. Conventional histo- and cytopathology are being complemented by molecular pathology, describing the expression level or mutational status of key oncogenes. The detection of various specific gene events during the differentiation of germ-cell tumours is only one typical example of this development. Cells harbouring genes affected by translocation or inversion can now be detected with unprecedented sensitivity by PCR-assisted amplification in a frequency of 10^{-6}–10^{-5}, a technique applied for monitoring of response, bone-marrow purging, and relapse prediction. A clearly undesirable aspect of this progress is an unwarranted tendency to replace conventional cell biological parameters with more sophisticated molecular-biological assays. However, conventional parameters such as mitotic index, S-phase values, and other histological and cytological findings still have demonstrated prognostic value and are, in essence, the net result of the underlying oncogenetic changes.

The achievements of the molecular biology of DNA repair, drug transport, and survival probability will most probably result in new definitions of how cancer cells can be selectively killed and, hopefully, in improved patient stratification and adapted therapy.

Although these and other developments are of obvious importance, the major goal still is to design more efficient and less toxic therapeutic strategies, specifically aiming at the genetic defects in cancer cells. The prospects of various forms of gene therapy of cancer are currently under critical review. It will take a long time and much research effort before they can be applied to the benefit of large groups of patients.

References

Bishop, J.M. (1991). Molecular Themes in Oncogenesis. *Cell*, 64, 235–48.

Borst, P. (1991). Genetic mechanisms of drug resistance. A review. *Acta Oncologica*, 30, 87–105.

Chan, H.S., Grogan, T.M., DeBoer, G., Haddad, G., Gallie, B.L., and Ling, V. (1996). Diagnosis and reversal of multidrug resistance in paediatric cancers. *European Journal of Cancer*, 32A, 1051–61.

Cote, R.J., Esrig, D., Groshen, S., Jones, P.A., and Skinner, D.G. (1997). p53 and treatment of bladder cancer. *Nature (scientific correspondence)*, 385, 123–25.

Gottlieb, T.M. and Jackson, S.P. (1994). Protein kinases and DNA damage. *Trends in Biochemical Science*, 19, 500–03.

Grundy, P. and Coppes, M. (1996). An overview of the clinical and molecular genetics of Wilms' Tumour. *Medical and Pediatric Oncology*, 27, 394–97.

Jacks, T. and Weinberg, R.A. (1996). Cell cycle control and its watchman. *Nature*, 381, 643–44.

Loeb, L.A. (1994). Microsatellite instability: marker of a mutator phenotype in cancer. *Cancer Reviews*, 54, 5059–63.

Morgan, D.O. (1995). Principles of CDK regulation. *Nature*, 374, 131–34.

Norris, M.D., Bordow, S.B., Marchall, G.M., Haber, P.S., Cohn, S.L., and Haber, M. (1996). Expression of the gene for multidrug-resistance-associated protein and outcome in patients with neuroblastoma. *New England Journal of Medicine*, 334, 231–38.

Rabbitts, T.H. (1994). Chromosomal translocations in human cancer. *Nature*, 372, 143–49.

Smets, L.A., Slater, R., Van Wering, E.R., Van der Does- Van den Berg, A., Hart, A.A., *et al.* (1995). DNA index and %S-phase cells determined in acute lymphoblastic leukaemia of children: A report from studies ALL V, ALL VI and ALL VII (1979–1991) of the Dutch Childhood Leukaemia Study Group and the Netherlands Workgroup on Cancer Genetics and Cytogenetics. *Medical and Pediatric Oncology*, 25, 437–44.

Vogelstein, B. and Kinzler, K. (1993) The multistep nature of cancer. *Trends in Genetics*, 9, 138–41.

Waldman, T., Lengauer, C., Kinzler, K.W., and Vogelstein, B. (1996) Uncoupling of S phase and mitosis induced by anticancer agents in cells lacking p21. *Nature*, 381, 713–16.

4 Principles of cancer chemotherapy in children

R. Riccardi, A. Lasorella, and R. Mastrangelo

Chemotherapy has made a fundamental contribution to the treatment of childhood cancer and has led to a marked increase in the cure rate of most of these diseases. The antineoplastic drugs currently used in clinical practice exert their cytotoxic effect by interfering with the synthesis or function of DNA. Most of these drugs are cell-cycle specific, i.e. they are active only in a given phase of the cell cycle. Figure 4.1 indicates schematically the site of action of commonly used anticancer drugs in paediatric oncology. DNA damage may either result in tumour-cell necrosis or may activate a specific, genetically determined mechanism leading to a form of programmed cell death. The latter process of apoptosis appears to have an important role in determining and modulating the cytotoxicity of many anticancer drugs.

The extent of tumour control achieved by chemotherapy is related to a number of different factors such as the antitumour spectrum of the drug, dose and schedule used, pharmacokinetics, tumour biology, cell kinetics, adequacy of drug delivery, and host tolerance. In the past two decades, the refinement of doses and schedules and the proper timing of surgery and radiotherapy, together with rigorous evaluation of results and rational planning of treatment, have led to current practice in chemotherapy.

Adjuvant chemotherapy

Initial results obtained with single-drug chemotherapy have subsequently been improved by combination chemotherapy, i.e. the combined, simultaneous use of antineoplastic drugs with different mechanisms of action and limited overlapping of side-effects, followed by an adequate rest interval. The results obtained with combination chemotherapy may be related to a number of factors, including tumour heterogeneity, in terms of sensitivity to the drugs, and synergy of the drugs included in the combination. Although tumour control by chemotherapy has been achieved in the presence of disseminated disease, the clinical setting in which combination chemotherapy has made a major impact is in those children who show no evidence of residual tumour after initial treatment. Following complete surgical resection, most forms of cancer have an high probability of developing distant metastases unless prophylactic chemotherapy is used. Combination chemotherapy in this setting is termed adjuvant chemotherapy. The fundamental value of

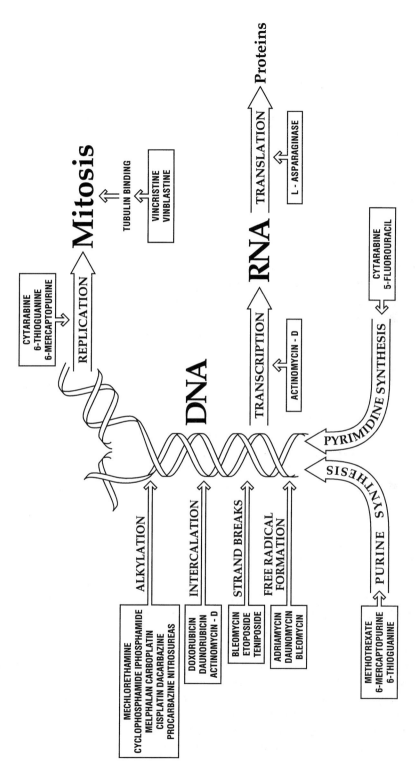

Fig. 4.1 Schematic representation of the action of commonly used antineoplastic agents.

adjuvant chemotherapy has been demonstrated in a number of prospective randomized trials in childhood tumours, suggesting the undetected presence of micrometastases at the time of surgery. The efficacy of adjuvant chemotherapy is most likely to be related to the following differences between micrometastases and clinically evident metastases:

(1) a reduced number of tumour cells to eliminate;

(2) most of the cells being in cycle and therefore susceptible to chemotherapy (Salmon 1979);

(3) all cells being exposed to an adequate drug concentration (no influence of lack of adequate blood supply in certain areas of the tumour);

(4) lower probability of emergence of resistant clones (Goldie and Coldman 1979).

Presurgical chemotherapy

Presurgical or neoadjuvant chemotherapy has been utilized to overcome such surgical problems as intraoperative rupture of Wilms' tumour, and to avoid mutilating surgery in patients with osteosarcoma. This form of neoadjuvant chemotherapy followed by standard postsurgical treatment has shown results superior to the previous standard approach (Lemerle *et al.* 1983). One major advantage is that surgery is easier to perform and often allows complete removal of the tumour, with a lower incidence of surgical sequelae. Interestingly, in Wilms' tumour, the decrease in tumour size and the lower incidence of regional involvement that follow chemotherapy improve prognosis by increasing the proportion of stage I tumours (Lemerle *et al.* 1983). In addition, response to treatment, usually based upon the use of more than one drug, can be evaluated in the individual patient, thus providing useful information for postsurgical treatment. The validity of this approach has been extensively tested in osteogenic sarcoma. However, the contribution of any single agent to combination chemotherapy is not known. To test the activity of a single antineoplastic agent, the drug can be administered at diagnosis for a short period of time in the presence of evaluable tumour before starting combination chemotherapy. This therapeutic window was initially used by Mastrangelo *et al.* (1984) with corticosteroids in acute lymphoblastic leukaemia (ALL). The response to glucocorticoids alone was evaluated at the end of the third day of treatment on the basis of the change in the total peripheral blast count. Not only was this up-front therapy able to discriminate between responders and nonresponders, but it also turned out to be a new and important prognostic factor in ALL (Riehm *et al.* 1987). The up-front therapeutic window has been utilized in a number of clinical studies (Mastrangelo *et al.* 1995) and it has been suggested as a model for anticancer drug evaluation since it predicts the true activity of the agent better than standard phase II studies (Horowitz *et al.* 1988).

High-dose chemotherapy

Experimental, transplantable tumour systems (Frei and Canellos 1980) and clinical experience support the therapeutic advantage of high-dose chemotherapy in inherently sensitive tumours. However, the definition of high-dose chemotherapy has rapidly changed and still remains a dynamic concept. As supportive care of cancer patients has become more comprehensive and more effective, particularly with the introduction of haematopoietic growth factors, it is possible to adopt dose escalation without a marked increased in haematological toxicity. When high-dose chemotherapy is used with bone marrow transplantation, or with peripheral blood stem cell (PBSC) support, it is usually called megadose chemotherapy. The alkylating agents are the best candidates for dose escalation since their extramedullary toxicity at high doses is relatively mild. Since tumour recurrence following high-dose chemotherapy is a major problem, it is important to take into account the real antitumour activity of the single drug included in the treatment proto-col. Chemosensitive tumours that are not cured by conventional dose are the best candidates for megadose chemotherapy.

At present, high-dose chemotherapy followed by autologous bone marrow or PBSC reinfusion in children is employed mainly for the treatment of metastatic neuroblastoma, advanced Ewing's sarcoma, relapsed brain tumours, and refractory lymphomas. Allogeneic bone marrow transplan-tation is performed mainly to treat refractory leukaemia, or after induction therapy in patients at high risk of relapse.

Clinical pharmacology

The main goal of clinical pharmacology studies with antineoplastic drugs is to increase the efficacy of cancer treatment while limiting toxic effects. Pharmacokinetics and pharmacodynam-ics are the two closely related aspects of clinical pharmacology. Pharmacokinetics is the study of a drug and its metabolites in the different areas of the body as a function of time; pharmacody-namics describes the effects of the antineoplastic agent on the tumour and the extent of damage caused to normal tissues. Pharmacokinetic parameters, usually derived from serial measurements of plasma levels, indicate the fate of the drug within the body. The most commonly used pharma-cokinetic terms for describing the rate of absorption, the metabolism, distribution, and the rate of excretion of a given drug are the following:

1. Area under the curve (AUC): area under the plasma concentration-time curve, quantifying the total drug exposure expressed as concentration x time.

2. Bioavailability: the amount of drug absorbed, expressed as percentage of the dose adminis-tered. In general, this is used to evaluate absorption of orally administered drugs.

3. Clearance: the rate of drug elimination. This includes all removal mechanisms, including the metabolic process, renal, and biliary excretion. It is expressed as mL/min.

4. Half-life: time required to reduce by half the drug concentration. The initial rapid distribu-tion phase in plasma is usually termed alpha and the terminal elimination phase, beta.

5. Volume of distribution: the theoretical volume of plasma necessary to dissolve the dose administered to give the observed plasma concentration. This defines a characteristic of the drug, not the volume of a physiological compartment.

Recently the influence of pharmacokinetics on tumour response and toxicity has been reviewed in greater detail (Rodman *et al.* 1993). Pharmacokinetic parameters have been shown to be closely related to tumour response in only a very few studies in children. Children with a higher systemic clearance of methotrexate (MTX) have a higher probability of relapse (Evans *et al.*

1984). A larger number of clinical studies showed a clear relationship between pharmacokinetic parameters and toxic effects (Table 4.1).

Therapeutic drug monitoring in other medical disciplines such as cardiology and neurology has been essential in obtaining optimum therapeutic effect by avoiding under- and overdosage caused by interpatient, pharmacokinetic variability. In oncology, despite a low therapeutic index and the risk of life-threatening toxicity, with the exception of MTX during high-dose MTX therapy, therapeutic drug monitoring is not yet routine. The lack of simple and sensitive drug assays and a predefined therapeutic range, as well as the lack of correlation between plasma levels and intracellular levels of active metabolites, are some of the reasons why drug monitoring in the individual patient has had limited clinical application. Therefore, despite a vast number of pharmacokinetic and pharmacodynamic studies, drug dosage is still calculated for virtually all antineoplastic agents on body surface area (BSA) or on body weight in smaller children. The only notable exception is carboplatin, a drug in which a simple dosing formula has been suggested in adults to obtain a predefined free or ultrafilterable (UF) carboplatin AUC (Calvert *et al.* 1989). This is possible because carboplatin is almost exclusively excreted by the kidney. UF AUC correlates linearly with GFR and UF AUC is the major determinant of carboplatin myelotoxicity. The adult dosing formula has been modified for children by Newell *et al.* (1993) taking into account GFR and the non-renal elimination: Dose (mg) = target AUC × GFR + 0.36 × body weight (kg). This formula has not been tested prospectively and relies on precise radioisotopic measurement of GFR. It may be useful in patients with decreased renal function. A mean AUC of 6 mg/ml/min is achieved with a dose of 600 mg/m². This may be a reasonable target AUC when carboplatin is employed in combination with other antineoplastic agents.

Increased dose intensity (in terms of mg/m² per week) appears as a favourable variable of cancer chemotherapy in a number of clinical studies both in adults and children (Ozols *et al.* 1993). Even if the validity of this approach has not yet been confirmed by prospective randomized studies in children, the highest dose intensity of chemotherapy compatible with host tolerance should be attempted.

Altered drug pharmacokinetics caused by organ dysfunction may represent an important cause of increased toxicity. In the presence of altered excretion, dose reduction should be adopted to avoid overwhelming toxicity. Finally, dose calculation espressed per unit of BSA may result in increased toxicity in infants, since small children have a higher BSA per kg compared with

Table 4.1 Clinical studies demonstrating a pharmacokinetics-toxicity relationship

Drug	Pharmacokinetic parameter	Effect
Anthracyclines	Peak level	Cardiotoxicity
Busulfan	AUC	Veno-occlusive disease
Cisplatin	Peak	Nephrotoxicity
Carboplatin	AUC	Bone marrow toxicity
Methotrexate	Systemic clearance	Bone marrow toxicity
Teniposide	AUC	Bone marrow toxicity
Vincristine	AUC	Neurotoxicity

adults. In children under 1 year of age or with a BSA of less than 0.5 m^2, dose calculation is usually based on body weight rather than BSA. Woods *et al.* (1981) were the first to suggest the need to calculate chemotherapy on body weight following the observation of life-threatening neuropathy and hepatotoxicity in infants treated with vincristine dosed on the basis of BSA. Several other cases of chemotherapy-related overwhelming toxicity in infants have been reported. It is now common practice to utilize per kg dosage in infants in the absence of specific pharmacokinetic and pharmacodynamic studies.

McLeod *et al.* (1992) were able to compare, although in a limited number of patients, the disposition of anticancer drugs in infants under 1 year of age and children over 1 year. It appears that with etoposide, teniposide, and cytarabine, dosing based upon BSA results in a similar, body weight systemic exposure for both age-groups. This suggests that calculation of dose based upon (BW) may result in under-dosing of these compounds in children under 1 year. MTX clearance following high dose MTX with leucovorin rescue tends to be lower in children under the age of one; however dose reduction was not necessary in this age-group. Conversely, systemic exposure to adriamycin appears to correlate with normalized body weight dosage rather than with BSA (McLeod *et al.* 1992). Overall, it appears that dose calculation based upon body weight may be justified with some drugs, while it may result in lower systemic exposure with other compounds. It may be wise to always use per kg dosing in infants when administering the first dose and, in the absence of severe toxicity, to increase the dose of subsequent administration with selected antineoplastic agents.

Central nervous system pharmacology

CNS pharmacology is of great interest to the paediatric oncologist since CNS leukaemia is the most common complication of ALL, and brain tumours are the most frequent solid neoplasms in children. The testes and CNS have long been considered pharmacological sanctuaries, since isolated relapses can be seen in these sites in patients with ALL. In the interstitium of the testes, however, where the leukaemic cells are characteristically found, a pharmacological barrier has not been demonstrated (Riccardi *et al.* 1982), while in the CNS, the blood-brain barrier (BBB) constitutes a physiological barrier formed by the endothelium of brain capillaries. The pharmacokinetics of antineoplastic agents in the CNS are markedly different from other areas of the body. The BBB prevents most of the antineoplastic agents from penetrating the CNS in therapeutic concentrations. This barrier, which is not uniformly intact in brain tumours, appears to function in at least some areas of the tumour. Molecular size, liposolubility, and electrical charge are the physicochemical characteristics that influence drug penetration in the CNS (Roll and Zubrad 1962). Protein binding is an additional factor since a protein-bound drug forms a complex which is too large to cross the BBB. Recent investigation showed that the development and the maintenance of the BBB derives from a quite complex interaction between endothelial cells and trophic factors produced by astrocytes. Multidrug resistance through p-glycoprotein plays a central role in the maintenance of the BBB by contributing to the active process of extruding a number of potentially toxic substances from brain endothelial cells (Schinkel *et al.* 1994). At standard doses, most of the antineoplastic agents do not cross the BBB in therapeutic amounts. The limited penetration of the CNS can be overcome by high-dose systemic therapy. High-dose MTX and high-dose Ara-C reach adequate

CSF levels and are capable of exerting an antitumour effect in the CNS. CSF drug-level monitoring may be useful in determining the percentage of drug crossing the intact BBB; however this information cannot be transferred to brain tumour treatment since the BBB is altered in most tumours, and CSF levels do not reflect the tissue levels. Tissue levels may be the best way to evaluate the penetration of a given antineoplastic agent within a tumour mass. In the case of etoposide, for example, the tumour tissue levels are in the 20% range of peak plasma levels, and approximately 20 times higher than those in the CSF. We have obtained similar results by evaluating CSF and tumour tissue levels in children treated with carboplatin (Riccardi *et al.* 1992).

Drug resistance

Drug resistance remains a major obstacle to the successful treatment of tumours. Both pharmacological and cellular factors may be responsible for drug resistance. Adequate drug exposure of tumour cells is crucial for antineoplastic activity. Drug concentration depends mainly on dose and infusion duration, drug inactivation or activation. Drug exposure may be limited by tumour localization (e.g. in the CNS) or by limited blood supply in some areas of the tumour. However, even if optimal tumour cell exposure is achieved, a number of cellular factors may be responsible for drug resistance. Decreased transport of the drug into the cell, defective metabolism of the drug to its active compound, increased drug inactivation, enhanced cellular repair mechanisms, altered target molecules, changes in the intracellular nucleotide pools for antimetabolites, activation of salvage pathways, and multidrug resistance (MDR) represent known mechanisms of chemoresistance.

MDR consists of the appearance of novel cancer cell variants which display resistance not only to the previously effective drug but also to other chemically unrelated antineoplastic drugs to which the cells had not previously been exposed. Interestingly, this type of resistance can be at least partially reversed in experimental systems using specific compounds. Drugs involved in MDR are large, hydrophobic molecules derived from natural products (vinca alkaloids, anthracyclins, actinomycin D, and others) and in general do not share common cytotoxic targets within cells. The common feature of MDR cells is the low intracellular drug concentration that appears to be maintained by the increased activity and expression of an energy-dependent drug efflux pump identified as a glycoprotein of 170 kDa molecular weight embedded in the plasma membrane (Morrow and Cowan 1988). P-glycoprotein is coded by a family of distinct structural genes (*mdr*) that upon transfection are able to confer a complete MDR phenotype to drug-sensitive cells. Numerous studies have very recently been conducted to assess p-glycoprotein overexpression in human tumours. Among treated patients with neuroblastoma, the nonresponsive tumours were found to have significantly higher levels of MDR RNA. Moreover, in children with soft-tissue sarcoma, high p-glycoprotein levels appear to be an adverse prognostic factor, while Wilms' tumours have a very low expression of the *mdr* gene.

Experimental work has identified a number of compounds, such as verapamil or cyclosporin, that can reverse drug resistance. These drugs are now being employed in some clinical trials in adults, but the results at present are still controversial (Lum *et al.* 1993).

In recent years, studies directed toward a better understanding of tumour sensitivity to chemotherapy have identified apoptosis as a major determinant of antitumour effect. Interestingly, several gene products such as p53, c-Myc, bcl-2, and bax, which are involved in tumourogenesis, appear to control the apoptotic process in tumour cells. Chemotherapeutic agents may activate apoptosis in damaged tumour cells. In the presence of an altered apoptotic pathway (i.e. lack of p53, amplification of c-Myc), tumour cells acquire drug resistance. Drug resistance in such cases involves different, unrelated antineoplastic agents and may explain the occurrence of the *de novo* clinical resistance. Figure 4.2 illustrates schematically the possible fate of tumour cells exposed to an adequate concentration of anticancer drug. Cells may be severely damaged and undergo necrotic death, may enter into apoptosis, or in the presence of specific genetic alteration, progress into cell cycle leading to a tumour which is resistant to chemotherapy (Lowe *et al.* 1993).

Side-effects

The common acute toxicities of antineoplastic agents are shown in Table 4.2. These side-effects are closely related to the antiproliferative action on normal, actively dividing tissues such as bone marrow and mucosal epithelial cells. At therapeutic doses, myelodepression, alopecia, and mucositis are usually predictable toxicities of most cytostatic drugs. Nausea and vomiting due to a direct effect on the gastrointestinal tract and/or stimulation of the chemoreceptor trigger zone in the fourth ventricle used to be a major side-effect of cancer chemotherapy. The use of inhibitors of $5HT_3$ receptors has greatly reduced the incidence of this disturbing side-effect. Although harmful

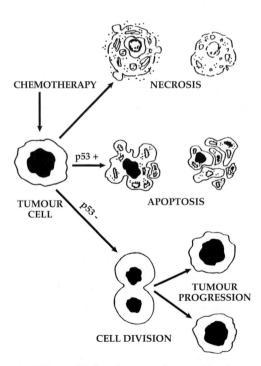

Fig. 4.2 Schematic representation of the possible fate of tumour cells exposed to adequate concentration of anticancer drug. Cells may be severely damaged and undergo necrotic death, may enter into apoptosis, or, in the presence of specific genetic alteration, progress into cell cycle leading to a tumour which is resistant to chemotherapy.

Table 4.2 Dose, schedule, toxicity, and route of elimination of commonly used antineoplastic agents

Drugs	Route	Dose mg m^{-2} and schedule	Major side-effects	Elimination
Alkylating agents				
Busulfan	PO	22–6 daily	BM, NV, pulmonary fibrosis	M
Carboplatin (CDBCA)	IV	175 wk × 4 q2–4 wk 560–1200 q4 wk	BM	R
Cisplatin (CDDP)	IV	50–200 over 4–6 h infusion qd × 5 q3–4 wk	NV, renal, A, NT, BM (mild)	R, M
BCNU (Carmustine)	IV	200–250 q6 wk	BM, NV, pulmonary fibrosis	M
CCNU (Lomustine)	PO	100–150 q6 w	BM, NV, pulmonary fibrosis	M
Cyclophosphamide (Cytoxan)	IV PO	400–2000 q3–4 wk 100 daily	BM, haemorrhagic cystitis, NV, A, infertility	M
Iphosphamide w/mesna	IV	1800 qd × 5q 3–4 wk 3000 qd × 3 q3–4 wk	BM, NV, A, haemorrhagic cystitis renal	M
Dacarbazine (DTIC)	IV	250 d × 5 q3–4 wk	NV, hepatic toxicity, flue-like syndrome, BM (mild)	M, R
Mechlorethamine (nitrogen mustard)	IV	6 q wk × 2q 4 wk	BM, NV, phlebitis, A, mucositis vesicant	M
Melphalan (L-PAM)	IV	10–40 q3–4 wk	BM, NV	M
Procarbazine (Natulan)	PO	100 qd × 10–14	NV, infertility, BM (moderate)	M
Antibiotics				
Bleomycin	IV, IM, SC	10–20 U weekly	Pulmonary fibrosis, liver, skin, Raynaud's phenomenon, hypersensitivity	R
Dactinomycin (actinomycin D)	IV	0.9–1.5 (max dose 2) q3–4 wk 0.45 qd × 5 q3–4 wk	BM, NV, mucositis, vesicant	R, B
Daunorubicin (daunomycin, DNR)	IV	30–45 qd × 3 qwk × 3	BM, mucositis, NV, A, cardiac (acute and chronic), vesicant	B, M
Doxorubicin (adriamycin, ADR)	IV	60–90 q3wk 30 qwk × 4	Same as daunorubicin	B, M

Table 4.2 *Continued*

Drugs	Route	Dose mg m⁻² and schedule	Major side-effects	Elimination
Antimetabolites				
Cytosine arabinoside (cytarabine, Ara-C)	IV, SC	100–200 continuous infusion 5–7 days	BM, NV, mucositis	M
	IV	2–3 gr, 2–3 h infusion q12h × 6	BM, NV, conjunctivitis, mucositis, gastrointestinal, cerebellar NT	
Methotrexate (MTX)	PO, IM	7.5–30 qwk	BM, mucositis, hepatic, rash	R
	IV	3–33 gr, 3–42 h infusion with leucovorin rescue q2–3 wk	renal hepatic, NT	
6-Mercaptopurine (6-MP)	PO	75–100 daily	BM, hepatic	M
6-Thioguanine (6-TG)	PO	75–100 daily	BM, mucositis, hepatic	M
Plant alkaloids				
Etoposide (VP-16)	IV	60–120 qd × 3–5 q3–6 wk	BM, A, NV, mucositis, mild peripheral NT	M, R
Teniposide (VM-26)	IV	70–180 qd × 3	same as Etoposide	M, R
Vinblastine (Velbe)	IV	3–6 qwk	BM, A	M, B
Vincristine (oncovin, VCR)	IV	1–2 qwk × 4–6 (dose max 2)	peripheral NT with pain, A, SIADH, vesicant	M, B
Miscellaneous				
Prednisone	PO, IV	60 daily	immunodepression, inhibition of skeletal growth, myopathy, hypertension	M
Dexamethasone	PO, IV	6–8 daily	same as Prednisone	M
L-Asparaginase	IV, IM	100–20 000 U qd × 10–20	hypersensitivity, NT, thrombosis or haemorrhage by inhibition of factors' synthesis, hepatic, pancreatitis	M

Abbreviations: IV, Intravenous; IM, intramuscular; PO, per os; SC, subcutaneous; A, alopecia; BM, myelosuppression; NV, nausea and vomiting; NT, neurotoxicity; SIADH, syndrome of inappropriate antidiuretic hormone; M, metabolic or spontaneous chemical decomposition; R, renal excretion; B, biliary excretion.

and disabling, acute side-effects of cytostatic drugs are almost always reversible. Organ-related toxicities are of major concern because they often limit dosage of subsequent treatment and may be responsible for long-term sequelae in potentially curable patients. The information derived from pharmacokinetic studies which have clearly demonstrated a relationship between pharmacokinetic parameters and toxicity of several drugs (Table 4.1) is very important in predicting, and probably reducing, the side-effects of chemotherapy. Scheduling is in some cases a major determinant of toxicity because it may influence the most critical pharmacokinetic elements (e.g. peak plasma levels, AUC). In addition, in combination or sequential chemotherapy regimens, specific drug toxicity may increase because of subclinical organ dysfunction resulting from a previously administered drug. The most frequent organ-related toxicities are discussed below.

Renal toxicity

Deterioration of renal function is a not infrequent occurrence in patients receiving cancer therapy. The antineoplastic agents commonly associated with renal toxicity and their respective clinical features are summarized in Table 4.3.

Hepatotoxicity

Liver dysfunction is a relatively frequent event during cancer treatment. Table 4.4 lists the most commonly used drugs causing hepatotoxicity.

Neurotoxicity

Neurological symptoms and signs are a disturbing side-effect of many antineoplastic agents. Neuropathy is the most frequent dose-limiting toxicity of vincristine. Peripheral neurotoxicity involves both sensory and motor structures, with consequent pain. In addition to pain, there may be loss of deep tendon reflexes and paraesthesia of the fingers and toes. Footdrop and wristdrop are symptoms of advanced neuropathy. Cranial motor nerves are occasionally affected (hoarseness and diplopia), and whereas constipation is frequent, severe autonomic neuropathies are unusual but may be responsible for paralytic ileus or urinary retention.

Ototoxicity of cisplatin is related to cumulative dose and results in decreased acuity at frequencies above 2000 Hz. With the administration of higher individual doses of cisplatin, peripheral neuropathy, which resembles the neuropathy of vitamin B deficiency, is also seen.

Although quite rare in children, the serious side-effect of cerebral and cerebellar dysfunction may be observed in patients receiving high doses of Ara-C. Symptoms include ataxia, dysarthria, nystagmus, and somnolence. This toxicity appears to be dose related, and the risk is increased at total doses per cycle exceeding 24 g/m^2. More recently, a new, potentially life-threatening complication of high dose Ara-C was reported in three children who developed bulbar and pseudobulbar palsy early in the course of treatment. Occasionally somnolence, disorientation, lethargy, seizures, and rarely coma are observed following therapy with iphosphamide.

Table 4.3 Renal toxicity of commonly used antineoplastic agents

Drug	Toxicity	Complications	Onset	Prevention	Reversibility
Cisplatin	Tubular damage	$\downarrow Mg^{2+}$, $\uparrow BUN$, creatinine	7–14 days	Hydration, diuretics; avoid concurrent nephrotoxic agents	Usually resolves over 3–4 weeks
High-dose methotrexate	Precipitates in tubules	Prolonged serum methotrexate levels	Within 24 h	Hydration, alkalinize urine; avoid concomitant administration of salicylates and sulphamethoxazole	Resolves over 2–3 weeks
Iphosphamide	Acute renal failure	$\uparrow BUN$, $\uparrow$ creatinine		Hydration; avoid concurrent nephrotoxic agents	Reversible with drug discontinuation
	Renal tubular dysfunction	Proteinuria, glycosuria, aminoaciduria, impaired phosphate reabsorption			
Cyclophosphamide	Free water excretion	Hyponatraemia	Within 24 h		Reversible with drug discontinuation
Vincristine	SIADH	Hyponatraemia	Within 24 h		Reversible with drug discontinuation

$\downarrow$ decreased $\uparrow$ increased

Table 4.4 Liver toxicity of commonly used antineoplastic agents

Drug	Dysfunction
High-dose methotrexate	Acute reversible increase in liver enzymes
Methotrexate	Hepatic fibrosis-cirrhosis
Cytosine arabinoside	Reversible intrahepatic cholestasis
6-Mercaptopurine	Reversible intrahepatic cholestasis
Actinomycin D	Hepatomegaly, jaundice, and ascites (veno-occlusive disease)
High-dose busulfan	Veno-occlusive disease

Significant neurotoxicity due to intrathecal MTX is not uncommon. The most common type is meningeal irritation or arachnoiditis which starts 2–34 h after treatment and lasts for 12–72 h. There may be severe headache, stiff neck, vomiting, lethargy, fever, and inflammatory pleocytosis of the CSF. The symptoms appear to be related to cumulative dose. A far less common and less acute side-effect is transient or permanent paraplegia. This syndrome may be related to delayed clearance of MTX from the CSF. Late sequelae of intrathecal MTX without concomitant irradiation are rare. The combination of intrathecal MTX and cranial irradiation used for CNS prophylaxis of ALL may be associated with computed tomographic brain scan abnormalities and minimal neurological sequelae. Very rarely, fatal necrotizing leukoencephalopathy has also been observed; in particular, the highest rate of leukoencephalopathy is observed following combined use of intrathecal MTX, intravenous MTX, and cranial irradiation. The clinical onset is insidious, with limb spasticity, ataxia, and, at a more advanced stage, coma. Computed axial tomography demonstrates cortical thinning, ventricular enlargement, and diffuse intracerebral calcification.

Cardiac toxicity

The anthracyclines are the agents most frequently associated with cardiac problems. They can occasionally cause acute toxicity in the form of arrhythmias occurring shortly after the administration of the drug. The chronic cardiomyopathy is related to cumulative dose of anthracyclines. The incidence of cardiomyopathy increases significantly after a cumulative dose of 450 mg/m^2 for adriamycin and 600 mg/m^2 for daunorubicin (Daunomycin). However, there is evidence of cardiac damage after much lower doses (Hausdorf *et al.* 1988). Congestive heart failure usually appears within 1 year of anthracycline therapy but can occur up to 10 years after treatment. Moreover, subclinical abnormalities of left ventricular function, including increased afterload and decreased contractility, are a common and often progressive condition in anthracycline-treated, long-term survivors of childhood cancer (Lipshultz *et al.* 1991). The incidence of these abnormalities appears to increase with follow-up irrespective of the anthracycline cumulative dose. Therefore, prolonged, probably life-long, cardiac follow-up is recommended in anthracycline-treated, long-term survivors. Factors which may increase the risk of anthracycline-induced congestive cardiomyopathy include:

(1) previous mediastinal irradiation;

(2) host factors (age under 1 year, female sex, liver dysfunction);

(3) schedule of administration (bolus injection). The additive effect of high-dose cyclophosphamide, iphosphamide, actinomycin, and dacarbazine is questionable.

The most sensitive method of assessing anthracycline-induced cardiomyopathy is the evaluation of pathological alterations in the myocardium by endomyocardial biopsy. Non-invasive functional studies such as echocardiography and radionuclide angiography, although commonly used, are unable to predict cardiac toxicity reliably. It is advisable, however, to discontinue anthracyclines if the ejection fraction on echocardiography is less than 50%, or after a decrease from the baseline of more than 10%.

An increasing number of reports suggest that dexrazoxane (ICRF-187) may reduce anthracycline-induced cardiotoxicity in children (Wexler *et al.* 1996). However, these studies only assessed early cardiotoxicity and it is currently not clear whether ICRF-187 treatment will reduce late cardiotoxicity. Moreover, additional information is needed on the effect of ICRF-187 on the response of most neoplasms to chemotherapy and on its acute and delayed side-effects.

Pulmonary toxicity

Bleomycin is the most notorious agent for pulmonary toxicity, but its use is infrequent in children. The lesion consists of interstitial pneumonitis with inflammatory infiltrates in the alveoli, interstitial, and intra-alveolar oedema, pulmonary hyaline membrane formation, and subsequent interstitial fibrosis. Progression to fibrosis may occur even after withdrawal of the drug. These changes are dose related. At doses above 450 IU/m^2 the incidence is 10–20%. Both high oxygen pressure and pulmonary irradiation may accelerate lung damage.

Pulmonary toxicity can be associated with other antineoplastic agents. Alkylating agents, in particular carmustine and busulfan, may also cause interstitial pneumonitis.

Acknowledgements

This work was supported by Associazione Italiana per la Ricerca sul Cancro.

References

Calvert, A.H., Newell, D.R., Gumbrell, L.A., O'Reilly, S., Burnell, M., Boxall, F.E., *et al.* (1989). Carboplatin dosage: Prospective evaluation of a simple formula based on renal function. *Journal of Clinical Oncology*, 7, 1748–1756.

Evans, W.E., Crom, W.R., Stewart, C.F., Bowman, W.P., Chen, C.H., Abromowtich, M., *et al.* (1984). Methotrexate systemic clearance influences the probability of relapse in children with standard risk acute lymphocytic leukaemia. *Lancet*, i, 359–362.

Frei, E. and Canellos, G.P. (1980). Dose: a critical factor in cancer chemotherapy. *American Journal of Medicine*, 69, 585–594.

Goldie, J.H. and Coldman, A.J. (1979). A mathematic model for relating the drug sensitivity of tumours to their spontaneous mutation rate. *Cancer Treatment Reports*, 63, 1727–1733.

Hausdorf, G., Morf, G., Bernon, G., Erttman, R., Winkler, K., Landbeck, G., *et al.* (1988). Long-term doxorubicin cardiotoxicity in childhood: non-invasive evaluation of the contractile state of diastolic filling. *British Health Journal*, 60, 309–315.

Horowitz, M.E., Etcubanas, E., Christensen, M.L., Houghton, J.A., George, S.L., Green, A.A., *et al.* (1988). Melphalan in children with newly diagnosed rhabdomyosarcoma: A model for anticancer drug development. *Journal of Clinical Oncology*, 6, 308–314.

Lemerle, J., Voute, P.A., Tournade, M.F., Rodary, C., Delemarre, J.F., Sarrazin, D., *et al.* (1983). Effectiveness of preoperative chemotherapy in Wilms' tumour: results of an International Society of Paediatric Oncology (SIOP) clinical trial. *Journal of Clinical Oncology*, 1, 604–609.

Lipshultz, S.E., Colan, S.A.D., Gelber, R.D., Perez Atayde, A.R., and Sallan, S.E. (1991). Late cardiac effects of doxorubicin therapy for acute lymphoblastic leukemia in childhood. *New England Journal of Medicine*, 324/12, 808–815.

Lowe, S.W., Ruley, H.E., Jacks, T., and Housman, D.E. (1993). p53-Dependent apoptosis modulates the cytotoxicity of anticancer agents. *Cell*, 74, 957–967.

Lum, B.L., Fisher, G.A., Brophy, N.A., Yahanda, A.M., Alder, K.M., Kaubisch, S., *et al.* (1993). Clinical Trials of Modulation of Multidrug Resistance. Pharmacokinetic and Pharmacodynamic Considerations, *Cancer*, 72(11) Suppl. 3502–3514.

Mastrangelo, R., Riccardi, R., and Corbo, S., (1984). Prediction of clinical response to glucocorticoids in children with acute lymphoblastic leukemia. *European Paediatric Haematology and Oncology*, 1, 33–36.

Mastrangelo, R., Lasorella, A., Riccardi, R., Colosimo, C., Lavarone, A., Tornesello, A., *et al.* (1995). Carboplatin in Childhood Medulloblastoma/PNET: Feasibility of an *In Vivo* Sensitivity Test in an 'Up front' Study. *Medical and Pediatric Oncology*, 24, 188–196.

McLeod, H.L., Relling, M.V., Crom, W.R., Silverstein, K., Groom, S., Rodman, J.H., *et al.* (1992). Disposition of antineoplastic agents in the very young child. *British Journal of Cancer*, 66, S23–S29.

Morrow, C.S. and Cowan, K.H. (1988). Mechanisms and clinical significance of multidrug resistance. *Oncology* 2, 55–68.

Newell, D.R., Pearson, A.D., Balmanno, K., Price, L., Wyllie, R.A., Keir, M., *et al.* (1993). Carboplatin pharmacokinetics in children: the development of the paediatric dosing formula. The United Kingdom Children's Cancer Study Group. *Journal of Clinical Oncology*, 11(12), 2314–2323.

Ozols, R.F., J.T. Thigpen., Dauplat, J., Colombo, N., Piccart, M.J., Bertelsen, K.., *et al.* (1993). Dose intensity. *Annals of Oncology*, 4 (suppl.4), 49–56.

Riccardi, R., Vigersky, R.A., Barnes, S., Bleyer, W.A., and Poplack, D.G. (1982). Methotrexate levels in the interstitial space and seminiferous tubule of rat testis. *Cancer Research* 42, 1617–1619.

Riccardi, R., Riccardi, A., Di Rocco, C., Carelli, G., Tartaglia, R.L., Lasorella, A., *et al.* (1992). Cerebrospinal fluid pharmacokinetics of carboplatin in children with brain tumours. *Cancer Chemotherapy and Pharmacology*, 30, 21–24.

Riehm, H., Reiter, A., Schrappe, M., Berthold, F., Dopfer, R., Gerein, V., *et al.* (1987). Corticosteroid-dependent reduction of leukocyte count in blood as a prognostic factor in acute lymphoblastic leukemia in childhood (therapy study ALL-BFM 83). *Klin Padiatr*, 199/3, 1S1–160.

Rodman, J.H., Relling, M.V., Stewart, C.F., Synold, T.W., McLeod, H., Kearns, C., *et al.* (1993). Clinical Pharmacokinetics and Pharmacodynamics of Anticancer Drugs in Children. *Seminars in Oncology*, 20(1), 18–29.

Roll, D. and Zubrad, C. (1962). Mechanism of drug absorption and excretion. Passage of drugs in and out of the central nervous system. *Annual Review of Pharmacology*, 2, 109–128.

Salmon, S.E. (1979). Kinetics of minimal residual disease. *Recent Results Cancer Research*, 65, 5–15.

Schinkel, A.H., Smit, J.J.M., van Tellingen, O., Beijnen, J.H., Wagenaar, E., van Deemter, L., *et al.* (1994). Disruption of the Mouse mdrla P-glycoprotein gene leads to a deficiency in the blood brain barrier and to increased sensitivity to drugs. *Cell* 77, 491–522.

Wexler, L.H., Andrich, M.P., Venzon, P., Berg, S.L., Weaver-McClure, L., Chen, C.C., *et al.* (1996). Randomized Trial of the Cardioprotective Agent ICRF-187 in Pediatric Sarcoma Patients Treated with Doxorubicin, 14(2), 362–372.

Woods, W.G., O'Leary, M., and Nesbit, M.E. (1981). Life-threatening neuropathy and hepatotoxicity in infants during induction therapy for acute lymphoblastic leukemia. *Journal of Pediatrics*, 98, 642.

5 Radiotherapy

M. Gaze

The classic injunction 'first do no harm' is somewhat trite for those treating cancer in children. All modalities of treatment have the capacity to cause damage which can sometimes prove fatal. The only certain way of ensuring no treatment-related morbidity or mortality is not to treat. Those who do treat malignant disease in childhood, therefore, must recognize that survivors will have to live with any damage caused by treatment for decades. A better aphorism would be 'take care to minimize the injuries you cause when trying to cure a child with cancer, and seek new ways of reducing treatment-related morbidity further'.

This chapter reviews the damage which radiation treatment can cause and discusses various factors which relate to the degree of harm done by irradiation. Examples are given of how modern radiotherapeutic practice uses this knowledge to minimize late treatment-related morbidity without compromising the chances for cure.

Adverse effects of radiation therapy in children

Acute and late effects

Acute effects which occur during a course of treatment or in the subsequent few weeks are generally tolerable and settle down with time. Examples include cutaneous erythema and diarrhoea following small bowel irradiation. Acute effects are usually due to depletion of a stem cell pool with rapid turnover in an organ with a hierarchical cellular organization. Some acute effects such as myelosuppression, pneumonitis, or hepatitis can be life-threatening, and may limit the dose which may be given safely to a particular organ. Late effects, which come on many months or years after treatment, are often progressive and usually irreversible. They may be due either to parenchymal cell damage or vascular endothelial cell damage in the affected organ. The possibility of development of late effects causes a lot of anxiety, and in many cases it is the likelihood of causing a severe late effect which is a dose-limiting factor.

Likelihood of late effects

Late effects may be divided into binary effects, graded responses, and continuous variables. With binary or stochastic effects, that is to say all or none responses to injury, the likelihood of occurrence, but not the severity, is related to the total radiation dose and other factors. Radiation myelitis and the induction of second malignant neoplasms are examples. With graded responses, a particular endpoint of normal tissue damage may be absent or be designated as mild, moderate, or severe. These are often scored as 0, 1, 2, or 3 respectively. Both the incidence and the severity of an adverse reaction can be described with this sort of system. While it is useful to rank the severity of morbidity encountered, these data are non-parametric and it cannot be assumed that grade 2 effects are twice as bad as grade 1 effects. Mean morbidity scores should not be derived from these data, as that would confuse the likelihood of a late effect occurring with its severity. Continuous variables are usually laboratory data, such as the glomerular filtration rate, as an index of renal damage (Bentzen and Overgaard 1993).

Growth of bone and soft tissue

One of the principal features which distinguishes children from adults is the fact that they are still growing. Radiation treatment may interfere with this process directly by its effects on the epiphyseal growth plates, for example, and also indirectly by its effects on the hypothalamic-pituitary axis, which often leads to growth hormone deficiency (Spoudeas 1994). The impairment of growth caused by radiation is not immediately apparent, but becomes progressively greater as the unaffected parts of the body grow. It is often not until after the pubertal growth spurt that the full extent of the damage is revealed. Growth difficulties lead not only to a short height in adulthood, but may also result in disproportion between body parts or deformities such as scoliosis. Late effects on growth cause not just cosmetic difficulties but also functional problems, and both these may lead to secondary psychological and social disturbances.

The epiphyseal growth plates are the most sensitive part of bone to irradiation. Doses as low as 10–12 Gy may impair chondroblast function and have an adverse effect on bone growth. In younger children, doses greater than 25 Gy to the upper part of the femur may lead to slippage of the capital epiphysis. Avascular necrosis of the femoral or humeral heads can occur after radiotherapy, more commonly when the patient also receives corticosteroid-containing chemotherapy. Spinal deformities such as scoliosis and kyphosis may result from spinal irradiation, especially if vertebral bodies are irradiated asymmetrically rather than uniformly. The likelihood of spinal deformity is increased if there has been flank surgery, and if there is radiation-induced hypoplasia of the paraspinal musculature. Treatment of orbital rhabdomyosarcoma and other head and neck malignancies can result in facial bone hypoplasia and consequent asymmetry of the face. Doses as low as 20 Gy before eruption of the second set of teeth may lead to impaired dental development. In addition, patients who have radiation-induced xerostomia are at increased risk of dental caries.

Doses above about 15 Gy may prevent full muscular development. Patients receiving radiotherapy to the neck for Hodgkin's disease may be left with thin, scrawny necks (Barrett *et al.* 1990). Children undergoing 20 Gy flank irradiation for Wilms' tumour will develop hypoplastic paraspinal musculature and narrow waists as they grow up. They may also have damage to part of the uterine wall muscle predisposing to foetal loss. Female breast development may be impaired after chest wall radiotherapy.

Central nervous system

Maturation of the central nervous system (CNS) in early life involves the development and branching of axons with the formation of new synapses, rather than an increase in the number of neurons. Much of this process is complete by three years, but it continues at a lower rate into the pubertal years. Radiotherapy affects this process by causing death of oligodendrocytes which leads to demyelination. In addition, radiation can destroy vascular endothelial cells.

The somnolence syndrome is an early or intermediate effect seen after a month or two in about half the patients who receive cranial irradiation. It is characterized by drowsiness, apathy, and irritability. It is self limiting after a few weeks and is attributed to transient demyelination.

High-dose (above about 60 Gy) radiotherapy to the brain may, sometimes many years later, lead to cerebral necrosis which can exert a mass effect and be mistaken for recurrent tumour. This complication is only rarely seen as doses used are usually kept within brain tolerance. Occasionally, re-irradiation is given for tumour recurrence, accepting that there will be a substantial risk of necrosis.

Lower doses, while producing no obvious structural changes in the brain, may have profound neuropsychological sequelae. Children who have received 18 or 24 Gy whole-brain radiotherapy for leukaemia are likely to have intelligence quotients within the normal range, although lower than those of unirradiated controls. There may be particular problems with short-term memory, and speed of processing of new information may be reduced (Halberg *et al.* 1991).

Lhermitte's syndrome is an electric-shock-like sensation in the legs when the neck is flexed, caused by a transient myelopathy associated with demyelination occurring about three months after radiotherapy to the spine. Radiation myelitis is a devastating complication of treatment, but is rarely seen because great care is always taken to keep the spinal cord dose within what are believed to be safe limits. Because of this, it is possible that safe limits may, in fact, be greater than generally recognized. This possibility, however, does not give the radiotherapist licence to exceed recognized norms. It is usually considered safe to give 35 Gy to the whole spinal cord and 45 Gy to a limited length (Halperin *et al.* 1994).

The eye

The lens of the eye is one of the most radiosensitive structures in the body, and radiation doses greater than about 6 Gy may lead to cataract formation. Damage to the lacrimal gland may occur at doses greater than about 40 Gy. The retina is also a dose-limiting structure, and radiation retinopathy can lead to blindness. It is not seen below about 45 Gy, and is rare below 55 Gy delivered with conventional fraction sizes (Harnett and Hungerford 1991).

The heart

Radiotherapy to the heart can result in a cardiomyopathy. This effect is thought to be more likely in younger children and is compounded by the use of anthracyclines. There is anxiety that patients who received cardiac irradiation in childhood may be at increased risk of developing coronary artery disease in adult life, and at an earlier age than usual. Up to 25 Gy given to the whole heart is considered safe, and higher doses to part of the heart may not be harmful.

The lungs

Acute pneumonitis may develop within 3–6 months of radiotherapy. It is characterized by cough and dyspnoea. A pleural reaction and diffuse infiltrate may be visible on chest radiography. Lung function tests show a restrictive abnormality. Irradiation of the whole of both lungs to a dose of about 14 Gy with conventional fractionation is generally considered to be safe, although this will result in a measurable reduction in lung function. The use of chemotherapy, especially bleomycin and actinomycin D, lowers the lung tolerance to radio-therapy. Smaller areas of lung can safely be irradiated to higher doses, but some pulmonary fibrosis will result (Travis 1991).

The liver

Abdominal pain, weight gain, ascites, and jaundice are the features of radiation hepatitis. The concomitant use of actinomycin D makes hepatitis more likely with low-dose hepatic irradiation. Late effects include atrophy of the liver with fibrosis. Veno-occlusive disease of the liver is a rare but severe complication of total body irradiation. Regenerating liver after partial hepatectomy is more sensitive than normal. The whole liver will usually tolerate 15 Gy. Smaller areas may take 30 Gy.

The kidneys

Irradiation of the kidneys may result in hypertension, anaemia, and chronic renal failure. Renal doses should therefore be kept below about 15 Gy. Contralateral renal hypertrophy after nephrectomy is inhibited by radiotherapy, and caution should be exercized if irradiating a single kidney.

Factors affecting the likelihood and severity of radiation injury

The incidence and severity of adverse reactions to radiotherapy among children treated for cancer are related to:

(1) the use of radiotherapy;

(2) the total dose given;

(3) the dose per fraction;

(4) the volume of tissue irradiated;

(5) the type of tissue irradiated;

(6) the type of radiation used;

(7) the use of chemotherapy in addition;

(8) age at time of treatment.

Knowledge of these factors allows for new strategies to be devised which may reduce adverse effects without compromising chances for cure. It is preferable for the safety of any reduction in therapy to be tested in a randomized trial. In rare diseases, it is sometimes possible to evaluate less intense treatment schedules in sequential cohorts of patients, but the validity of the data is less certain than that obtained from a randomized trial, as other, perhaps unrecognized, factors may be in operation.

The use of radiotherapy

Clearly, the first aim when faced with a child with cancer is to cure the disease. If radiotherapy, with its attendant side-effects, is necessary to achieve this, then so be it. If, however, cure can be achieved without the need for radiotherapy, then so much the better. With the introduction of new cytotoxic drugs, and with a better understanding of their use, it has been possible to remove the need for radiotherapy in many instances.

Sequential, randomized trials organized by the United States National Wilms' Tumor Study Group (NWTS) and the International Society of Paediatric Oncology (SIOP) have shown that radiotherapy is not needed in Stage I and Stage II Wilms' tumour (D'Angio *et al.* 1976, 1981, 1989). It is possible that radiotherapy may not be needed in some subgroups of patients with Stage III disease, but this remains unproven.

Similarly in Hodgkin's disease, the introduction of effective and relatively non-toxic combination chemotherapy has meant that, in the United Kingdom at least, radiotherapy is not used as a first-line treatment in children with Stage II, III, and IV disease.

Clinical studies have shown that for children with acute lymphoblastic leukaemia who are at low risk of developing CNS disease, CNS-directed therapy with intrathecal and intravenous chemotherapy is as effective and less toxic than craniospinal or cranial irradiation. Current studies are evaluating the need for CNS radiotherapy in children at higher risk.

The total dose given

In the pioneering days of radiotherapy, the dose prescribed was often the maximum tolerated dose. It has become apparent that for the more radiosensitive childhood tumours, lower doses are just as likely to cure the disease with a lower incidence of late effects.

The doses of 40–50 Gy which were used for Wilms' tumour in the 1940s have been replaced by doses as low as 10 Gy, thanks to sequential NWTS and SIOP studies (Gross and Neuhauser 1950).

Similarly, the doses used for intracranial germinoma have been reduced from 55 Gy to 40 Gy.

In the first Intergroup Rhabdomyosarcoma Study (1972–78), radiation doses up to 65 Gy were employed. Currently, doses of 40–50 Gy are thought to be adequate when radiotherapy is indicated (Maurer *et al.* 1988).

The dose per fraction

The late effects of radiation therapy are critically dependent on the dose per fraction. This is because normal tissues have a substantial capacity for repair of sublethal damage caused by low doses of radiation, but this capacity is swamped when a threshold is exceeded. The likelihood of adverse effects in late responding tissues is proportional to the square of the dose per fraction. A small increase in dose per fraction will greatly increase the late effects, even if the total dose is no greater (Joiner 1993).

For example, the incidence of cataracts in leukaemic patients after single-fraction (often 10 Gy) total body irradiation is approximately 80%, whereas after fractionated irradiation (usually 14.4 Gy in eight fractions of 1.8 Gy) it is only about 20%.

In paediatric practice it has therefore become conventional to limit the fraction size to 1.8 Gy, or exceptionally 2 Gy, in radical treatments. In the palliative setting, where one can be certain that the child will not live to experience late effects, hypofractionation (the use of a smaller number of large fractions) provides good results without the need for many attendances for treatment.

The volume of tissue irradiated

If the volume of normal tissue irradiated can be kept to a minimum, then late effects will be fewer.

Craniospinal irradiation used to be advised following surgery for ependymoma because of the possibility of cerebrospinal-fluid-borne metastases affecting parts of the CNS remote from the primary tumour. The advent of magnetic resonance imaging to detect CNS spread coupled with the realization that first relapse in most instances was local, with distant metastases being a late or secondary event, has lead to local radiotherapy to the tumour bed being the preferred treatment in most instances.

The propensity for CNS spread of parameningeal rhabdomyosarcomas meant that whole-brain irradiation, with its attendant neuropsychological sequelae, used to be considered necessary. Currently, irradiation of any continuous intracranial extension of the primary tumour and the adjacent skull base and basal meninges is considered adequate. Whole cranial irradiation is now only used if there is diffuse intracranial disease.

The volume of normal tissue adjacent to a tumour, which is inevitably irradiated with the tumour, can now be minimized by use of modern radiotherapy planning techniques used in conjunction with the latest imaging modalities. For example, in conformal therapy radiation fields are shaped with great precision, so that the shape of the high-dose radiation volume conforms to the shape of the tumour (Tait and Nahum 1994).

Stereotactic radiotherapy is a type of conformal radiotherapy which enables irradiation of a spherical or ovoid volume encompassing a brain tumour with narrow margins. First the head is fixed in a stereotactic frame with a set of external fiducial markers, and the tumour is localized by computed tomography or magnetic resonance imaging with computed tomography image fusion. Then a finely collimated radiation beam is moved in an arc around the patient's head, focused on the tumour coordinates. Other, non-coplanar arcs are focused on the same point. The tumour receives a high dose while the radiation dose to the rest of the brain is kept very low. A single treatment, sometimes called radiosurgery, is more suited to the treatment of benign intracranial lesions such as arteriovenous malformations. Tumours are better treated with fractionated stereotactic radiotherapy which entails multiple treatments of conventional fraction size and requires a relocatable frame (Brada and Graham 1994).

The development of multileaf collimators has enabled rotation therapy, with radiation fields of continuously variable size and shape, to be used. This dynamic conformal therapy offers the prospect of treating larger, irregularly shaped tumours with greater normal tissue sparing than was previously possible. This technique must still be regarded as experimental, and it remains to be seen whether it does allow a reduction in normal tissue morbidity with preservation of the local tumour control rate. It also offers the prospect of permitting dose escalation, with the aim of improving local control rates while keeping normal tissue morbidity unchanged compared with conventional treatment.

The type of tissue irradiated

As mentioned earlier, the likelihood of an adverse effect occuring depends on the type of tissue or organ being irradiated. Careful radiotherapy planning and precision treatment techniques now enable some radiosensitive structures to be kept out of the way while nearby tumours are being irradiated. An example is the use of a small, finely collimated, lateral radiation beam to treat a retinoblastoma at the back of the eye, while sparing the lens.

When treating an extremity soft tissue or bone sarcoma, it is essential to spare a strip of skin and subcutaneous tissue at one side of the limb if at all possible. This allows lymphatic drainage of the distal part of the limb to continue unimpeded. Without it, fibrosis of the lymphatic channels will lead to the development of lymphoedema.

The type of radiation used

In current radiotherapy practice, high-energy (megavoltage) photons are the most commonly used type of radiation. Low-energy (orthovoltage) radiation, which was formerly the most widely available type, has several disadvantages. The most important of these is that it is absorbed to a much greater extent in tissues such as bone, which contains relatively high atomic-number elements such as calcium. Because of this, children treated with orthovoltage radiation had a much higher likelihood of developing serious skeletal deformities. In addition, orthovoltage radiation, unlike megavoltage radiation, has no skin-sparing effect, and so both acute and late skin reactions tended to be more pronounced.

Electrons differ from photons in that, instead of being exponentially attenuated as they pass through tissue, they tend to penetrate well for a certain distance, depending on their energy, and then the dose falls off very rapidly at deeper levels. This makes electrons very suitable for treating superficial tumours, while sparing the dose to underlying, critical, normal structures. For example, superficial lesions of the chest wall can be treated without giving excess radiation to the lungs or myocardium, and cervical nodes involved with nasopharyngeal or thyroid carcinoma can be boosted to high dose without exceeding spinal cord tolerance.

Heavy-particle radiotherapy with neutrons and protons has not found a place in paediatric radiotherapy. Use of fast neutron beam therapy in adults has, by and large, been associated with an excessive level of late normal tissue morbidity, including necrosis without a significant improvement in cure rates.

The use of chemotherapy with radiotherapy

Certain chemotherapy drugs can potentiate the damage caused by radiotherapy. This may require doses of either chemotherapy or radiotherapy to be modified, or lead to a preference to treat with either one modality or the other, rather than to use combined therapy.

Anthracyclines such as doxorubicin may cause a cardiomyopathy, and the incidence is dose related. In the treatment of Wilms' tumour, the total dose of doxorubicin is usually limited to 360 mg/m^2, but if the heart is irradiated, as in whole-lung irradiation for pulmonary metastases, the dose should be kept to 300 mg/m^2.

In Hodgkin's disease, second malignant neoplasms are more likely to develop following combined chemotherapy and radiotherapy than if either modality alone is used (Chapter 10). For this reason, in the United Kingdom, it is regarded as preferable to use radiotherapy alone in Stage I disease and chemotherapy alone for more advanced disease, in the first instance. The use of the other modality can then be reserved for patients who do not respond, or who relapse after initial treatment.

Age at time of treatment

The developing tissues and organs of younger children are, in general, more susceptible to the adverse effects of radiation. This is particularly true of the CNS. For that reason there has been an increasing tendency to try to delay the use of radiotherapy in younger children, or even avoid it altogether (Duffner *et al.* 1993). If radiotherapy is deemed necessary in young children, an arbitrary dose reduction is usually applied, although there is no evidence that tumours in infants are more radiosensitive than those in older children. As growth and maturation are continuous processes, it is difficult to be certain about what constitutes being too young for radiotherapy. Most studies of the use of chemotherapy to delay the need for radiotherapy in very young children with malignant brain tumours have taken 3 years as the cut-off. It has to be said that this approach must still be regarded as experimental.

It must be remembered that radiotherapy is not 'contraindicated' in younger children, merely that it is better to delay or avoid it if possible.

Administration of radiotherapy

Ionizing radiation can be administered in one of three ways to treat patients with cancer. Firstly, a radiation beam may be directed from an machine towards the tumour. Secondly, radioactive materials may be implanted directly into the tumour, or inserted into a natural body cavity such as the uterus, on a temporary or permanent basis. Finally, unsealed, radioactive isotopes may be administered. Given orally or intravenously, some drugs are physiologically or pharmacologically concentrated in tumour tissue. Alternatively, unsealed sources may be directly inserted into a tumour cyst or natural space such as the peritoneum.

External-beam radiotherapy

External-beam therapy accounts for the majority of radiotherapy treatments in both adults and children. A wide variety of treatment machines is available to deliver external-beam radiotherapy. There has been a continuing evolution of radiotherapy technology, and modern machines are increasingly sophisticated, enabling more precise and complex treatments. One of the most important attributes of a treatment machine is the energy of the beam produced, as this governs the depth of penetration into the body. The energy is measured in kV (low energy) or MV (high energy). Most commonly, high-energy or 'megavoltage' radiation (about 4–10 MV) is used. The radiation usually comprises X-rays or 'photons' from a machine called a linear accelerator or 'linac'. Linacs can be used to provide beams of electrons as well as photons. Gamma rays produced by cobalt (^{60}Co) units are composed of another type of high-energy photon. They have similar powers of penetration to X-rays produced by a 2 MV linear accelerator. The increasing capability and sophistication of modern linacs means that cobalt units can no longer be considered satisfactory alternatives to linear accelerators.

Radiotherapy treatment planning

The basic principle of radical external-beam radiotherapy is to give as high a radiation dose as necessary to a tumour to be certain of killing it, while keeping the dose to surrounding normal tissues as low as possible to avoid damaging them. Radiotherapy planning has to be undertaken before treatment can start, and this may require three or four hospital visits. Planning may involve preparation of an immobilization device, especially for a brain, head and neck, or extremity tumour. This device, which is usually a plastic shell made from a plaster cast of the patient, keeps the part of the body in the same position from day to day, enabling the treatment volume to be kept as small as possible. It bears marks to guide the radiographers who deliver the treatment, and means that the patient's skin does not need to be marked.

In the next part of the planning process, the tumour location is identified from diagnostic imaging which may include a CT scan specially performed for planning purposes. A number of beams are then chosen which encompass the tumour completely. These may be shaped to keep them as small as possible. Diagnostic X-rays are taken on a radiotherapy planning simulator to check that the proposed field arrangement gives the desired result. All the data are entered into a radiotherapy planning computer, and a final plan is decided upon (Lichter 1993). This ensures that all the tumour, and any areas of potential spread which are to be treated, receive an adequate dose, while the dose to normal tissues is kept to a minimum, paying special attention to the need to protect critical structures such as the eyes and spinal cord.

Anaesthesia or sedation?

An essential prerequisite for accurate and sophisticated radiotherapy is that the patient lies still. Most children older than about three years of age can, with patience and perseverance, be encouraged to cooperate. Younger children, however, almost always require anaesthesia. For daily radiotherapy, a light, general anaesthetic is given first thing in the morning after fasting overnight. The child then wakes up rapidly after treatment and is able to eat and go home. This is preferable to sedation, when a drowsy child may still wriggle when stimulated, but go to sleep for hours afterwards and fail to eat properly throughout a prolonged course of radiotherapy.

Brachytherapy

The principal advantage of intracavitary or interstitial radiotherapy, or 'brachytherapy', is that the source gives a very high radiation dose to the immediately adjacent tissues, but only a small dose beyond a couple of centimeters or so away. Brachytherapy has an established place in the treatment of some adult tumours, particularly gynaecological cancer. It is, however, less used in paediatric practice, although there may be advantages to its use in some patients with sarcomas, particularly rhabdomyosarcoma.

Unsealed sources

Radioactive chemicals which are selectively taken up by tumour tissue may be injected or ingested. This is sometimes known as biologically targeted radiotherapy. It was hoped that monoclonal antibody technology would enable this form of treatment to be used successfully against previously uncurable tumours. Sadly, this dream has not been realized. Radionuclide therapy is rarely used alone, but may form an important part of the strategy against selected tumours in conjunction with other treatment modalities.

Perhaps the best example is the use of oral radioactive iodine (^{131}I) in the management of thyroid cancer. Following surgery, an ablative dose of radioiodine is given which is taken up with great avidity by any remaining normal thyroid tissue and destroys it. Metastatic thyroid carcinoma takes up radioiodine less well than normal tissue, but second and subsequent therapeutic doses of radioiodine are concentrated in metastases, as competition from normal tissue has been abolished by the initial ablative dose.

The catecholamine analogue mIBG, when labelled with radioiodine, can be used for imaging and therapy of neuroendocrine tumours such as phaeochromocytoma and neuroblastoma (Hoefnagel and Lewington 1994).

Unsealed radionuclides can also be physically (rather than biologically) targeted into a tumour, in much the same way as interstitial therapy with removable implants is given. An example is the instillation of yttrium (^{90}Y) colloid into brain-tumour cysts using stereotactic localization. This can be valuable for patients who continue to have problems after surgery and external-beam radiotherapy.

Conclusions

Radiotherapy plays an important part in the management of some children with cancer. Patients must be carefully selected, taking into account the possible risks of radiation treatment and likely benefits. Knowledge of the response of developing tissues to radiation, coupled with the use of sophisticated, modern equipment and techniques, may allow morbidity to be minimized. The possibility of reducing the use of radiotherapy in certain clinical situations should continue to be tested in randomized trials.

References

Barrett, A., Crennan, E., Barnes, J., and Radford, M. (1990). Treatment of clinical stage I Hodgkin's disease by local radiotherapy alone—a UKCCSG study. *Cancer*, 66, 670–674.

Bentzen, S.M. and Overgaard, J. (1993). Clinical manifestations of normal tissue damage. *Basic Clinical Radiobiology*. Steel GG (Ed). London, Edward Arnold. pp. 89–98.

Brada, M. and Graham, J.D. (1994). Stereotactic radiotherapy in the treatment of glioma and other intracranial lesions. *Current Radiation Oncology* 1. Tobias JS and Thomas PRM (Eds). London, Edward Arnold. pp. 85–100.

D'Angio, G.J., Evans, A.E., Breslow, N., Beckwith, B., Bishop, H., Feigl, P., *et al.* (1976). The treatment of Wilms' tumour: results of the National Wilms' Tumour Study. *Cancer*, 38, 633–646.

D'Angio, G.J., Evans, A., Breslow, N., Beckwith, V., Bishop, H., Farewell, V., *et al.* (1981) The treatment of Wilms' tumor: results of the second National Wilms' Tumor Study. *Cancer*, 47, 2302–2311.

D'Angio, G.J., Breslow, N., Beckwith, J.B., Evans, A., Baum, H., de Lorimier, A., *et al.* (1989). Treatment of Wilms' tumor: results of the third National Wilm's Tumor Study. *Cancer*, 64, 349–360.

Duffner, P.K., Horowitz, M., Krischner, J., Friedman, H.S., Burger, P.C., Cohen, M.E., *et al.* (1993). Postoperative chemotherapy and delayed radiation in children less than two years of age with malignant brain tumours. *New England Journal of Medicine*, 328, 1725–1731.

Gross, R.E. and Neuhauser, E.B.D. (1950). Treatment of mixed tumors of the kidney in childhood. *Pediatrics*, 6, 843–852.

Halberg, F.E., Kramer, JH, Moore, I.M., Wara, W.M., Matthay, K.K., and Albin, A.R. (1991). Prophylactic cranial irradiation dose effects on late cognitive function in children treated for acute lymphoblastic leukaemia. *International Journal of Radiation Oncology, Biology and Physics*, 22, 13–16.

Halperin, E.C., Constine, L.S., Tarbell, N.J., and Kun, L.E. (1994), *Pediatric Radiation Oncology*. Second edition. New York, Raven Press. pp. 485–554.

Harnett, A.N. and Hungerford, J.L. (1991). Ocular morbidity in radiotherapy. *Complications of Cancer Management*. Plowman PN, McElwain T, and Meadows A (Eds). London, Butterworth Heinemann. pp. 361–378.

Hoefnagel, C.A. and Lewington, V.J. (1994). MIBG Therapy, In. Murray IPC and All PJ Eds. Nuclear Medicine in Clinical Diagnosis and Treatment. Churchill Livingstone, Edinburgh

Joiner, M.C. (1993). The linear-quadratic approach to fractionation. *Basic Clinical Radiobiology*. Steel GG (Ed). London, Edward Arnold. pp. 55–64.

Lichter, A.S. (1993). Clinical experience with a three-dimensional treatment planning system. *Current Radiation Oncology* 1. Tobias JS, Thomas PRM (Eds). London, Edward Arnold. pp. 36–50.

Maurer, H.M., Beltangady, M., Gehan, E.A., Crist, W., Hammond, D., Hays, D.M., *et al.* (1988). The Intergroup Rhabdomyosarcoma Study-I: a final report. *Cancer*, 61, 209–220.

Spoudeas, H.A. (1994). Endocrine consequences of irradiation for childhood malignancy. *Current Radiation Oncology* 1. Tobias JS and Thomas RPM (Eds). London, Edward Arnold. pp. 137–159.

Tait, D.M. and Nahum, A.E. (1994). Conformal therapy and its clinical application. *Current Radiation Oncology* 1. Tobias JS, Thomas PRM (Eds). London, Edward Arnold.pp 51–68.

Travis, E.L. (1991). Lung morbidity of radiotherapy. *Complications of Cancer Management*. Plowman PN, McElwain T, and Meadows A (Eds). London, Butterworth Heinemann. pp. 232–249.

6 The supportive care of children receiving treatment for cancer

M. Yule

The last two decades have witnessed a dramatic improvement in the survival of children with malignant disease (Birch *et al.* 1988). While much of this achievement has been attributed to the development of multiagent chemotherapy schedules, the introduction of these regimens has been accompanied by parallel improvements in radiotherapy, surgery, and supportive care. Recent increases in the dose intensity of chemotherapy and the widespread use of high-dose therapy with haematopoetic stem-cell support have necessitated further refinements in antimicrobial and nutritional therapy. One of the reasons why centralization of care within the United Kingdom improved patient survival was that it ensured that children receiving chemoradiotherapy were cared for by physicians who could anticipate and treat the inevitable complications of such therapy (Stiller 1988). Prolonged periods of isolation from family and friends need intensive psychosocial support in order that a cured child may function effectively in society.

Infection

Infection is the most frequent cause of morbidity and mortality in children receiving chemotherapy for malignant disease (Ninane and Chessels 1981). The risk of serious infection is increased by altered mucosal and skin barriers, by compromized cellular and humoral immunity, and by malnutrition. Severe prolonged neutropaenia as a consequence of chemotherapy is the most important factor in determining the risk of serious bacterial or fungal infection (Bodey *et al.* 1966). This reduction in neutrophil number is often accompanied by damage to the gastrointestinal tract and skin.

Following injury to these barriers and in the presence of neutropaenia (absolute neutrophil count less than $1 \times 10^9 \, 1^{-1}$), resident microorganisms may become either locally invasive or progress to septicaemia. Such infections typically occur at areas of the gastrointestinal tract (oropharynx, oesophagus, and anorectal regions) and the respiratory tract (paranasal sinuses and lungs), and are usually produced by gram-negative bacilli, gram-positive cocci, or fungal species. Mucosal barriers at these sites may also be damaged by radiotherapy. Microorganisms may originate either from the patient or the hospital environment. The widespread use of central venous catheters, which are indispensible both for delivering chemotherapy and also as a means of obtaining repeated blood samples for analysis, provide a further portal of access for bacteria, especially coagulase-negative *Staphylococci*, into the circulation (Viscoli *et al.* 1988).

The prevention of infection

Exposure to environmental microorganisms may be minimized by isolation and careful attention to hygiene by medical and nursing staff. The use of laminar air flow and a 'clean diet' has only been shown to benefit children undergoing prolonged periods of neutropaenia such as following allogeneic bone marrow transplantation (BMT). The benefit of oral, non-absorbable antibiotics, such as gentamicin and polymixin, is unproven. Recent studies utilizing systemic antibiotics, such as ciprofloxacin, as prophylaxis in neutropaenic patients have shown a reduction in the infection rate with sensitive bacteria, but only at the cost of an increasing emergence of multi-resistant species such as *Streptococcus faecalis*. Preservation of the integrity of the skin and the maintenance of good dental hygiene are also important in reducing infection rates (Peterson and Overholser 1981). Digital examination of the rectum or the insertion of thermometers should be avoided in order to protect the anal mucosa.

The managment of the febrile neutropaenic child

In the presence of neutropaenia, the localizing symptoms and signs of infection are often absent, and most reliance in determining ongoing infection is placed upon the detection of fever. In the clinical assessment of a neutropaenic child, a temperature of 38°C or greater for two hours must be assumed to represent infection, and merits empirical antibiotic therapy (Albano and Pizzo 1988). Untreated infections in the presence of neutropaenia disseminate rapidly and often end fatally. The initial choice of antibiotic should be determined by the prevailing local environmental flora, the incidence of multiresistant microorganisms, and the presence or absence of an indwelling central venous catheter. In the 1960s and early 1970s, gram-negative bacteria such as *Klebsiella pneumoniae* and *Pseudomonas aeruginosa* were the most common microorganisms infecting neutropaenic cancer patients. More recently there has been an increase in the incidence of infection with gram-positive cocci, such as *Staphlococcus aureus* and *Streptococus viridans*. In clinical practice, uncertainty as to the nature of the infecting organism has lead to the widespread use of combination antibiotic therapy as first-line treatment of the febrile neutropaenic patient (often an aminoglycoside plus a broad spectrum penicillin) following appropriate cultures. Combination therapy may not always be necessary following the introduction of the carbepenems, imipenem, and meropenem (Barza 1985). Possible first-line antibiotic combinations are described in Table 6.1.

In the face of a persisting fever despite 48 hours of broad-spectrum antibiotic treatment, most clinicians would add a glycopeptide antibiotic, such as vancomycin, in order to ensure complete coverage of gram-positive species and multiresistant *Streptococcus faecalis* (Granowetter *et al.* 1988). Persisting fever at 72 hours or beyond is an indication for empirical, anti-fungal therapy with amphotericin B and a thorough search for an underlying viral infection (EORTC International Antimicrobial Therapy Cooperative Group, 1989). Children with persisting fever

Table 6.1 Examples of first-line antibiotic therapy used for the treatment of febrile neutropaenia in children

Antibiotic(s)	Advantages	Disadvantages
Imipenen	single agent anaerobic activity	poor CNS penetration nausea and vomiting neurotoxicity
Ceftazidime/ Amikacin	? synergistic excellent antipseudomonal activity	nephrotoxicity ototoxicity need to monitor serum levels
Piperacillin/ Gentamycin	? synergistic anaerobic activity	nephrotoxicity ototoxicity need to monitor serum levels hypokalaemia
Ceftriaxone	single agent once daily dosing ? suitable for outpatient therapy	insufficient gram-positive cover
Ciprofloxacin	single agent ? convert to oral formulation for outpatient therapy	selects for multiresistant organisms insufficient gram-positive cover

accompanied by respiratory symptoms should receive erythromycin or clarithramycin to treat possible *Mycoplasma pneumoniae*. Infections with anaerobic bacteria are unusual in neutropaenic patients but should be considered if there is evidence of severe mucositis. Antibiotics with significant activity against anaerobes include metronidazole, augmentin, and the carbepenems.

There is considerable variation between centres with regard to the duration of antibiotic treatment required. While some clinicians would consider an early discharge or as little as 72 hours of antibiotics in patients who respond rapidly, others continue with treatment until neutrophil recovery. Proven septicaemia should be treated with a more prolonged course of antibiotics (usually 7 days) than culture negative episodes. Because of the difficulty in obtaining laboratory confirmation of fungal infection, treatment with amphotericin B should be continued for the duration of neutropaenia. Proven, systemic, fungal infections require at least 3 weeks of amphotericin B therapy. Persistent fever despite all these measures is often secondary to central venous catheter colonization, and may improve dramatically following its removal.

Fungal infections

The recent increase in invasive fungal infections has paralleled the use of chemotherapy regimens which are followed by prolonged periods of neutropaenia, and the introduction of BMT. Invasive fungal infections are associated with considerable mortality and account for up to 30% of fatal infections in children with acute leukaemia (Barson and Brady 1987). The most common infecting organisms are *Candida* species, which are responsible for both mucocutaneous and systemic candidiasis (Hawkins and Armstrong 1984). Invasive disease often follows prolonged periods of neutropaenia and treatment with broad-spectrum antibiotics. Infection is more common in children with central venous catheters, particularly when they are being used to provide total parenteral nutrition (Bodey 1986). Many centres routinely prescribe oral, non-absorbable antifungals, such as nystatin or miconazole, during periods of neutropaenia. While these may be successful in preventing oral candidiasis, any benefit in the prevention of invasive disease is unproven.

Three different clinical presentations of invasive candidiasis have been described (Bodey 1986). Some children present with sudden onset of fever, tachycardia, tachypnoea, and hypotension. A second group presents with an insidious onset of fever in the absence of any specific complaints. Lastly, some children present with a steady deterioration in their clinical condition, with or without fever. The diagnosis of systemic candidiasis is difficult as blood cultures are not a reliable means of detecting disseminated disease (Meunier and Klastersky 1988). Only 10% of affected individuals exhibit typical, macronodular, erythematous skin lesions. Infection may also be suggested by the presence of fluffy infiltrates in the optic fundus. Amphotericin B is the only drug with proven efficacy against all common fungal pathogens and is the treatment of choice in invasive candidiasis (Hawkins and Armstrong 1984). It should be started at the earliest clinical suspicion of invasive fungal disease or in the presence of neutropaenic fever which has not responded to 72 hours of broad spectrum antibiotic therapy. The incidence of chills and renal toxicity following amphotericin B may be reduced by substituting the expensive liposomal preparation at a dose ratio of 1:3–5. Fluconazole, a new triazole antifungal, is being increasingly used as prophylaxis against infections with *Candida* species (Grant and Clissold 1990).

Aspergillus species, particularly *Aspergillus fumigatus*, are the second most common cause of invasive fungal infection in the immunocompromised child (Hawkins and Armstrong 1984). *Aspergillus* spores are ubiquitous in distribution and are often found circulating in environmental air. Spores are constantly inhaled, with colonization usually occurring in the lungs or paranasal sinuses of patients. Exposure to the spores can be reduced by the use of laminar air flow. Growth occurs by extension to adjacent air spaces and invasion of the bronchial walls. *Aspergillus* invasion typically produces a necrotizing bronchopneumonia with cavitation and abscess formation accompanied by fever, dyspnoea, and cough (Gerson *et al.* 1985). Vascular invasion can result in haemorrhagic pulmonary infarction and dissemination to other organs. Rhinocerebral infection occurs less often than pulmonary infection, and progresses through the soft tissues, cartilage, and bone producing necrotic lesions in the palate and nose. Amphotericin B therapy should be started at the earliest clinical or radiological suspicion of infection (Barson and Brady 1987). Any additional benefit of nebulized amphotericin B is unproven. The use of itraconazole as prophylaxis against *Aspergillus* infection is limited by the absence of a parenteral formulation and its propensity to inhibit the metabolism of other drugs (Murphy *et al.* 1995).

Viral infections

The use of increasingly intensive chemotherapy has been accompanied by a reduction in host defences against several viral pathogens. The most common viral pathogens affecting immunosuppressed children are the herpes viruses, which include herpes simplex virus (HSV), varicella-zoster virus (VZV), cytomegalovirus (CMV), and Epstein-Barr virus (EBV). These agents are ubiquitous and can be responsible for illness following primary infections or reactivation of endogenous virus. Unlike bacterial and fungal infections which follow episodes of neutropaenia, viral reactivation occurs as a result of deficient cell-mediated immunity. The lymphotoxic nature of most cytotoxics acts to inhibit cell-mediated immunity in children receiving chemotherapy.

HSV can result in local infections, most commonly gingivostomatitis, but also conjunctivitis, vesicular skin lesions, pneumonia, and encephalitis. The healing of superficial infections is pro-longed in neutropaenic patients, and superinfection with bacteria and fungi often occurs, causing severe pain (Pizzo 1981). These lesions usually represent reactivation of endogenous virus. Reactivation of HSV occurs in up to 80% of bone marrow recipients and may be associated with a fatal outcome. Tissue culture isolation of HSV from infected tissues or secretions remains the most reliable means of diagnosis. The current treatment of mucocutaneous infections is with acy-clovir, which may be applied topically to speed healing in mild lesions, but usually requires sys-temic administration in more severe cases (Saral 1988). Prophylactic acyclovir reduces the incidence of recurrent HSV infections both in BMT recipients and in children with leukaemia undergoing induction therapy (Saral *et al.* 1981). Severe, mucocutaneous HSV infection is exquisitely painful and requires opiate analgesia.

Primary infection with VZV results in chickenpox. Although this infection is usually self limit-ing in normal children, VZV infection in the immunosuppressed can lead to a fulminant illness with visceral dissemination of the virus (Feldman *et al.* 1975). Untreated VZV pneumonitis may be fatal in up to 7% of affected children, and can be identified by the presence of diffuse, ill-defined, nodular densities on chest X-ray (Hughes 1987). Superimposed bacterial infection occurs in nearly one-half of cases. The presence of antibodies to VZV can be used to determine the susceptibility of patients to this virus, and should be performed in all children prior to starting treatment. Following exposure to VZV, susceptible children should receive VZV immune globu-lin within 96 hours of exposure to community cases (Immunization Practices Advisory Committee, 1984). Oral acyclovir may be a safer and less painful alternative. Children who develop established disease should be treated with intravenous acyclovir for 7–10 days.

CMV infection is common at all ages, but serological evidence of infection is more common in children with cancer, possibly as a result of post-transfusion infection (Cox and Hughes 1975). The isolation of CMV from body sites is common in immunocompromised patients and does not necessarily indicate active disease. The clinical signs of active CMV infection include fever, rash, hepatosplenomegaly, retinitis, pneumonia, and a variety of neurological signs. Lymphocytosis with atypical lymphocytes may occur. Several factors are associated with a particularly high rate of CMV infection. These include bone marrow transplantation from a CMV-antibody positive donor into a seronegative recipient, the presence of graft-versus-host disease. and the use of anti-thymocyte globulin. CMV pneumonitis is heralded by fever and increasing respiratory distress and may be manifest as diffuse, bilateral interstitial infiltrates on chest X-ray (Hughes 1987). Establishing the role of CMV as the aetiologic agent in a symptomatic child may be difficult. Documentation of seroconversion or the presence of a CMV-specific antibody supports the diag-nosis of a primary infection (Rasmussen *et al.* 1982). The identification of CMV early antigen in fresh specimens of urine can be a useful indicator of systemic infection. CMV may also be detected in blood using the polymerase chain reaction, although this technique has a high rate of false positive results. Isolation of the virus from affected viscerae, which may require bronchoalveolar lavage in the case of pulmonary infection, is often necessary. Both gancyclovir and trisodium phosphonoformate (foscarnet) are active in the treatment of established disease, but prolonged courses of therapy are necessary to eradicate the infection, and relapses following the completion of treatment are common (Koretz *et al.* 1986). The use of acyclovir prophylaxis, continuing to 30 days after transplant, in bone marrow recipients leads to a significant reduction in the rate of CMV infection (Meyers *et al.* 1988).

EBV infections in immunocompromised children may result in a spectrum of lymphoproliferative disorders ranging from benign, polyclonal B-cell hyperplasias to monoclonal B-cell lymphomas. Common respiratory virus infections with the respiratory syncitial virus, the influenza viruses, the parainfluenza viruses, and the adenoviruses are usually well tolerated by immunosuppressed patients, although the duration of viral excretion is often prolonged (Engelhard *et al.* 1986). The role of ribavirin, an antiviral nucleoside analogue with a broad spectrum of activity, has yet to be defined. Historically, measles pneumonitis and encephalitis presented a significant risk to immunosuppressed children; however the incidence of this infection has decreased dramatically following an effective vaccination programme. Exposure to an individual with active disease should be followed by treatment with human normal immunoglobulin.

Protozoal infections

The most important protozoal pathogen in children receiving chemotherapy is *Pneumocystis carinii*. This poorly understood organism is a important cause of pneumonia in cancer patients, particularly children who experience prolonged immunosuppresion, such as those receiving maintenance chemotherapy for lymphoblastic leukaemia (Wong 1984; Masur 1989*a*). Although infection in adolescents follows the reactivation of dormant cysts in the lung, it is not clear whether pneumonia in the younger child is a consequence of reactivation or primary infection. Clinically, *Pneumocystis carinii* pneumonitis is characterized by fever, cough, and dyspnoea, which is usually accompanied by the presence of diffuse pulmonary infiltrates on the chest X-ray (Walzer 1988). Diagnosis requires the identification of the organism in a clinical specimen, often fluid, obtained during bronchoalveolar lavage. Sputum induction with nebulized, hypertonic saline may also facilitate diagnosis in the older child. High-dose intravenous cotrimoxazole is the treatment of choice for established infection (Masur 1989*b*). A deterioration in the clinical condition of the patient may be seen during the first 2–5 days of treatment as a result of the patient's inflammatory response to protozoal lysis. Failure to respond to 7 days of cotrimoxazole is an indication to add intravenous pentamidine. The use of corticosteroids in infected children remains controversial. The incidence of *Pneumocystis carinii* pneumonia has been dramatically reduced by prophylactic cotrimoxazole given twice a day for 3 days per week in children receiving prolonged courses of chemotherapy (Hughes *et al.* 1987). Nebulized pentamidine is a useful alternative to cotrimoxazole in patients who are unable to tolerate the drug.

Toxoplasma gondii is an obligate, intracellular protozoan whose definitive host is the cat. Human infection occurs either congenitally, or by ingestion of sporulated oocysts or poorly cooked meats containing viable tissue cysts. Following the development of cellular immunity to toxoplasma and resolution of the acute infection, viable toxoplasma cysts persist in the brain and cardiac muscle of the host for life (McCabe and Remington 1990). Toxoplasmosis in immuno-compromised patients may be due to a newly acquired infection or, more commonly, be the result of reactivation of latent infection, and often presents with a variety of neurological symptoms (Wong 1984). Central nervous system disease, including encephalitis or cerebral abscess, is the most common site of infection. The diagnosis is based upon seropositivity in a patient with characteristic signs on a computed tomographic scan of the brain. Most cases will respond to a prolonged course of pyrimethamine and sulfadiazine given in combination with folic acid.

Blood product transfusion

In addition to producing immunosuppression as a consequence of failure of white cell production, most cytotoxics also inhibit red cell and platelet production. While granulocyte transfusions are no longer widely used, many patients require platelet transfusions, and almost all will at some stage need red cell transfusions. Blood product transfusion should not be undertaken lightly as it is not without risk. Red cell transfusions are thought to be responsible for the current mini-epidemic of hepatitis C infection. All blood products should be CMV-negative and carefully screened for viral infection. Formerly, all blood products administered to children receiving chemotherapy were irradiated to reduce the incidence of transfusion-related, graft-versus-host disease from donor lymphocytes. This risk has been exaggerated, and irradiated blood products are not thought to be necessary, other than following myeloablative therapy prior to BMT or in children with Hodgkin's disease (Webb 1995).

It is unnecessary to increase the haemoglobin concentration to normal levels; the aim should rather be to achieve a red cell concentration which is compatible with a moderate level of physical activity. Most centres accept a haemoglobin concentration of less than 8 g dl^{-1} as an indication for transfusion. Lower levels may be appropriate in children following BMT in order to stimulate erythropoiesis. Regular administration of the erythropoeitic stem-cell factor, erythropoietin, reduces the need for red cell transfusion, but requires supplemental iron therapy. The cost-effectiveness of erythropoietin in children is currently under evaluation.

Platelet transfusions are necessary for thrombocytopaenic patients who are actively bleeding. In most cases, prophylactic platelet transfusions are an inappropriate use of a limited resource. Prophylaxis may be useful under certain conditions, for example after BMT, during episodes of sepsis, and in patients receiving chemotherapy for either neuroblastoma or intracranial tumours, in whom the risk of spontaneous haemorrhage may be greater. Repeated transfusions may lead to alloimmunization, reducing the therapeutic effect of transfused platelets. Under these circumstances, the use of compatible, single-donor transfusions may be appropriate. Potential 'thrombopoietins' are currently undergoing clinical trials in adults.

Colony-stimulating factors

Laboratory studies on human bone marrow cultures have identified a variety of growth factors which are important in sustaining myelopoiesis *in vitro*. Two of these, granulocyte-stimulating factor (G-CSF) and granulocyte-macrophage colony-stimulating factor (GM-CSF), have been synthesized using recombinant DNA technology and are in widespread clinical use. As the name suggests, GM-CSF stimulates the division of a more primitive haematopoietic stem cell than G-CSF, which results in an increase in the circulating number of both macrophages and granulo-cytes, rather than granulocytes alone. In addition to increased circulating numbers, both colony-stimulating factors increase the functional activity of their target cells (Metcalf 1990). The adverse effects of treatment including fever, skin rashes, arthralgia, bone pains, and pleurisy, are more severe with GM-CSF.

Both agents have been introduced into clinical practice in a number of settings. Continuous treatment with colony-stimulating factors has been shown in the majority of studies to reduce the incidence of febrile neutropaenia in patients receiving chemotherapy. The cost-benefit analysis of using these expensive drugs in this situation has yet to be clearly demonstrated. At present there is no evidence that initiating treatment with growth factors at the onset of sepsis reduces the severity or duration of that event. Treatment with G-CSF or GM-CSF reduces the duration of neutropaenia and also the morbidity of high-dose chemotherapy procedures (Monroy et al. 1987; Baethmann et al. 1994). Both agents are also widely used in patients who fail to engraft, or who lose a graft after BMT (Nemunaitis et al. 1990).

Colony-stimulating factors may be used to shorten the duration of chemotherapy-induced neu-tropaenia, enabling treatment to be delivered at shorter time intervals, and providing a practical means of increasing dose intensity. Treatment may also recruit a higher proportion of leukaemic cells into the active phase of the cell cycle, thereby increasing their sensitivity to cytotoxic drugs (Cannistra et al. 1989). Lastly, growth factors may be used, either alone or in combination with myelosuppressive chemotherapy, to facilitate a successful haematopoietic stem-cell harvest from peripheral blood (Ravagnani et al. 1990). Although G-CSF and GM-CSF have found their way into many clinical applications, there remains an urgent need to define their current role in the therapeutic armamentarium in terms of overall patient benefit.

Nutrition

Protein-calorie malnutrition is a common problem in children with cancer, with up to 40% of patients becoming malnourished during therapy (van Eys 1979). The underlying aetiology is complex and includes poor dietary intake, cancer cachexia, and the gastrointestinal complications of chemo- and radiotherapy which are manifest as anorexia, vomiting, stomatitis, and malabsorption (Costa and Donaldson 1979; Kein and Camitta 1983). Abdominal or pelvic irradiation may lead to strictures, fistulas, and altered peristalsis, which may also reduce dietary intake. All children should undergo a nutritional assessment as part of their initial evaluation, which should include a dietary assessment, anthropometric measurements, and laboratory estimates of albumin and transferrin. The early involvement of a trained dietician is invaluable in optimizing energy and amino acid intake. Prevention is considerably easier than cure, and nutritional support should be anticipated for child-ren who are expected to undergo intensive therapy regimens. Intervention is required in children who lose more than or equal to 10% of their initial body weight during treatment.

When the gastrointestinal tract is functioning, the enteral route is preferred for nutritional support as it is simpler, safer, and more economical than parenteral nutrition. The initial step involves dietary counselling and the selection of calorifically rich foods. This is followed by the use of high-calorie oral supplements which, unfortunately, may result in diarrhoea. Children often dislike drinking these supplements and tire of taking the same products on a long-term basis. If this approach fails to provide adequate calories, nasogastric tube feeding should be started immediately. Enteral tube feeding may also help to maintain the integrity of the intestinal mucosa and prevent the gastrointestinal toxicity of chemo-radiotherapy (Donaldson 1977). The technique of nasogastric tube feeding can often be taught to the child's parents who can then continue the programme at home. Contraindications to tube feeding include a nonfunctional gastrointestinal tract, intestinal obstruction, gastrointestinal bleeding, persistent nausea and vomiting, and severe diarrhoea. A gastrostomy may be useful in children who will not tolerate a nasogastric tube. There are numerous commercial formulas which supply all essential nutrients and are available specifically for tube feeding. Elemental formulas provide these nutrients in simpler forms that do not require further digestion prior to absorption, and may be useful in children with abnormal gastrointestinal function. Such formulas have a high osmolarity and may cause diarrhoea.

Parenteral nutrition should only be used for children whose gastrointestinal dysfunction precludes adequate nutritional support via the enteral route. It may be indicated for patients who are being treated with very intensive treatment regimens known to produce a high incidence of nutritional failure such as BMT. Prolonged parenteral nutrition may lead to metabolic disturbances including glucose intolerance, electrolyte disturbances, hyperlipidaemia, and liver dysfunction. These complications can be minimized by careful biochemical monitoring. In order to reduce the incidence of local thrombophlebitis, parenteral nutrition solutions are usually delivered via a central venous catheter.

Analgesia

Because of the difficulty of recognizing pain in young children, their symptoms have often been undertreated. Careful attention must be paid in order to suspect pain as a primary cause of irritability and withdrawal. The pain of malignant disease is constant and there is no place for the prescription of analgesia 'as required' As part of their treatment, children repeatedly undergo painful proceedures such as lumbar punctures and bone marrow aspirates. The discomfort experienced during these proceedures can be minimized by careful psychological preparation and the prescription of adequate analgesia (Zeltzer et al. 1989). Established scales of analgesics from paracetamol, escalating via codeine and nonsteroidals, to potent opiates such as diamorphine should be followed until adequate pain relief is achieved in each case. Membrane-stabilizing drugs such as carbamazepine and amytriptiline can be useful in persisting neuralgia which, if severe, may require nerve blockade. Neutropaenic mucositis is exquisitely painful and should be treated with opiate infusions and appropriate antimicrobials.

Antiemetics

The use of 5-hydroxtryptamine antagonists has revolutionized the treatment of cytotoxic-induced emesis in children (Zoubek et al. 1993). There is little to choose between ondansetron, granisetron, and tropisetron in terms of their pharmacological properties. Headache is less of a problem with

these drugs in children than in adults. It should be remembered that cytotoxic drugs with low eme-
togenic potential, such as methotrexate and the vinca alkaloids, do not usually require treatment
with these relatively expensive drugs. 5-Hydroxytryptamine antagonists are not optimal therapy
for the delayed emesis seen following cisplatin and oxazaphosphorine treatment, which may be
better controlled using a combination of metoclopramide and dexamethasone. If vomiting persists
despite adequate treatment with 5-hydroxytryptamine antagonists, it may be worth adding dexamethasone (effect is maximal after 24 hours of therapy), cyclizine, chlorpromazine, or metoclopramide (Hahlen *et al.* 1995). Lorazepam remains a useful adjunct for anticipatory vomiting.

Vaccination

While vaccination policies vary from centre to centre, there are some broad areas of agreement
(Table 6.2). No child should be vaccinated within 1 year of completing chemotherapy. For children
treated in the United Kingdom, patients who had not completed their primary course of oral polio,
pertussis/diphtheria/tetanus, and *Haemophilus influenzae* B at the time of diagnosis should have all
three doses repeated. Patients who had completed their initial course should have antibody levels
measured 1 year after treatment, and if these are subprotective they should then receive a further
booster dose. It may be more appropriate to use the killed form of polio vaccine following a period
of intensive chemotherapy. All recommendations are flexible and what is appropriate for a child who
received a 3-month course of chemotherapy is very different from that for a patient following BMT.

Psychosocial support

This is an extremely complex subject which is worthy of a volume in itself. Although mood
changes and difficulties in peer-relations are common in patients during treatment, particularly

Table 6.2 Vaccination recommendations following the treatment of malignant disease

Interval from treatment	Recommendation
1 Year	In children who have not completed a course of polio, diphtheria/pertussis/tetanus, and *Haemophilus influenzae* B REPEAT ENTIRE COURSE USING KILLED POLIO VACCINE
	Measure antibody levels in children who have completed a primary course of polio, diphtheria/pertussis/tetanus, and *Haemophilus influenzae* B REIMMUNIZE ONLY IF LEVELS ARE SUBPROTECTIVE
18 Months	Measles/mumps/rubella vaccine in previously untreated children
24 Months	BCG vaccine in previously untreated children (May NOT be appropriate following matched, unrelated BMT)

adolescents, the proportion of children who develop frank psychiatric illness is low (Stehbens 1988). The needs of individual families are diverse and the considerable financial burden faced by the parents of children undergoing protracted treatment should also not be ignored. Provision should be made for families and patients to express their anxieties and uncertainties at all times. Certain critical periods are particularly stressful for patients and their families. These include diagnosis, waiting for the results of investigations, and coming off treatment. Children should be encouraged to continue with a normal life as far as possible during treatment. If school attendance is not possible, children should continue with their work while in hospital. It is important to encourage feelings of independence and self-confidence in patients in order to facilitate their successful return to society.

References

Albano E.A. and Pizzo P.A. (1988). Infectious complications in childhood acute leukemias. *Pediatric Clinics of North America*, 35, 873–901.

Barson W.J. and Brady M.T. (1987). Management of infection in children with cancer. *Haematology/Oncology Clinics of North America*, 1, 801–39.

Barza M. (1985). Imipenem; First of a new class of beta-lactam antibiotics. *Annals of Internal Medicine*, 103, 552–60.

Birch J.M., Marsden H.B., Morris Jones P.H., Pearson D., and Blair V. (1988). Improvements in survival from childhood cancer in results of a population based study over 30 years. *British Medical Journal*, 296, 1372–6.

Bodey G.P. (1986). Fungal infections and fever of unknown origin in neutropaenic patients. *American Journal of Medicine*, 80, 112–9.

Bodey G.P., Buckley M., and Sathe Y.S. (1966). Quantitative relationships between circulating leukocytes and infection in patients with acute leukaemia. *Annals of Internal Medicine*, 64, 328–40.

Baethmann M., Peters C., Laws H.J., Luder M., Hanenberg H., Gadner H., *et al.* (1994). Comparison of G-CSF versus GM-CSF after myeloablative. radiochemotherapy and haematopoietic stem cell rescue in children with solid tumours. *Bone Marrow Transplantation,* 14, Supplement 1, S15–6.

Cannistra S.A., Groshek P., and Griffin J.D. (1989). Granulocyte-macrophage colony stimulating factor enhances the cytotoxic efects of cytosine arabinoside in acute myeloblastic leukemia and in the myeloid blast crisis phase of chronic myeloid leukemia. *Leukemia*, 3, 328–34.

Costa G. and Donaldson S.S. (1979). Effects of cancer and cancer treatment on the nutrition of the host. *New England Journal of Medicine*, 300, 1471.

Cox F. and Hughes W.T. (1975). Cytomegaloviraemia in children with acute lymphocytic leukaemia. *Journal of Pediatrics*, 87, 190–4.

Donaldson S.S. (1977). Nutritional consequences of radiotherapy. *Cancer Research*, 37, 2407–12.

Engelhard D., Marks M.I., and Good R.A. (1986). Infections in bone marrow transplant recipients. *Journal of Pediatrics*, 108, 335–46.

EORTC International Antimicrobial Therapy Cooperative Group. (1989). Empiric antifungal therapy in febrile granulocytopenic patients. *American Journal of Medicine*, 86, 668–72.

Feldman S., Hughes W.T., and Daniel C.B. (1975). Varicella in children with cancer; 27 cases. *Pediatrics*, 56, 388–97.

Gerson S.L., Talbot G.H., and Lusk E. (1985). Invasive pulmonary *aspergillosis* in adult leukemia; clinical clues to its diagnosis. *Journal of Clinical Oncology*, 3, 1108–16.

Granowetter L., Wells H., and Lange B. (1988). Ceftazidime with or without vancomycin versus cephalothin, carbenicillin and gentamicin as the initial therapy for the febrile neutropaenic pediatric cancer patient. *Pediatric Infectious Disease*, 7, 165–170.

Grant S.M. and Clissold S.P. (1990). Fluconazole. A review of its pharmacodynamic and pharmacokinetic properties and therapeutic potential in superficial and systemic mycoses. *Drugs*, 39, 877–916.

Hahlen K., Quintana E., Pinkerton C.R., and Cedar E. (1995). A randomised comparison of intravenously administered granisetron versus chlorpromazine plus dexamethasone in the prevention of ifosfamide-induced emesis in children. *Journal of Pediatrics*, 126, 309–13.

Hawkins C. and Armstrong D. (1984). Fungal infections in the immunocompromised host. *Clinical Haematology*, 13, 599–630.

Hughes W.T. (1987). Pneumonia in the immunocompromised child. *Seminars in Respiratory Infection*, 2, 177–83.

Hughes W.T., Rivera G.K., and Schell M.J. (1987). Successful intermittent prophylaxis for *Pneumocystis carinii* pneumonitis. *New England Journal of Medicine*, 316, 1627–32.

Immunization Practices Advisory Committee, (1984). Varicella-zoster immune globulin for prevention of chickenpox. *Annals of Internal Medicine*, 100, 859–62.

Kein C.L. and Camitta B.M. (1983). Increased whole-body protein turnover in sick children with newly diagnosed leukemia and lymphoma. *Cancer Research*, 43, 5586–92.

Koretz S.H., Buhler W.C., and Brewin A. (1986). Treatment of serious cytomegalovirus infection with 9-(1,3-dihydroxy-2-propoxymethyl) guanine in patients with AIDS and other immunodeficiencies. *New England Journal of Medicine*, 314, 801–5.

Masur H. (1989*a*). Prevention of *Pneumocystis carinii* pneumonia. *Reviews in Infectious Disease*, 11, S1664–8.

Masur H. (1989*b*). Pneumocystis pneumonia from bench to clinic. *Annals of Internal Medicine*, 111, 813–26.

McCabe R.E. and Remington J.S. (1990). *Toxoplasma gondii*. In *Principles and Practice of Infectious Disease*, Eds Mandell G.L., Douglas R.G. and Bennett J.E. 3rd Edition, Churchill Livingston, New York.

Metcalf D. (1990). The colony stimulating factors; discovery, development, and clinical applications. *Cancer*, 65, 2185–95.

Meunier F. and Klastersky J. (1988). Recent development in prophylaxis and therapy of invasive fungal infections in granulocytopenic cancer patients. *European Journal of Cancer and Clinical Oncology*, 21, 539–44.

Meyers J.D., Reed E.C., and Shepp D.H. (1988). Acyclovir for prevention of cytomegalovirus infection and disease after allogeneic bone marrow transplantation. *New England Journal of Medicine*, 318, 70–5.

Monroy R.L., Skelly R.R., Mac Vittie T.J., Davis T.A., Sauber J.J., and Clark S.C. (1987). The effect of recombinant GM-CSF on the recovery of monkeys transplanted with autologous bone marrow. *Blood*, 70, 1696–9.

Murphy J.A., Ross L.M., and Gibson B.E. (1995). Vincristine toxicity in five children with acute lymphoblastic leukaemia. *Lancet*, 346, 443.

Nemunaitis J., Singer J.W., Buckner C.D., Epstein C., Hill R., Storb R., *et al.* (1990). Use of recombinant human granulocyte-macrophage colony stimulating factor in graft failure after bone marrow transplantation. *Blood*, 76, 245–53.

Ninane J. and Chessels J.M. (1981). Serious infections during continuing treatment of acute lymphoblastic leukaemia. *Archives of Disease in Childhood*, 56, 841–4.

Peterson D.G. and Overholser C.D. (1981). Increased morbidity associated with oral infection in patients with acute nonlymphocytic leukaemia. *Oral Surgery*, 51, 390–3.

Pizzo P.A. (1981). Infectious complications in the child with cancer. II. Management of specific infectious organisms. *Journal of Pediatrics*, 98, 513–23.

Rasmussen L., Kelsall D., and Nelson R. (1982). Virus specific IgG and IgM antibodies in normal and immunocompromised subjects infected with cytomegalovirus. *Journal of Infectious Diseases*, 145, 191–9.

Ravagnani F., Siena S., and Bregni M. (1990). Large-scale collection of circulating haematopoietic progenitors in cancer patients treated with high-dose cyclophosphamide and recombinant human GM-CSF. *European Journal of Cancer*, 26, 562–4.

Saral R., Burns W.H., and Laskin O.L. (1981). Acyclovir prophylaxis of herpes simplex infections; a randomised double-blind controlled trial in bone marrow transplant recipients. *New England Journal of Medicine*, 305, 63–7.

Saral R. (1988). Management of mucocutaneous herpes simplex lesions in immunocompromised patients. *American Journal of Medicine*, 85, 57–60 (Supplement 29).

Stehbens J.A. (1988). childhood cancer. In Routh D., Ed. *Handbook of Pediatric Psychology*, Guildford. New York. pp. 135–61.

Stiller C.A. (1988). Centralisation of treatment and survival rates for cancer. *Archives of Disease in Childhood*, 63, 23–30.

van Eys J. (1979). Malnutrition in children with cancer: Incidence and consequence. *Cancer*, 43, 2030–5.

Viscoli C., Garaventa A., and Boni L. (1988). Role of broviac catheters in infections in children with cancer. *Paediatric Infectious Diseases Journal*, 7, 556–60.

Walzer P.D. (1988). Diagnosis of *Pneumocystis carinii* pneumonia. *Journal of Infectious Disease*, 157, 629–32.

Webb, D.K.H. (1995). Irradiation in the prevention of transfusion associated graft-versus-host disease. *Archives of Disease in Childhood*, 73, 388–9.

Wong B. (1984). Parasitic diseases in immunocompromised hosts. *American Journal of Medicine*, 76, 479–86.

Zeltzer L.K., Jay S.M., and Fisher D.M. (1989). The management of pain associated with paediatric procedures. *Pediatric Clinics of North America*, 36, 941–64.

Zoubek A., Kronberger M., Puschmann A., and Gadner H. (1993). Ondansetron in the control of chemotherapy-induced and radiotherapy-induced emesis in children with malignancies. *Anti-Cancer Drugs*, 4, 17–21 (Supplement 2).

7 Late and very late effects of therapy—towards lifetime follow-up of cured patients

J. Lemerle, O. Oberlin, F. de Vathaire, F. Pein, and F. Aubier

Between the 1950s and 1980s, the overall cure rate of children treated for cancer or leukaemia has increased, and reached 80–90% for some tumours such as Wilms', nonmetastatic neuroblastoma, and all lymphomas. In 1950, the mere fact that a child survived after cancer treatment was considered a major achievement.

Gradually, long-term survivors became a significant group, and were increasingly faced with difficult and unexpected problems. Most of these late effects, essentially due to radiotherapy at that time, appeared and worsened during growth. Curing more patients and, even more importantly, without sequelae, then became, and still is, the goal to be achieved. Wilms' tumour is a good example of what is now commonly considered a 'success story' in paediatric oncology. Surgery, radiotherapy, and actinomycin alone cured 50% of the patients. This figure improved very significantly only when pre-and postoperative systematic chemotherapy reduced the incidence of overt metastases. Cautiously studied and tested in the SIOP trials, among others (D'Angio *et al.* 1989; Tournade *et al.* 1993), chemotherapy has brought us to the present situation in which 80–90% of all Wilms' tumour cases are cured, with only 20–25% having undergone any irradiation and thus at risk of developing either abdominal, spinal, or pulmonary sequelae.

The same kind of effort towards quality of cure, as well as high cure rates, is now the basis of most protocols designed to treat childhood malignancies.

However, as long as new drugs are used, it is possible that new adverse effects will be identified. Furthermore, we are now witnessing 'very late' complications of therapy, up to 20 or 30 years after treatment.

Organs and functions impaired by cancer therapy in children

The first problems recognized were directly related to radiotherapy, given then with orthovoltage machines. Then chemotherapeutic agents were found to have specific longterm toxicity. Finally, things became increasingly complex with the generalized use of combined treatments and the possible mutual enhancement of specific toxicities. All organs can be injured by radiotherapy given during childhood, either in terms of growth or function or both. The damage, as discussed in Chapter 5, is correlated with several factors, particularly:

(1) the total dose given, the fractionation schedule, and overall treatment time;

(2) the volume involved;

(3) the age of the patient at the time of treatment, with damage being worse in younger children;

(4) the time elapsed between radiotherapy and observation. Growth impairment becomes more and more visible as the child grows, and cannot be fully assessed before the end of somatic growth.

Chemotherapy, at the moment, seems to be responsible more for immediate toxic effects than for long-term sequelae. However, it is too early for us to state that the long-term effects of chemical agents are strictly confined to those which are already well known. With new drugs being used, and the fact that an observation period of several decades is needed, many questions are still outstanding.

Functional, morphological, and cosmetic sequelae

The sequelae of surgery are obvious. Sequelae of radiotherapy may be severe and enhanced by concomitant chemotherapy. The appropriate local treatment should be that which produces the least sequelae.

After radiotherapy, soft tissues, muscles, muscle sheaths and vessels, and also the skin, may undergo sclerosis, retraction, and finally necrosis due to a deficient blood supply. This will impair the function, but also the growth, of adjacent bones and joints. The bone itself can become sclerotic and necrotic resulting in fractures, especially of the limbs. Growth plates in young children are particularly sensitive and irradiation (or surgical removal) of these zones accounts for bone-growth impairment. When the irradiation is not perfectly symmetrical, growth defects will result in bones which are short and curved. This is particularly obvious for cases involving vertebrae; spinal deformities invariably arise. Bone and soft tissue alterations are dose related: little damage is observed when the total dose is less than 10 Gy, but significant damage is seen above 20 Gy, especially in the young child (Donaldson 1992).

Limbs

Limb shortening is common after radiotherapy. In many cases it can be corrected surgically by lengthening another bone, e.g. the femur when the tibia is too short, and also by slowing down growth of the opposite limb. In a few cases, damage is so considerable that amputation and an appropriate prosthesis may be necessary. Prevention is more efficient than surgical correction of joint deformities or dysfunction. It can often be achieved using early and prolonged physiotherapeutic procedures.

Thorax

Trunk irradiation may impair normal breast development. Unilateral irradiation will result in breast asymmetry which may need surgical correction during adulthood. In Hodgkin's disease, when doses as high as 35–45 Gy were given to 'mantle' fields, deformities such as thin neck, short clavicles, and narrow shoulders were seen.

Apart from these essentially cosmetic injuries, which should not be underestimated due to the psychological impact they may have on the young adult's perception of his/her body image, the alteration of the thoracic wall and of the spine by radiotherapy are of critical importance.

A fractionated dose of 20 Gy to the whole thorax for metastases from Wilms' tumour invariably resulted, in adulthood, in a reduction of 25–50% in vital capacity, or even more if the child was very young during irradiation or if additional boosts had to be given. This was due to a combination of impaired growth of the bony thoracic wall and of more complex factors such as soft tissue injury and insufficient lung development.

Spinal irradiation-related vertebral sequelae largely depend on the spinal level involved, and on the radiotherapy schedules/doses given. Thoracic irradiation, or spinal irradiation for medulloblastoma, which are both perfectly symmetrical, produce only a growth defect resulting in predictable stature loss with reduced sitting height, but very seldom scoliosis. On the other hand, unilateral abdominal irradiation for Wilms' tumour will result in scoliosis and kyphosis, or rarely lordosis. This is due to the unavoidable combination of two major factors: unilateral sclerosis and reduced growth of soft tissues of the involved lumbar fossa, and also slightly asymmetrical irradiation of the spine, in order to spare the remaining kidney, which will result in asymmetrical growth (Mayfield *et al.* 1981).

The treatment of scoliosis should be prevention. For the majority of Wilms' tumours, radiotherapy is no longer needed when primary chemotherapy downstages lesions and leads to a predominance of stages I and II.

When radiotherapy has to be delivered to the spine of a child, there should be careful follow-up, especially at the pubertal growth spurt: frontal and lateral radiographs should be obtained at least every 6 months. If a spinal curve reaches 10–20, the prescription of a brace should be considered, especially in the case of kyphosis.

Face

Radiotherapy of the face may have cosmetic and functional consequences. Such is the case when the mandible and the temporo-mandibular joint are involved, causing permanent trismus. These may be preventable if brachytherapy can be used following chemotherapy. Chemotherapy alone, as proposed in a SIOP rhabdomyosarcoma protocol, is of course, the best option when applicable.

Endocrine sequelae—growth and reproduction

All endocrine glands can be damaged by cancer therapy. The most frequent problems are effects on growth, pituitary and thyroid glands, reproduction, and the offspring of those who had cancer during childhood.

Growth hormone and other pituitary hormones

Growth hormone (GH) deficiency is frequent after radiotherapy to the pituitary, although prolonged hydrocephalus is also an important factor. Its consequences can be worsened by thyroid hormone deficiency, vertebral radiotherapy, and early puberty (Brauner *et al.* 1989). With doses under 20 Gy, GH deficiency is unusual, while it is almost always present over 45 Gy. Age is also important, young patients being more sensitive to radiation. The time elapsing between a 35–45 Gy dose of cranial irradiation and a significant drop in GH levels is 18–24 months. Growth alterations vary according to the tumour and to the treatment administered. In the case of medulloblastomas, high-dose (25–35 Gy) irradiation to the spine arrests growth rapidly just before the drop in GH levels. In these cases, GH replacement therapy has little effect, nor does puberty. These patients end up with low sitting height and comparatively long lower limbs.

In leukaemias, chemotherapy alone does not modify growth velocity. 50% of cases which receive 24 Gy to the brain develop low GH levels. This proportion reaches 100% if TBI is added (Sanders *et al.* 1988). These patients are also likely to have early puberty due to cranial irradiation (Brauner *et al.* 1984). GH treatment in leukaemias treated without TBI is more efficient than in the case of medulloblastomas. It should be started when low GH levels are associated with slowing down of growth.

In optic nerve gliomas, early puberty is very frequent before any treatment. GH deficiency is constant soon after treatment, due to the high doses of radiation used. Thus, treatment should often combine an LHRH analogue and GH.

Secretion of other pituitary hormones is less frequently altered by cancer treatment. Thyroid-stimulating hormone (TSH) secretion is rarely impaired, nor is adrenocorticotrophic hormone (ACTH). Cranial irradiation can, however, speed up puberty, for reasons which remain obscure, and it can also inhibit gonadotrophin secretion.

Thyroid-stimulating hormone (TSH)

Thyroid irradiation usually induces thyroid hypofunction, exceptionally hyperthyroidism, and depends on the dose received (Constine *et al.* 1984). Most frequently it is compensated and only indicated by high TSH levels with normal thyroid hormone levels and no clinical symptoms. A high TSH level may persist for as long as 2 years after irradiation, and will return to normal in one-third of cases. Treatment of isolated, raised TSH is controversial, but usually done for the unproven reason that a permanently high TSH level could stimulate oncogenesis in the thyroid. Thyroid tumours after irradiation are considered in another section of this chapter.

Reproduction

Testicular sequelae can be induced by irradiation and/or by chemotherapy. Radiotherapy produces Leydig cell hypofunction at low doses, starting at 5–6 Gy, which is almost constant after 24 Gy given for testicular leukaemic involvement. At the normal age of puberty, high luteinizing hormone (LH) and low testosterone blood levels reflect this disorder.

Spermatogenesis is impaired by doses of 3–10 Gy given to the testes during childhood.

Aubier *et al.* (1989) have shown that 38% of boys previously treated for solid tumours who were post pubertal had either azoospermia or elevated follicle-stimulating hormone (FSH) or both after chemotherapy. All had normal puberty and most, normal LH levels. Among chemotherapy drugs, alkylating agents are associated with infertility, the risk of which is correlated with dose. Pubertal status at the time of chemotherapy does not influence the outcome. Adriamycin, vincristine, and actinomycin D are not toxic to spermatogenesis.

Prevention of male infertility related to chemotherapy is difficult and so far can only be obtained by limiting the use of alkylating agents, whenever possible. Semen preservation in adolescents and young adults is often tried, but with rather disappointing results.

In girls, ovarian function can also be altered by radiotherapy and chemotherapy. In children, a fractionated dose of 20 Gy seems to produce permanent ovarian failure consistently. When single fraction TBI is considered, the toxic dose is as low as 10 Gy.

The toxicity of chemotherapy is not well documented in girls, but is obviously much lower than in boys. However, ovarian failure has been reported after high doses of alkylating agents, and is usually gradual and incomplete. Cases of premature menopause are reported. Apparently, an older age at the time of chemotherapy is a poor prognostic factor for ovarian function.

The offspring of children treated for cancer

The risk of inherited cancer is well documented in the case of retinoblastoma (see Chapter 20). In the case of other tumours having affected one of the parents, the only clear data reported are negative (see Chapter 1).

The rate of congenital malformations is similar to that of the general population.

Today there is limited information on the offspring of patients treated with aggressive, multi-agent chemotherapy during the past 10–15 years. It seems to be appropriate to follow the opinion expressed by Mulvihill in 1992 with respect to genetic counselling. 'If there is a pregnancy, the existing data do not indicate a risk of congenital or genetic problems above the 4% risk of a baby with a major malformation that any pregnancy has' (Mulvihill and Byrne 1992).

Neuropsychological late effects

Will a person who experienced a cancer during childhood become a 'normal' adult? It is not easy to provide a straightforward answer to this question, since 'normality' is difficult to define and, also, 'cancer' covers a wide variety of diseases which have been treated in very different ways according to the cases and period. Furthermore, few objective, well defined, and comprehensive studies have been done on the subject, and as far as psychology is concerned, many studies are either simplistic or merely reflect wishful thinking on the part of the observer rather than every-day reality.

Neurological late effects of a given tumour (e.g. cord or thalamic tumours) are well known and may be anticipated at the time of diagnosis. But it is most often difficult to predict the progression of symptoms which depends on many factors, such as deterioration of nervous tissue, duration of symptoms before treatment, effectiveness of treatment, etc.

'Psychological' late effects must first be considered in young adults who are cured with no major physical disability. In this context, our general impression is that a large majority of patients, no matter how difficult the experience they have been through, have 'healed' and recovered apparently completely. They are normal adults, who are well adjusted to social and professional life. This includes patients with serious sequelae such as limb amputation, or even sterility. One major exception is long-term survivors who sustained considerable damage to the CNS caused by the disease or the treatment or both, for example in leukaemia or brain tumours. They often have 'neuropsychological' sequelae.

Radiotherapy, with or without the additional toxicity of drugs, mainly methotrexate, is the main cause of CNS lesions. The total dose given, fractionation, and young age are important factors to be considered. Massive necrosis of areas of the brain is avoided by limiting total doses. Leucoencephalopathy, of various degrees, is far more frequent in patients treated for leukaemia or brain tumours. It can sometimes appear on MRI as hypodense, periventricular images, with or without micro calcifications. These defects are considered due to the effects of radiation on the microvasculature. Clinical symptoms of therapy-induced brain damage are not constantly observed and may vary from one case to another according to many factors (seizures, neurological local symptoms, intellectual regression, etc.). The most frequent symptoms seen in cured patients are intellectual, psychological, and functional anomalies, which may worsen with time.

Many studies have been conducted on cured leukaemic patients, and it is now widely admitted that prophylactic cranial irradiation produces dose-related intellectual damage. This can be a low IQ, difficulties in learning, and poor memory. The incidence of such disorders differs from one study to another, but they are always present whatever the patient population.

Brain tumour sequelae are a more complex problem, since an increase in intracranial pressure and neurosurgery may have damaged the brain before the paediatric oncologist and radiotherapist intervene. In addition, the location of the tumour, the area irradiated, and the doses given vary considerably. An important factor in the risk of sequelae, common to leukaemia and brain tumours, is the young age at treatment. Radiotherapy is particularly harmful if administered before the end of the myelination process. Intellectual outcome of children who underwent surgery with additional whole-CNS irradiation was poorer than in those receiving irradiation only to the posterior fossa (Hoppe-Hirsch *et al.* 1995). Post-operative complications, mostly related to brain-stem lesions, were predictive of a poor intellectual outcome in both groups.

The IQ is a valuable but general test which does not adequately define the functional status of most long-term survivors of medulloblastoma. These young adults may have severely impaired physical, social, emotional, and intellectual lives. This is particularly marked in children treated before the age of five, but is less obvious in children treated as teenagers (Spunberg *et al.* 1981).

So far, 'rehabilitation' efforts have met little success in this population of patients, and no spontaneous improvement is ever seen. Attempts are made to postpone radiotherapy in children under the age of three to five, by using sequential chemotherapy and, in some cases, high-dose chemotherapy with ABMT.

Systematic studies with promising early results have been undertaken to analyse precisely the variety of cognitive defects that can occur in these children, and to try to attempt more selectively targeted rehabilitation (Moore *et al.* 1992).

Little has been achieved so far with chemotherapy in the field of brain tumours, but many efforts are being made in most institutions and cooperative groups to find drugs or combinations of drugs efficient enough to replace radiotherapy, without these serious side-effects.

Thoracic and pulmonary late effects

In Hodgkin's disease, bleomycin has been used on a large scale in children. This drug can induce pulmonary fibrosis when a cumulative dose of 200 mg/m^2 is exceeded. This effect is aggravated by radiotherapy, and adults as well as children have suffered from severe lung fibrosis following treatment with the ABVD protocol (containing bleomycin) given with mantle field radiotherapy which, in children, involves a significant lung volume. Other drugs are known to induce lung fibrosis: methotrexate (small doses repeated for years), BCNU, busulfan, and even cyclophosphamide.

Experience of the effect of thoracic irradiation involving both lungs has been acquired during treatment of lung metastases from Wilms' tumour (Benoist *et al.* 1982). The effect of radiation is enhanced by actinomycin D given at the time of irradiation and/or after lung irradiation. Respiratory function studies, in most patients who have received 20 Gy to both lungs, show an abnormally low vital capacity and total pulmonary volume. These findings are more severe if the child is young at the time of irradiation, and they usually worsen as the child grows. Vital capacity values of 50–75% of the normal values based on the patient's height are commonly observed at the end of growth. In a limited number of cases (XRT boosts added, radiation acute pneumonitis, fibrosing drugs added) the patients become symptomatic and a small minority will die.

These severe and disabling sequelae may be avoided by restricting radiation doses to less than 15 Gy and omitting drugs which may compound the adverse effects of radiation such as actinomycin D. The SIOP Wilms' Tumour Study provides a protocol for lung metastases which combines chemotherapy with surgery and cures 75% of the cases, with radiation being used only in 20% of them (De Kraker *et al.* 1987). The number of drugs now available to treat Wilms' tumour is so great that it is practically always possible to avoid radiation pneumopathy and lung sequelae.

Heart and vessels

Cardiac sequelae of radiation have been documented in long-term survivors of Hodgkin's disease who had received up to 45 Gy to the heart (Gottdiener *et al.* 1983). Sudden deaths were observed and coronary disease, pericarditis, and chronic pancarditis with a variety of valvular alterations. Since lower doses of radiation have been used, the role of chemotherapy in cardiac complications in children has become more important.

Anthracycline-related cardiac toxicity was immediately recognized as soon as these drugs were used at high cumulative doses. Early toxicity was infrequent and it has long been considered that the benefits of anthracycline therapy largely outweigh its drawbacks.

In the early 1990s, however, impressive data were reported on delayed cardiac problems in long-term survivors. It is now clear that the risk increases with time after therapy and with the patient's growth. It has been shown that anthracyclines induce a loss of myocardial myocytes by necrosis followed by fibrosis. In children, after the age of 6 months, the total number of myocytes will not increase, and the only way the myocardium has to adapt to new needs is by hypertrophy of the existing normal fibers. Anthracycline therapy induces linear dose-related myocardial degeneration which is constant over the cumulative dose of 240 mg/m^2, and which reduces the capacity of the myocardium to adapt to new needs: the progressive increase in the after-load caused by puberty, rapid growth periods, pregnancy, and sport, etc.

Late appearing toxicity, 10–20 years after therapy, is now seen with increasing frequency, as cohorts of long-term survivors increase in number (Steinherz *et al.* 1993).

The major risk factors are cumulative dose of anthracyclines, young age at therapy, life style, and most importantly, the duration of observation. A further predictive factor is an abnormal ultrasound examination during or at the end of therapy.

Cardiac changes are hidden for years unless screening is undertaken in patients at risk, using ultrasound to measure shortening fraction, angioscintigraphy to measure left ventricle ejection fraction, and echo-Doppler to measure after-load (end-systolic wall stress).

Clinically, late cardiac toxicity is revealed by congestive heart failure (CHF), arrhythmia, and sudden death. Prevention and treatment of CHF is a difficult problem. Monitoring of patients at risk is by ultrasound. ECG is of little use. Prevention is of course best achieved by reducing the anthracycline doses and administering drugs in continuous (6 h, 24 h, 48 h) infusion instead of by bolus injection. Cardioprotectors are also being tested. In patients who have already received high doses, follow-up and monitoring should be systematic, and lifestyle counselling is warranted. When abnormalities appear on ultrasound, specific treatment is still controversial and should be discussed for each patient. Conversion enzyme inhibitors should probably be used, rather than cardiotonic drugs.

It must be stressed that in the major, long-term, follow-up studies which are ongoing (Donaldson *et al.* 1975) as many as 50% of the patients who have received a significant dose of anthracycline during childhood (mainly adriamycin) exhibit cardiac dysfunction to a certain degree after 15 years of follow-up. Some have already died or have received a heart transplant. These patients must be followed up indefinitely, so that we can learn more about this iatrogenic disease. It should also be remembered that very often adriamycin was probably the effective drug which cured the tumour.

Large and small vessels alike are particularly exposed to radiation injury. Proliferation of the endothelium of vessel walls gradually leads to complete vessel obstruction. These lesions in small vessels probably account for many very late sequelae due to radiotherapy. Large vessels can also be affected by this slow process, which can be very severe when it affects brain, abdominal, or renal vessels. In very young children, normal growth of vessels can also be stunted, as is the case in other organs.

Gastrointestinal tract, liver

Chemotherapy alone has never been shown to be responsible for long-term sequelae in the gastrointestinal tract in children.

Sequelae arising from abdominal irradiation are most often due to whole-abdominal irradiation. Treatment, whose side-effects may be potentiated by concurrent or subsequent chemotherapy, first produces acute radiation enteritis. Weeks or months later, intestinal obstruction or repeated subacute obstruction may occur, which may complicate treatment, especially if surgery is to be considered. In the long run, 10–20 years or more later, these young adults may continue to have frequent chronic, subacute, or even acute problems, such as obstruction or intestinal perforation due to mesenteric vessel thrombosis. The patients may be intolerant of fat, milk, gluten, and fibre-containing food. Usually they do not grow or gain weight normally (Donaldson *et al.* 1975).

These sequelae are prevented by limiting abdominal radiation doses to 20 Gy, especially in very young children, and sensitizing agents such as actinomycin D should not be added. A gluten-free diet, without milk, fat, or fibre, is routinely advised during abdominal irradiation and the following weeks, as there is a clinical impression that this is beneficial.

Chemotherapy-induced, veno-occlusive disease of the liver is well known, especially after high-dose chemotherapy with ABMT, even without total-body irradiation. It is an acute, sometimes severe, or even lethal condition. It does not seem to be followed by chronic dysfunction of the liver in long-term survivors. So called 'radiation hepatitis' is a variant of the above-described condition, and is most often related to combined treatment. Apart from permanent atrophy of an irradiated part of the liver, which is compensated by hypertrophy, resulting occasionally in a bizarre shaped liver, we are not aware of significant late effects in the liver.

Urinary tract

Kidneys are severely affected by doses of radiation exceeding 15–20 Gy, which should never be given to both kidneys. Late renal failure and/or hypertension can occur if this recommendation is not respected.

Some drugs such as platinum compounds and iphosphamide may cause early or late nephrotoxicity. Very long-term effects of these drugs in children are poorly documented, but persistent renal failure has been reported, and cases of permanent post-iphosphamide therapy Fanconi syndrome are known to occur. Limiting doses, good hydration, bladder protection with mesna in the case of iphosphamide and high-dose cyclophosphamide will limit long-term effects of alkylating drugs.

Second malignant tumours in children

Second malignant tumours (SMN) or second primaries are, by definition, different from metastases or recurrences of the primary. In a given child, they are histologically different from the first primary, and occur after it. There are also a few cases in which two different tumours are diagnosed at the same time in the same child.

These SMN are closely related to the treatment of the primary which, (a) having become more effective has allowed more patients to live long enough to present with SMN, and (b) plays a role in the aetiology of most SMN.

Incidence

Taking into account different studies, the cumulative risk of developing SMN among survivors varies from 3.7–12% 25 years after treatment of a first cancer in childhood. The two, main, multicentre, international studies which are considered here are the LESG (Late Effects Study Group) study of a cohort of patients from 10 centres in the USA and 3 in Europe (Meadows *et al.* 1985) and a European one involving 8 centres and including 4568 children (De Vathaire *et al.* 1989) with a follow-up ranging from 2–46 years, (mean 13 years). Among these patients, 144 developed at least one SMN.

The risk of SMN can be formulated as a 'relative risk' (RR), which is the ratio of observed cancers in a group of patients to the number expected in a comparable group of the general population. In the European study, RR is 12 at 25 years. It is similar for the first 2 decades (13 and 15, respectively), but decreases to eight in the third decade, and to three over 30 years after the diagnosis of the primary.

Types of second cancers and relationship with the treatment of the first tumour

In the European study, among the 144 SMN, sarcomas are the most frequent (61 cases), followed by carcinomas (37 cases) involving mainly the breast and thyroid (14 of each). Then come skin tumours (19 cases), brain tumours (15 cases), leukaemias (14 cases), and miscellaneous (11).

Sarcomas are mainly osteosarcomas (31/61), chondrosarcomas (11/61), and soft-tissue sarcomas (19/61). The mean time to occurrence is 11 years, but can be as long as 46 years. The mean age at which sarcomas occur is 17 years. The overall incidence at 25 years is 2.8%. Secondary sarcomas usually occur within a radiation field, and are dependent on the total dose of radiation received previously. In retinoblastoma, however, secondary osteosarcoma may develop in a non-irradiated area, and this is explained by the role played by a genetic predisposition, common to retinoblastoma and osteosarcoma. Chemotherapy with alkylating agents increases the risk of secondary sarcoma.

Benign adenomas are much more frequent than carcinomas in previously irradiated children (3/4 cases with a nodule in the thyroid). Thyroid tumours are differentiated carcinomas. The median interval is 16 years. Even very small doses of radiation can be responsible for second thyroid tumours, which all occur in previously irradiated areas. Chemotherapy does not seem to play a significant role. A young age and neuroblastoma as a first tumour are significant risk factors. The RR is related to the dose of radiation to the thyroid, which is 7-fold higher after 20 Gy and 20-fold after 40 Gy. The probability of developing such SMN was 4.4% at 26 years in the LESG study.

Breast cancers developed in 14 of the 2000 girls in the European study, at a median age of 27 years, 3–33 years after the primary. The relative risk is 16 compared to the general population. With the small numbers and comparatively short follow-up, a relationship was found with previous chemotherapy, but not with radiotherapy in this study. This relationship has also been shown in other studies.

An excess of leukaemias, mainly AML, has been observed in survivors of childhood cancers, as well as in patients treated as adults for Hodgkin's disease and other tumours.

The mean latency of AML is 3.5 years (2–12), which is much shorter than that of secondary solid tumours. Chemotherapy, especially with alkylating agents, is associated with a significant risk of leukaemia, with a strong dose/effect relationship. Radiation therapy does not increase the relative risk, which reaches 24 in the group which has received the highest dose of an alkylating agent. The epipodophyllotoxins, etoposide and teniposide, have more recently been identified as risk factors for secondary leukaemias. These are usually monoblastic or myelomonoblastic, with a specific mutation on chromosome 11, at the 11q23 locus. Cumulative doses and the drug administration schedule seem to play a role in the occurrence of these leukaemias.

The type of first cancer

As expected, the risk of a second cancer and its type vary with the type of initial primary. In the European study, the lowest risk is after Wilms' tumour (RR:1) and the greatest after Ewing's sarcoma (RR:4.7); it is 3 in soft-tissue sarcomas, and 2.9 in Hodgkin's disease.

Predisposing conditions

We have already seen that in the case of retinoblastoma, the inherited forms lead to a high risk of a second osteosarcoma, within or outside the radiation field. In certain studies the RR is as high as 100 to nearly 1000. Other, genetically determined conditions predispose to multiple cancers. Among these are neurofibromatosis and naevoid basal cell carcinoma syndrome. In the Li Fraumeni syndrome, familial clustering of cancers is associated with multiple cancers in the individuals. A mutation of the *p53* gene is found in about 50% of these families and is likely to determine the predisposition to developing a single, as well as multiple, cancer in individuals belonging to affected families. Genetic predisposition and therapies received for a first cancer are two interrelated risk factors in these families.

What is a 'cured patient'? Long-term survival figures

Here we shall only consider patients with solid tumours and try to reply, at least in a very general way, to a question which is often asked: 'is it really possible to "cure" children with cancer?' Is it possible to assert that their life expectancy will become similar to that of the general population? Obviously, the following deals with a quantitative appraisal of survival, and not with the quality of life, which is a different problem.

We have reviewed the survival data of a cohort of 1733 patients aged below 16 at diagnosis, who were treated for a solid tumour in our institution (IGR) between 1942 and 1979, and had survived at least 5 years after diagnosis. In 1992, at the time of analysis, there was a median follow-up of 19 years (range 5–47), and a median age of 25 years (range 5–54) among survivors. There were 1562 survivors and 171 patients had died before August 1992.

The cause of death could be identified in 153 cases. It was recurrent primary tumour in 67 cases and SMN in 42. Medical conditions which could be related to treatment of the tumour were found in 33 cases. One patient committed suicide and 10 died in accidents.

From this material, the following statements can be made.

1. It is difficult to compare this population, which was treated as long ago as 50 years, with the population of cases we treat today. It represents a selection of patients who survived despite little or no chemotherapy and despite very aggressive radiotherapy in some cases. Many cases probably had only surgery and therefore can be considered as displaying the 'natural history' of these minimally-treated patients. Bearing in mind these reservations, we can embark on further statements.

2. 90% of the patients have survived 5–50 years. 10% have died after the first 5 years following treatment: when?, why?, who?
During the first 20 years, recurrences and therapy-related complications were the main causes of death. After 20 years, SMN were the main reason for death.
Those who survive in the greatest proportion are statistically well defined: they are the Wilms' and the neuroblastoma cases; the patients treated surgically; those who received treatments before 1960. These categories represent, at least partly, a selection of good cases, which were spared aggressive therapy.

3. The whole cohort has an excess mortality compared to the general population. But this excess varied with time and the type of tumour diagnosed. CNS and soft-tissue tumours still account for this excess 30 years after diagnosis. For all other tumours, this excess mortality falls to zero 22–30 years after diagnosis. This means that at least 70% of all the survivors of a solid tumour of childhood at 5 years recover a life-span which is similar to that of the general population after a maximum of only 30 years from diagnosis.

These data will probably evolve with time and it is difficult to predict in what way. They are, nonetheless, solid and allow us to affirm that it is indeed possible to 'cure' a patient with a solid tumour.

Informing families and patients, follow-up policies—looking forward to a long life

Today the vast majority of children with the diagnosis of cancer or leukaemia will survive and be cured. Cancer is no longer a death sentence: this is the first message that should be conveyed to the families of our patients.

1. Your child has a cancer...
    ... 'but there is a given probability for him/her being cured, at a given cost of treatment burden, complications, and sequelae. Please sign your name here.'

This is called 'informed consent', and is a caricature of the relationship between human beings which has more to do with courts, lawyers, and insurance fees than with medical practice. It is to be anticipated, and hoped, that it will not survive this century and will soon become a relic of the past only to be found in some dusty museum attesting to the 'hypocrisy in the olden days'.

It is easy, but not very helpful on the day of the diagnosis, to throw at parents a comprehensive list of all incidents, disasters, and disabilities which may threaten their baby. It is far more relevant, and also more difficult, to tell them repeatedly and gradually where you are trying to go in this given case. Life should be the first subject addressed, for this is the only point parents are interested in at this stage. Then, as time passes and hope is restored, a future can be considered, and good opportunities will arise for giving further details about what you know of this future. There is no set uniform policy to be followed, and occasionally parents will not allow you to put your hands on their child before they know 'everything' regarding the present and the future.

In all cases, however (and preferably as soon as possible), the appropriate time will come when the family is ready to receive all the available information and to hear your plans for the future, in terms of care and follow-up, and what you believe will happen to the child.

2. Your child is probably cured, but...
    ... 'we have to follow him/her up because of possible recurrences and late complications of treament.'

Then deal with the modalities of the follow-up suggested, which will depend on the case and on the institution's policy. Often you know the type of problems to expect: a Wilms' tumour cured by surgery and gentle chemotherapy is a case for which simple cure can be predicted; a medulloblastoma which required neurosurgery, intensive care, radiotherapy, and chemotherapy may entrain a whole series of problems, endocrine and growth problems, adjustment in school, social integration, etc. Another patient will have had aggressive, multimodality treatment with comparatively high doses of radiotherapy despite his young age, new drugs ... and his young mother has a breast carcinoma. Anything may happen to this child and his siblings, and even his grandparents: a multipurpose, close follow-up of the whole family, including a complete genetic check-up, is warranted. In the three cases, especially the third, a potential second primary will be discreetly borne in mind (Meadows and Fenton 1994). Apart from different problems which require vigilance in different cases, the ongoing research programmes in your institution or co-operative group will lead you to systematic screening, or organ-oriented investigations, to be performed at given intervals.

In all cases, good judgement is needed to decide between random, non-oriented investigations which are often pointless and may impair the quality of life of the former patient and his family, and on the other hand a follow-up programme based on experience and/or a specific aim.

A problem may arise when the 'child' is no longer a teenager and therefore no longer catered for in a paediatric clinic. It is very often observed that doctors who specialize in the treatment of adults know very little about cancers in children because they are so rare, and are puzzled when a young adult who had a cancer in childhood comes to them with a medical problem or a question.

Paediatric oncologists therefore, like all paediatricians, must establish links with their adult counterparts, and refer their patients to them. Ideally, combined clinics should be organized where patients are seen by both together. It sometimes happens that paediatric oncologists follow 'their' patients until the age of 40 or even longer. This has some drawbacks, but also major advantages for the oncologist who can, in this way, build up a unique experience of the very late effects of the treatments he/she administered 25 years earlier (Schwartz *et al.* 1994).

In all cases, the patient should be given a purposely designed, written summary of his paediatric oncology history, including an opinion on the specific points to be checked in the future, and the phone number of the paediatric oncology team which treated him. Finally, whatever the practical means, regular appointments or contact by mail, paediatric oncologists, or paediatric oncology institutions, should aim to keep in touch indefinitely with all the patients formerly entrusted to their care. In many cases this proves to be of mutual benefit (Schweisguth 1985).

References

Aubier, F., Flamant, F., Brauner, R., Caillaud, J.M., Chaussain, J.M., and Lemerle, J. (1989). Male gonadal function after chemotherapy for solid tumours in childhood. *Journal of Clinical Oncology*, 7, 304–309.

Benoist, M.R., Lemerle, J., Jean, R., Rufin, P., Scheinmann, P., and Paupe, J. (1982). Effects on pulmonary function of whole lung irradiation for Wilms' tumour in children. *Thorax*, 37: 175–180.

Brauner, R., Czernichow, P., and Rappaport, R. (1984). Precocious puberty after hypothalamic and pituitary irradiation in young children. *New England Journal of Medicine*, 311, 920.

Brauner, R., Rappaport, R., and Prevot, C. (1989). A prospective study of the development of G.H. deficiency in children given cranial irradiation and its relation to statural growth. *Journal of Clinical Endocrinology and Metabolism*, 68, 346–351.

Constine, L.S., Donaldson, S.S., McDougall, R., Cox, R.S., Link, M.P., and Kaplan, H.S. (1984). Thyroid dysfunction after radiotherapy in children with Hodgkin's disease. *Cancer*, 53, 878–583.

D'Angio, G.J., Breslow, N., Beckwith, J.B., Evans, A., Baum, H., de Lorimier, A., *et al.* (1989). The treatment of Wilms' tumour. The results of the Third National Wilms' Tumour Study, *Cancer*, 64, 349–363.

De Kraker, J., Voute, P.A., and Lemerle, J., for the SIOP Nephroblastoma Committee (1987). SIOP nephroblastoma stage IV study. A more individualized approach. *Medical and Paediatric Oncology*, 15, 323.

De Vathaire, F., Francois, P., Hill, C., Schweisguth, O., Rodary, C., Sarrazin, D., *et al.* (1989). Role of radiotherapy and chemotherapy in the risk of second malignant neoplasms after cancer in childhood. *British Journal of Cancer*, 59, 792–796.

Donaldson, S.S., (1992). Effects of irradiation on skeletal growth and development. In Green, D.M., D' Angio, G.J., editors: *Late effects of treatment for childhood cancer*, New York Wiley-Liss, pp. 63–70.

Donaldson, S.S., Jundt, S., Ricour, C., and Sarrazin, D. (1975). Radiation enteritis in children. *Cancer*, 35, 1167–1178.

Gottdiener, J.S., Katin, M.J., Borer, J.S., Bacharach, S.L., and Green, M.V. (1983). Late cardiac effects of therapeutic mediastinal irradiation: assessment by echocardiography and radionuclide angiography. *New England Journal of Medicine*, 308, 569–572.

Hoppe-Hirsch, E., Brunet, L., Laroussinie, F., Cinalli, G., Pierre-Khan, A., Renier, D., *et al.* (1995). Intellectual outcome in children with malignant tumours of the posterior fossa: influence of the field of irradiation and quality of surgery. *Child's Nervous System*, 11, 340–346.

Mayfield, J.K., Riseborough, E.J., Jaffe, N., and Nehme, M.E. (1981). Spinal deformity in children treated for neuroblastoma: the effect of radiation and other forms of treatment. *Journal of Bone and Joint surgery* 63A: 183–193.

Meadows, A.T., Baum, E., Fossati-Bellani, F., Green, D., Jenkin, R.D., Marsden, B., *et al.* (1985). Second malignant neoplasms in children: an update from the Late Effects Study Group. *Journal of Clinical Oncology*, 3, 532–538.

Meadows, A.T. and Fenton, J.G. (1994). Follow-up care of patients at risk for the development of second malignant neoplasms. In Schwartz, C.L., Hobbie, W.L., Constine, L.S., Ruccione, K.S. editors: *Survivors of childhood cancer, assessment and management* St Louis Mosby, p. 319–328.

Moore, B.D., Copeland, D.R., Reid, R., and Levy, B. (1992). Neuropsychological basis of cognitive deficits in long term survivors of childhood cancer. *Archives of Neurology*, 49, 809–817.

Mulvihill, J.J. and Byrne, J. (1992). Genetic counselling for the cancer survivor: possible germ cell effects of cancer therapy. In Green, D.M., D'Angio, G.J. editors: *Late effects of treatment for childhood cancer*, New York Wiley-Liss, pp. 113–120.

Sanders, J.E., Buckner, C.D., Sullivan, K.M., Doney, K., Appelbaum, F., Witherspoon, R., *et al.* (1988). Growth and development in children after bone marrow transplantation. *Hormone Research*, 30: 92–97.

Schwartz, C.L., Hobbie, W.L., and Constine, L.S. (1994). The establishment of the follow-up clinic. In Schwartz, C.L., Hobbie, W.L., Constine, L.S., Ruccione, K.S. editors: *Survivors of childhood cancer, assessment and management* St Louis Mosby, pp. 367–389.

Schweisguth, O. (1985). L'avenir des enfants guéris d'un cancer: morbidité ultérieure. *Archives Françaises de Pédiatrie* 42: 119–121.

Spunberg, J.J., Chang, C.H., Goldman, M., Auricchio, E., and Bell., J. (1981). Quality of long-term survival following irradiation for intra-cranial tumours in children under the age of two. *International Journal of Radiation Oncology, Biology Physics*, 7, 727–736.

Steinherz, L.J., Steinherz, P.G., and Heller, G. (1993). Anthracycline-related cardiac damage. In Bricker, J.T., Green, D.M., and D' Angio, G.J. editors: *Cardiac toxicity after treatment for childhood cancer*. Wiley-Liss New York, pp. 63–72.

Tournade, M.F., Com-Nougue, C., Voute, P.A., Lemerle, J., de Kraker, J., Delemarre, J.F., *et al.* (1993). Results of the Sixth International Society of Pediatric Oncology Wilms' Tumour Trial and Study: a risk-adapted therapeutic approach in Wilms' Tumour. *Journal of Clinical Oncology*, 11, 1014–1023.

8 Acute leukaemias

G. Gustafsson and S.O. Lie

The childhood leukaemias have, in many ways, served as a model for both the understanding of and therapy of malignant disorders in children. Malignant transformation of bone marrow progenitor cells leads to the most common childhood cancer which was, 30 years ago, almost universally fatal. There may be no better example of the results of multi-institutional and multi-national clinical research than childhood leukaemia. Our understanding of the biological features of these diseases has also increased greatly in recent years, and the two main types (acute lymphoblastic leukaemia, ALL; and acute myeloid leukaemia, AML) are today further subdivided into groups with their own distinct biological and prognostic characteristics.

In this chapter we will focus on epidemiology, pathological features, and clinical management. Examples will be drawn from the experiences of the Nordic Society for Paediatric Hematology and Oncology (NOPHO) which has run population-based registries and follow-up of all childhood leukaemias since 1981. The reader is also referred to some recent comprehensive articles (Riehm *et al.* 1990; Rivera *et al.* 1993; Lie 1995, Pui 1995; Barnard *et al.* 1996, Chessels *et al.* 1995; Lie *et al.* 1996; Reiter *et al.* 1994; Veerman *et al.* 1996).

Epidemiology

Acute childhood leukaemias constitute 25–30% of all childhood malignancies. The incidence rate is 4–4.5 annual cases per 100 000 children below 15 years of age. ALL constitutes 83% and AML 17% of the cases in developed countries. There is a moderate racial variation with higher rates in White compared to Black children. The incidence trend has been stable in the Nordic countries for the last 20 years. The male/female ratio is 1.15 in ALL and close to 1.0 in AML. The specific age peak at 2–5 years is typical for White children with ALL. This peak is mainly due to an excess of pre-B ALL cases in this age range. This peak is absent among Black people in developing countries, but is appearing among Black people in developed countries. There has been speculation that the peak is a result of some unknown environmental factors in industrialized countries.

The aetiology remains unknown in the vast majority of cases. However, children with some constitutional genetic defects (e.g. trisomy-21, Bloom's syndrome, Fanconi's anemia, and Ataxia telangiectasia) have an increased risk of leukaemia. There is also an increased concordance rate for leukaemia in monozygous twins diagnosed early.

Studies on environmental factors have focused both on exposures *in utero* and postnatally. The Children's Cancer Group (CCG) has run a case-control study of 204 patients and shown that paternal or maternal exposure to pesticides and petroleum products increases the risk of leukaemia in their offspring. A significant risk was associated with maternal use of marihuana (Neglia and Robison 1988).

High doses of radiation are leukaemogenic in adults, as documented after the atomic bomb explosions in Hiroshima and Nagasaki. *In utero* exposure to high-dose radiation has not lead to a significant increase in leukaemia incidence. The low-dose radiation after fall-out from atmospheric nuclear testing and from nuclear power plant accidents (e.g. Chernobyl) has so far not significantly increased the incidence of childhood leukaemias, but a lively debate continues.

Diagnostic X-ray examination of the abdomen used during the first trimester in pregnancy gave a five-fold increase in ALL during the 1940s, when this method was used routinely. Today, this examination is very rare and few cases can be explained by this factor.

Controversy persists about the risk of exposure to electromagnetic fields (EMF). Some studies have found no increase, but recent studies suggest a two-fold, non-significant increase of ALL among children living in proximity to high-voltage power lines (Savitz 1993). The number of exposed children is low so, even if there is a real risk, this factor accounts for a very small proportion of childhood ALL cases (see Chapter 1).

The most interesting hypothesis today concerning the aetiology of childhood leukaemia is a role for viral and/or bacterial infections as proposed by Greaves (Greaves and Alexander 1993). He suggests a two-step mutation in the immune system, the first during pregnancy or early infancy and the second during the first years of life as a consequence of an abnormal response to a common infection.

In recent years, particular attention has been paid to the development of secondary AML after aggressive chemotherapy. The risk of AML after Hodgkin's disease is well documented and is caused by alkylating agents. The leukaemic clone often shows chromosomal abnormalities involving numbers 5 and 7 and has a FAB-type M1/M2. A most disturbing relationship has recently been found between the use of epipodophyllotoxins and secondary AML. It is estimated that children with ALL treated with high doses of epipodophyllotoxins (VP-16 and/or VM-26) have a cumulative risk of 5–12% of developing a secondary AML (Winick *et al.* 1993; Smith *et al.* 1994). This AML is different from that seen after treatment with alkylating agents in that there is a shorter latency period and the majority of cases involve changes in chromosome 11q23 and are of FAB-type M4/M5. Myelodysplasia and secondary AML are also increasingly seen in patients receiving myeloablative therapy with autologous stem-cell transplantation. Actuarial risks as high as $18 \pm 9\%$ have recently been reported (Rohatiner 1994). Certainly, if these bone marrow 'lethal' therapies are going to increase in number, this is a problem of increasing concern.

Biology

In order to understand the pathogenesis of the acute leukaemias it is necessary to understand the present concept of normal haemopoiesis. It is widely accepted that all haemopoietic cells, including lymphocytes, orginate from a common multipotent stem cell and that the haemopoietic system can be divided into several compartments in a hierarchy of development. The mature cells seen in peripheral blood such as erythrocytes, polymorphonuclear granulocytes, monocytes, and platelets arise from bone marrow progenitors that are committed to differentiation along a single lineage. (Figs 1(a) and 1(b)).

It is clear that the majority of leukaemias are of monoclonal (unicellular) origin, representing cells with a mutational event at some stage in their early development. The malignant cell retains the capacity for self renewal, but not for maturation. Our classification of the leukaemias depends on where in normal haemopoietic development the mutation has taken place, and using immunologic, enzymatic, and molecular probes, it is possible to establish the cell lineage in most cases.

Blast cells are easy to recognize and very often the main distinction between lymphoid and myeloid blasts can be made by light microscopy. The French/American/British (FAB) classification from the mid 1970s has been applied to ALL with three subtypes (L1, L2, and L3) defined according to morphologic features. L3 is now defined as B-cell leukaemia and is clearly a separate entity. The distinction between L1 and L2 has not proved useful.

The modified (FAB) classifications from 1985 distinguished 7 distinct subgroups (M1–M7) based on conventional morphology, cytochemical, and immunological methods (Bennett *et al.* 1985). Recently M0 has been defined by the same working group as a very undifferentiated leukaemia. The characteristic features of each FAB group are given in Table 8.1.

Immunophenotype

As mentioned above, leukaemic cells are the result of a mutational event in early haemopoietic development. Immunophenotypic classification has been most helpful in classifying the

Table 8.1 FAB classification and childhood AML

FAB class	Histochemistry*	Cell-surface markers	Associated cytogenetic findings
AML M0	MP– NSE–	CD33+, CD13+, CD14+, HLA DR–	
AML M1	MP+	CD33+, CD13+, CD11+, HLA DR+	+8, –5, –7
AML M2	MP+	CD33+, CD13+, CD11+	t(8;21)
AML M3	MP+	CD33+, CD13+, CD11+	t(15;17)
AML M 4	MP+ NSE+	CD33+, CD13+, CD11+, HLA DR+	inv 16
AML M5	NSE+	CD33+, CD13+, CD11+, HLA DR+	t(1;11) t(9:11)
AML M6	PAS+ MP+	Glycophorine+ spectrin+, HLA DR+	
AML M7	PPO+	Clycoprotein IIb/IIIa (CD 41) or IIIa (CD 61)+	inv 3 or t(3;3), t(1;23)

Abbreviations:
* MP, myeloperoxidase; NSE, non-specific esterase; PPO, platelet peroxidase.

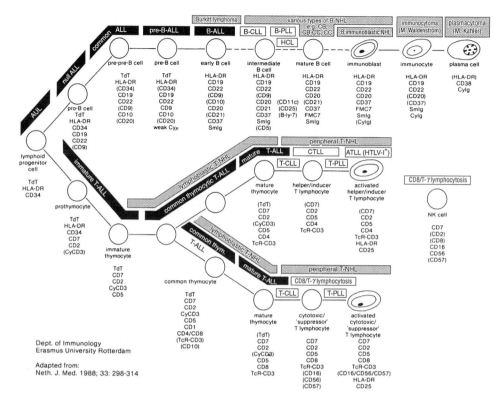

Fig. 8.1(a) Scheme of normal differentiation pathway during haematopoeisis. Hypothetical scheme of lymphoid differentiation.

leukaemias according to normally recognized maturation sequences. Usually a panel of lineage-associated antibodies must be used. Most groups now classify ALL into a B-cell precursor, a B cell, or a T-cell leukaemia. B-cell precursor includes CD19, CD20, CD22, and CD79. Mature B cells are characterized by immunoglobulins on their surface, while the T cells carry the immunophenotypes CD3, CD7, CD5, or CD2. The specific myeloid markers include CD13, CD14, and CD33. The presence of B-cell markers and/or T-cell markers can occasionally be detected in low concentration on myeloid leukaemic cells, but should not be present in large numbers. If the leukaemic cells express both myeloid and lymphoid antigens at the same time, the leukaemia is considered to be biphenotypic. In rare instances, different malignant cells express independently myeloid and lymphoid markers and the leukaemia is then considered to be bilineal. The origin of these hybrid leukaemias is unclear. The possible impact of the presence or absence of specific markers on prognosis is still unclear.

Genetic features

Clonal chromosomal abnormalities can now be identified in the majority of cases of acute childhood leukaemias (Sawyers 1997). It has turned out that such a karyotype carries both diagnostic and prognostic information.

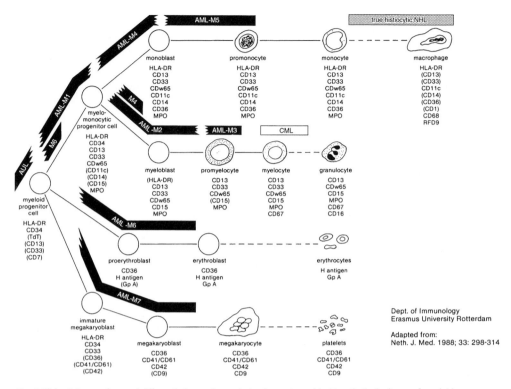

Fig. 8.1(b) Scheme of normal differentiation pathway during haematopoeisis. Hypothetical scheme of myeloid differentiation.

In ALL, the number of chromosomes (or DNA content) per leukaemic cell has been recognized as an important prognostic parameter (Trueworthy *et al.* 1992). In hyperdiploid disease (> 50 chromosomes per cell), the prognosis is very favourable in contrast to the dramatically poor prognosis in patients with hypodiploid disease (< 45 chromosomes per cell).

Specific chromosomal translocations in ALL include the classical t(8;14) in B cell ALL that brings c-*myc* on chromosome 8 under the control of the immunoglobulin regulatory sequences on chromosome 14. The *BCR-ABL* gene in CML and ALL results from the classic t(9;22) translocation that forms the Philadelphia chromosome. This translocation, with an extremely unfavourable prognosis, is identified in 5% of ALL cases in children compared to 25% in adults. Other important translocations in ALL are the t(1;19) and t(12;21).

Progress in cytogenetics has confirmed the value of the FAB classification of AML in that specific chromosomal translocations can be assigned to each group (Table 8.1). Translocation between chromosome 8 and 21 [t(8;21)] is almost exclusively found in M1 and M2. All cases of M3 should carry the translocation t(15;17) and M5 is associated with t(9;11). Finally, abnormalities of chromosome 16 are predominantly seen in M4 and are often associated with increased eosinophils in the marrow.

In infants, chromosomal changes involving 11q23 are very common (Chen *et al.* 1993). Many different chromosomes can participate in translocations involving this locus (Gu *et al.* 1992). The gene on chromosome 11 which is involved (called *MLL*, *HRX*, or *ALL-1*) has recently been characterized and it turns out to be closely related to a homeobox gene in *Drosophila* which, when mutated, gives rise to bizarre morphological malformations of the thorax and abdomen in these organisms.

Other gene products of the specific translocations have recently been identified (Cline 1994). In the translocation seen in the promyelocytic leukaemias (FAB M3) (t(15;17), the break point on chromosome 17 is in a gene encoding for the retinoic acid nuclear receptor alpha (RAR-α) and on chromosome 15 in a gene initially called *myl* and later renamed *PML* (Warrell *et al.* 1993). It is one of the most exciting developments in the biology of leukaemias that this leukaemia is responding to all-trans retinoic acid.

The gene product of the t(8;21) (q22;q22) translocation has also been detected recently. The chromosomal breakpoint on chromosome 21 involves a gene called *AML-1* and the probable candidate on chromosome 8 is a gene called *EOT*. As usual, this translocation results in the production of a chimeric gene and a message that eventually may lead to a malignancy. The tumour-suppressor gene *WT1* which is implicated in the development of some cases of Wilms' tumour has recently been shown to be detectable in all of 45 patients with AML examined (Inoue *et al.* 1994), and it seems that high expression is associated with a poor prognosis. The role of the tumour-suppressor gene *p53* has recently been reviewed (Imamura *et al.* 1994).

Risk factors

Thirty years ago, almost every child with leukaemia died of their disease, and consequently all had very high risk disease. However, after chemotherapy was introduced, and well before advances in cell biology and molecular genetics could define subsets of leukaemia, it was clear from clinical experience that childhood ALL could be divided into many prognostically distinct subtypes. The concept of risk-adapted therapy was therefore introduced in the late 1970s (Riehm *et al.* 1990). In the past, different study groups defined different risk groups, but there is now almost universal agreement on the following prognostic factors in ALL.

1. The most important prognostic factor is the treatment itself. It has been the fundamental goal of all randomized trials to identify the most effective therapy for the individual child by identifying subgroups with different prognosis.

2. The single most important prognostic factor gained from investigation is the white blood cell count (WBC) value at diagnosis. This is confirmed in almost all studies and is the basic factor for choosing treatment strategy in most ALL protocols. Tumour burden as defined by the BFM (Berlin, Frankfürt, Münster) group (WBC, enlargement of liver and spleen) is translated into a risk factor which has been used by many groups.

3. The age of the patient at diagnosis is important. Infants do poorly in all series, especially children < 6 months of age at diagnosis. Infant leukaemia is often associated with 11q23 rearrangements such as t(4;11) or t(11;19) and high white blood cell counts. The risk-adapted treatment for children > 10 years of age has now improved the prognosis for these children so that the cure rate is as good as for younger children.

4. The immunophenotype of the lymphoblasts at diagnosis has prognostic value. B-cell leukaemia (L3 in the FAB classification), with kappa and lambda antibodies on the surface of the

blasts, previously had a bad prognosis. With modern, specific, B-cell directed protocols, the prognosis has improved considerably.

T-cell leukaemia has also been associated with a poor prognosis and has consequently been treated as high-risk disease. Recent results with intensive therapy have shown that T-cell leukaemia with no other bad prognostic factors has a prognosis comparable to the pre-B-cell leukaemias. On the other hand, T-cell ALL with additional poor prognostic factors has a poor prognosis in spite of intensive therapy. It is an area of controversy if T-cell phenotype is a high risk factor per se, but most of these children are still treated with high-risk protocols. The prognostic significance of mixed lineage ALL, defined as the presence of CD13 and/or CD33 in addition to pre-B- or T-cell markers, is still a matter of dispute.

5. The prognostic value of gender is divergent in different studies and populations. Some studies report no difference in prognosis between boys and girls (Pui 1995) but other groups, especially from the UK (Chessels et al. 1995) and NOPHO (Lanning et al. 1992), have found a consistently higher relapse rate among boys. Why gender matters is unknown, but one suggestion is different tolerance to maintenance therapy due to sex differences in the metabolism of mercaptopurine and methotrexate (Hale and Lilleyman 1991).

6. Response to therapy as measured by the number of peripheral blasts after 1 week of prednisolone treatment (BFM model) or by remaining blasts in the bone marrow at day seven or 14 (Steinhertz et al. 1996) has identified 5–10% of children with a poor prognosis. It is still controversial whether more aggressive treatment can improve the prognosis for these children.

7. Chromosomal numbers or abnormalities have some prognostic significance in ALL. Hyperdiploidy (> 50 chromosomes) is found in 25% of cases and confers a good prognosis. The hypodiploid ALLs (3–5%), have a significantly worse prognosis compared to other groups. Specific translocations may be associated with an intermediate prognosis such as t(1;19). Translocation t(9;22) (in 5% of children) or t(4;11) (mostly seen in infants) identifies children with a bad prognosis.

In the present NOPHO stratification, these insights into the biology of ALL have led to three major risk groups based on factors such as WBC at diagnosis, age, immunophenotype, and chromosomal findings (Table 8.2).

In AML, risk factors have been much more difficult to identify due to the lack of effective therapy for more than 50% of children. However, with recent, more effective protocols, certain subgroups can be distinguished.

1. Age at diagnosis does not seem to be as important as in ALL. In the Nordic experience, infants actually tend to do better than older children.

2. High WBC is a risk factor in many, but not all, studies.

3. Children with FAB M3 (promyelocytic leukaemia) respond to retinoic acid and should be treated with a combination of this vitamin and chemotherapy.

4. Children with Down syndrome constitute more than 10% of all cases. Most of them have a FAB M7 and respond very favourably to adequate chemotherapy.

5. Chromosomal translocations are of increasing importance. Better prognosis is associated with t(8;21), t(15;17), and inversion 16. Ploidy has not been identified as an important prognostic factor.

6. Early response to therapy is emerging as a positive factor in AML as well.

Table 8.2 Risk groups in ALL

Standard risk (30% of total)	
WBC	$< 10 \times 10^9/l$
Age	$> 2 < 10$ years
No high-risk criteria	

High risk (35% of total)	
WBC	$> 50 \times 10^9/l$
and/or T-cell leukaemia	
Disease in CNS or testis at diagnosis	
Mediastinal tumour	
Slow responder	
Chromosomal translocation (9;22) (4;11) (22q-)	

Intermediate risk (35% of total)
All others

(Source: NOPHO protocols from 1992.) Infants and B-cell leukaemia excluded.
In other groups, standard risk = WBC $< 50 \times 10^9/l$.

Clinical management

The diagnosis of acute leukaemia in children in developed countries is usually straight forward. Lack of normal mature blood cells may result in anaemia, bleeding, and infection. More than 50% have hepatosplenomegaly, and/or lymphadenopathy. The incidence of central nervous system involvement at diagnosis in Nordic children is 3% in ALL and 4% in AML. Usually the CNS involvement is clinically silent. Chloromas (also called granulocytic sarcoma) are localized collections of leukaemic cells seen almost exclusively in patients with AML. These may occur at any site, including CNS, bone, skin, and orbit.

In countries with limited resources, where anaemia with repeated infections and malnutrition are prevalent, the diagnosis may be more difficult. Diagnosis must be confirmed by bone marrow examination, and morphologic, immunophenotypic, and genetic characteristics of the malignant cell should be determined if at all possible.

It should be emphasized that leukaemia may present as an acute emergency with life threatening complications such as infections, haemorrhage, or organ dysfunction secondary to leukostasis.

Sometimes the diagnosis of AML is preceded by a prolonged preleukaemic phase lasting several weeks or months. Usually this is characterized by a lack of one of the normal blood cell lineages, resulting in either a refractory anaemia, a moderate degree of neutropaenia, or thrombocytopaenia. Bone marrow examinations fail to detect a leukaemia, but there are definite morphological changes. This condition is often referred to as a myelodysplastic syndrome (MDS) and these have their own FAB classification (Hasle 1994). Usually it is a requirement for this diagnosis that there is a hypercellular marrow, but in our experience this is not always the case. Some children may be seen with a hypoplastic marrow that later develops into an acute leukaemia.

Therapy of ALL

Since the introduction of 'total therapy' as first described by Pinkel (1971), the prognosis in ALL has improved from < 5% survival before 1965, to 25–50% during the 70s, and 70% for children diagnosed in the 80s. The main reason behind this improvement is a global increase in intensity of treatment.

Modern therapy can be divided into four main phases: induction therapy, CNS-directed therapy, late intensification (not in standard risk patients), and maintenance therapy. The induction therapy, lasting 4–6 weeks, is based on three or four different drugs (prednisolone or dexamethasone, vincristine, L-asparaginase, and/or anthracycline). In intermediate and high-risk patients, induction is intensified with additional cytostatics to improve the quality of the remission. More than 95% of children will achieve remission during this phase.

The CNS-directed treatment includes frequent intrathecal injections of methotrexate, often in combination with repeated infusions of high-dose methotrexate (3–5 gr/m^2). In high-risk patients more than 5 years of age, it may be more effective to give cranial irradiation (18–24 Gy) instead of using high-dose systemic chemotherapy.

Maintenance treatment is based on mercaptopurine daily and methotrexate once a week, given orally, with pulses of other cytostatics during the first year of treatment.

The duration of therapy in most studies is 2–2.5 years, and there seems to be no advantage with a treatment exceeding 3 years. Individual doses of cytostatics are guided by WBC and/or monitoring of drug concentrations during maintenance therapy.

With modern intensive therapy, remission will be achieved in 98% of patients, 2–3% of the children will die in CCR (continuous complete remission), and 25–30% will relapse.

Thus, the main cause of treatment failure is relapse of the disease. The site of relapse is predominantly in bone marrow (20% of children), while CNS relapses occur in 3–4%, and testicular relapse in 2% of children. Early bone marrow relapses (within 18 months of diagnosis) have the worst prognosis (10–20% long-term survival), while late relapses occurring after cessation of therapy have a better prognosis, especially testicular relapse where 50–60% long-term survival can be expected.

The treatment of relapse must be more aggressive than the first-line therapy with inclusion of new drugs to overcome the drug resistance that has developed. For early relapses, BMT may offer the best chance of cure, especially for children with T-cell leukaemia who, after relapse, have a very bad prognosis with conventional cytostatic treatment. The overall survival after relapse is 20–40% in different series.

As an example, the ALL results from the Nordic countries for three time periods are shown in Fig. 8.2. Event-free survival has increased from 53% (1981–85), through 68% (1986–91) to the present 81% (1992–95). The main reason behind these improvements is more intensive therapy for all risk groups. As an example, our current protocols for standard and intermediate risk patients are shown in Figs 8.3 and 8.4. The probability of event-free survival after relapse for children diagnosed between 1986 and 1991 is shown in Fig. 8.5.

Our results are comparable to many other population-based studies. Some of these are listed in Table 8.3. It is remarkable that with different protocols and differences in risk stratification, the overall results are nearly identical.

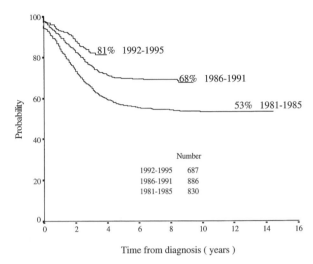

Fig. 8.2 Probability of event-free survival in Nordic children with non-B ALL in three different time periods.

Table 8.3 Results of some trials in childhood ALL

	Years of entry	**Number**	**Age (years)**	**p-EFS (%)**
ALL-BFM 86[1]	1986–90	998	< 18	72 + 2
NOPHO[2]	1986–91	886	< 15	68 + 2
DFCI[3]	1985–87	220	< 18	78 + 3
UKALL X[4]	1985–90	1612	< 15	62 + 2
				(71% with late intensification)
St. Jude[5]	1984–88	358	< 18	71 + 2
DCLSG[6]	12/1984–7/1988	291	< 15	72 + 3

[1] (Reiter *et al.* 1994)
[2] (Gustafsson *et al.* Unpublished thesis)
[3] (Schorin *et al.* 1994)
[4] (Chessels *et al.* Lancet 1995)
[5] (Rivera *et al.* 1993)
[6] Veerman *et al.* 1996)

Therapy of AML

Thirty years ago, almost every child with AML died and no risk groups could be identified. Today, survival figures of more than 40% are reported in many studies, including the Nordic population-based material (Lie 1995; Vormoor *et al.* 1996). The change came in the 1970s with the introduction of cytarabine (Ara-C) and anthracyclines. With different combinations of these

Standard risk criteria

☐ age over 2 and under 10
☐ white count < 10 at presentation
☐ no high risk factors

Management plan

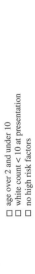

Week 0	Induction	Consolidation	Maintenance	2.5 yrs
	0	7	14	

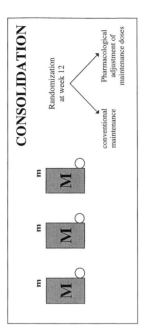

INDUCTION

Prednisolone

asparaginase
(Erwinia)

```
      A        A
      V    A   V    A
A     V    V   m    V
V     m                        (start
m                              consolidation)
week  0    1    2    3    4    5    6    7
```

Start **Prednisolone** 60 mg/m²/day

V = vincristine (Oncovin) 2 mg/m² (max.dose 2 mg) iv injection

A = adriamycin (Doxorubicin) 40 mg/m² iv infusion over 24 h

m = methotrexate intrathecally 2–3 years 10 mg, > 3 years 12 mg

CONSOLIDATION

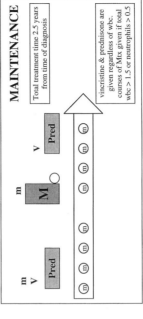

Randomization
at week 12

conventional
maintenance

Pharmacological
adjustment of
maintenance doses

 = methotrexate 5 g/m²/day infusion
and leucovorin rescue

m = methotrexate intrathecally 2–3 years 10 mg > 3 years 12 mg

MAINTENANCE

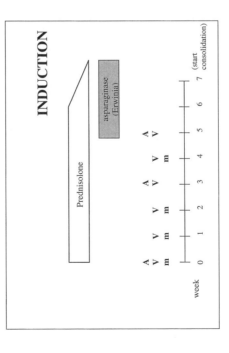

Total treatment time 2.5 years
from time of diagnosis

vincristine & prednisone are
given regardless of wbc.
courses of Mtx given if total
wbc > 1.5 or neutrophils > 0.5

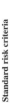 = ORAL MAINTENANCE

6 Mercaptopurine 75 mg/m²/day
Methotrexate 20 mg/m² once weekly

wbc should be maintained between 1.5–3.5 with dose ↑ if wbc > 3.5 and break in treatment if wbc
< 1.

transaminase > 10 x normal   half dose methotrexate first, then 6MP.

Fig. 8.3 Treatment protocol in non-B ALL (NOPHO-92) for children in standard-risk group.

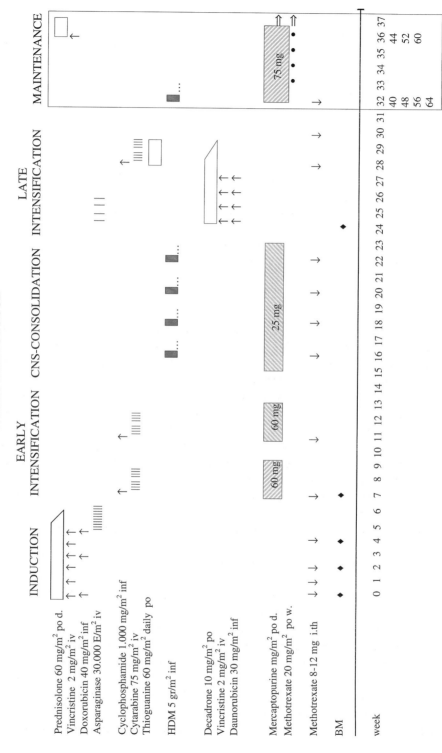

Fig. 8.4 Treatment protocol in non-B ALL (NOPHO-92) for children in intermediate-risk group.

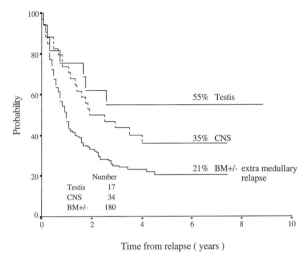

Fig. 8.5 Probability of event-free survival after relapse in Nordic children with non-B ALL diagnosed 1986–91 according to site of relapse.

drugs, remission could be induced in about 75–85% of the children. However, without further therapy most children relapsed within a year. The resistance of myeloblasts necessitated an intensity of therapy which certainly was at the limit of what a child could tolerate. Death in aplasia and even death in complete remission have been the price we have had to pay for the progress we have seen. For every child going into a modern AML protocol, the morbidity is very significant, and life-threatening complications have to be dealt with. Modern therapy of AML is therefore only justified in larger centres, as the children often need complex support and must be monitored at all times as an intensive care patient. Needless to say, the availability of psychosocial care and the need to handle the patient and the whole family in an environment of total care is a prerequisite, although this topic is outside the scope of this chapter.

The quality of remission has to be improved by intensive consolidation therapy. However, the intensity of remission may also influence the outcome regardless of the type of consolidation therapy used (Woods *et al.* 1996). Three methods of consolidation therapy have been extensively explored: intensive chemotherapy alone, autologous bone marrow transplantation, or allogeneic bone marrow transplantation from an HLA-identical donor. Direct comparison between these has been difficult because of selection pressures. For logistical reasons, it is often difficult to perform a BMT within the first 6 months of chemotherapy, and many high-risk patients have relapsed before this time. When 'intention-to-treat' analysis is used, the difference between transplantation arms and chemotherapy only becomes smaller. Today, it seems that autologous bone marrow transplantation does not seem to offer any advantage (Ravindranath *et al.* 1996; Woods *et al.* 1996), while allogeneic transplantation from an HLA-identical donor still seems to offer the best chance of cure. Clearly, with the emerging recognition of prognostic factors in AML as well, it is not difficult to foresee that within the near future, patients with high-risk factors (slow responders, unfavourable karyotype) will be elected for transplant when possible, while children with standard-risk disease will probably be treated with chemotherapy only. It is important to note that a matched transplant is an option for only about 20% of the children who enter complete remission. In the Nordic countries this option is even smaller due to the lower number of sibling donors.

Two types of AML deserve special comment:

Down's syndrome and acute myelogenous leukaemia

Down's syndrome (DS) is associated with a more than 10 times increased incidence of leukaemia. In our Nordic studies we were puzzled by the fact that a high proportion of the patients in our AML registry turned out to have DS (Slørdahl *et al.* 1993). Out of the first 236 children, 32 had DS (10 boys and 22 girls). Their age distribution was strikingly different from normal children, since 30 of the 32 were between 14 and 31 months of age at diagnosis. Nineteen had a myelodysplastic syndrome of 2–9 months duration prior to the development of leukaemia, and the majority of the leukaemias were classified as M7.

Acute promyelocytic leukaemia (M3)

M3 accounts for about 10–15% of children with AML. As described earlier, this disease is characterized by t(15;17) where the breakpoints are on the gene for the nuclear receptor for retinoic acid on chromosome 17 and the *PML* (promyelocytic leukaemia) locus on chromosome 15. The result of the fusion of these two genes results in the synthesis of a fusion transcript which generates a disease-specific fusion protein that in some way is involved in carcinogenesis (Warrell *et al.* 1993). In 1988, Chinese scientists reported that induction of complete remission could be achieved in M3 by the use of all-trans retinoic acid (ATRA) as a single agent (Huang *et al.* 1988). This was quickly verified by French and American groups. It is indeed almost unbelieveable that a vitamin alone can induce a complete remission in a disease like leukaemia. Of course, the involvement of the nuclear receptor for retinoic acid has something to do with the sensitivity of the leukaemia for this vitamin, although the molecular details are still unknown.

The great advantage of all-trans retinoic acid (ATRA) therapy is that the well known bleeding complications of M3 are avoided. What is very clear, however, is that the disease is not cured with this therapy alone, and that relapse is the rule unless the remission is consolidated with post-remission intensive chemotherapy. A randomized intergroup study in the USA is now exploring whether it is best to induce the remission with ATRA first and then consolidate with high-dose chemotherapy, or whether it is better to start with conventional induction chemotherapy.

It is important to note that ATRA toxicity in children is probably more severe than in adults. Most important is a distinctive respiratory distress/fluid overload disorder (the retinoic acid syndrome). Low-dose chemotherapy may reduce the complication, but more important is that it seems to be related to a subgroup expressing CD13 on the leukaemic cell surface.

Results of the Norpho studies

The results of three consecutive Nordic studies are shown in Fig. 8.6. NOPHO-88 was an intensification of NOPHO-84, with introduction of VP16 and mitoxanthrone (Lie *et al.* 1996). This very high-intensity protocol carried a high morbidity and did not lead to significant

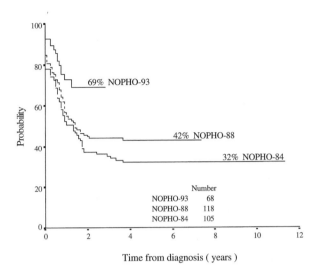

Fig. 8.6   Probability of event-free survival in Nordic children with AML in three consecutive protocols.

improvement. In our latest protocol (NOHPO-93), we have used the same blocks of therapy as in NOPHO-88, but give the first block only, and then wait until the bone marrow has repopulated. Seventy percent of children are then in remission and continue with the same therapy in a low-risk protocol, while the remaining 30% have identified themselves as having a high-risk disease and therefore need a more intensive therapeutic approach.

Some recently published studies are listed in Table 8.4. Different protocols obviously lead to rather similar results.

Future considerations

One hope for the future is that the therapy of the acute leukaemias in children should be more globally available to children. Probably not more than 20% of the children on this planet with leukaemia are offered a therapy that gives any chance of cure. Although cancer certainly does not belong to the top priorities in the list of childhood enemies, it is certainly a fact that the children are there. The modern, high-intensity protocols are expensive and carry a high risk of morbidity and even mortality. However, it is worth emphasizing that even less aggressive therapy in ALL may cure up to 50% of children. Such a protocol, which is based on modest induction and antimetabolite maintenance therapy, could be the place to begin with regard to children with cancer in countries with limited resources.

In the market economy countries, although the progress in treating ALL/AML has been dramatic, 20–25% of children with ALL and 30–40% of children with AML will still relapse, in spite of intensive therapy.

It is to be anticipated that more knowledge will allow a more precise categorization of the leukaemic disease based on chromosomal changes and molecular genetic techniques. The detection of minimal residual disease (MRD) with polymerase chain reaction is under intensive investigation in many groups at present (Steenbergen *et al.* 1995). The results so far are encouraging in

Table 8.4 Results of some trials in childhood AML

	CCG-251	CCG-213	POG-8498	CCG-2861	AIEOP	BFM-83	BFM-87	MRC-10	NOPHO-84	NOPHO-88
Years entered	1979–83	1986–89	1984–88	1986–89	1987–90	1982–86	1986–91	1988–93	1984–88	1988–92
Number evaluable	490	591	285	142	161	173	210	270	105	118
Death in aplasia	50	38	19	19	6 (+6)	12	11	25	8	14
Resistant disease	59	89	24	15	22	22	35		15	4
Complete remission number	381	439	242	108	127	139	164	245	82	100
(%)	78	77	85	76	79	80	78	91	78	85
DFS	40	39	45	40	31	61	52	56	43	56

(Source: Lie 1995.)

that children with slow response to therapy and persistence of leukaemic cells in small numbers may be identified as a group with a bad prognosis. However, it remains to be seen whether more intensive therapy for this group of children will improve their prognosis.

The development of an *in vitro* resistance assay may also identify resistant disease and lead to a more specific design of therapy in the individual child. Again, results are encouraging, but not yet in general use.

The possible role of bone marrow ablative therapy with stem cell support requires further study, but prospective, randomized, clinical trials have been exceedingly difficult to perform. It seems that bone marrow lethal therapy with autologous bone marrow or peripheral stem cell support has no convincing role in the therapy of acute leukaemias. Allogeneic transplant is still an option both in ALL, with resistant or relapsed disease, or in AML, where there is a donor. The problem today, however, is that the identification of children with high-risk disease does not necessarily translate into better therapy, since we simply do not have one.

Therapy-related death or complications are of great concern. In ALL, between 3 and 5% die from therapy-related complications, either during induction or remission. In AML, the number may reach 10%. Clearly, a substantial improvement can be reached if this complication rate can be reduced. Better supportive care and optimal use of growth factors may improve the problem, but it remains the fact that serious infections/complications are the rule rather than the exception during therapy of the acute leukaemias.

Long-term late effects are also of increasing concern, especially when it comes to the commonly used anthracyclines and the development of heart failure. Clearly, the risk of heart failure is very significant in children, especially in young girls, and must be continuously monitored. The proportion of children who need radiotherapy is now greatly reduced, and side-effects from this will consequently be of limited importance in the future. However, the use of prophylactic, cranial irradiation in the past has certainly both increased the risk of second malignant tumours and impaired the intellectual and cognitive development of the child.

The therapy of children with leukaemia today is a tough challenge for the child, the family, and the health service. There are very few signs to indicate that this burden is going to be smaller, but hopefully the results will continue to improve.

References

Barnard, D.R., Kalousek. D.K., Wiersma, S.R., Lange, B.J., Benjamin, D.R., Arthur, D.C., *et al.* (1996), Morphologic, immunologic, and cytogenetic classification of acute myeloid leukemia and myelodysplastic syndrome in childhood: a report from the Children's Cancer Group. *Leukemia*, 10, 5–12.

Bennett, J.M., Catovsky, D., Daniel, M.T., Flandrin, G., Galton, D.A., Gralnick, H.R., *et al.* (1985). Proposed revised criteria for the classification of acute myeloid leukaemia. *Annals of Internal Medicine*, 103, 620–9.

Chen, C.S., Sorensen, P.H., Domer, P.H., Reaman, G.H., Korsmeyer, S.J., Keerema, N.A., *et al.* (1993). Molecular rearrangements on chromosome 11q23 predominate in infant acute lymphoblastic leukemia and are associated with specific biologic variables and poor outcome. *Blood*, 81, 2386–93.

Chessels, J.M., Bailey, C., and Richards, S.M. for the Medical Research Council Working Party on Childhood Leukaemia. (1995). Intensification of treatment and survival in all children with lymphoblastic leukaemia: Results of UK Medical Research Council trial UKALL X. *Lancet*, 345, 143–8.

Cline, M.J. The molecular basis of leukaemia. (1994). *New England Journal of Medicine*, 330, 328–36.

Greaves, M.F., and Alexander, F.E. (1993). An infectious etiology for common acute lymphoblastic leukaemia in childhood? *Leukemia*, 7, 349–60.

Gu, T., Nakamura, T., Alder, H., Prasad, R., Canaani, O., Cimino, G., *et al.* (1992). The t(4;11) chromosome translocation of human acute leukaemias fuses the ALL-1 gene, related to drosophila trithorax, to the AF-4 gene. *Cell*, 71, 701–8.

Hale, J.P. and Lilleyman, J.S. (1991). Importance of 6-mercaptopurine dose in lymphoblastic leukaemia. *Archive of Disease in Children*, 66, 462–466.

Hasle, H. (1994). Myelodysplastic syndromes in childhood—classification, epidemiology and treatment. *Leukaemia and Lymphoma*, 13, 11–26.

Huang, M.E., Ye, Y.C., Chen, S.R., Chai, J.R., Lu, J.X., Zhoa, L., *et al.* (1988). Use of all trans retinoic acid in the treatment of acute promyelocytic leukemia. *Blood*, 72(2), 567–72.

Imamura, J., Miyoshi, I., and Koeffler, H.P. (1994). p53 in hematologic malignancies. *Blood*, 84, 2412–21.

Inoue, K., Sugiyama, H., Ogawa, H., Nakagawa, M., Yamagami, T., Miwa, H., *et al.* (1994). WT1 as a new prognostic factor and a new marker for the detection of minimal residual disease in acute leukaemia. *Blood*, 84, 3071–9.

Lanning, M., Garwicz, S., Hertz, H., Jonmundsson, G., Kreuger, A., Lie, S.O., *et al.* (1992). Superior treatment results in females with high risk acute lymphoblastic leukemia in childhood. *Acta Paediatric*, 81, 66–68.

Lie, S.O. (1995). Treatment of acute myeloid leukaemia in children. In *Bailliére's Clinical Paediatrics* (J.M. Chessels and I.M. Hann, eds.) 3, 757–78.

Lie, S.O., Jonmundsson, G., Mellander, L., Simes, M.A., Yssing, M., and Gustafsson, G. (1996). A population-based study of 272 children with acute myeloid leukaemia treated on two consecutive protocols with different intensity: Best outcome in girls, infants, and children with Down's syndrome. *British Journal of Haematology*, 94, 82–8.

Neglia, J.P. and Robison, L.L. (1988). Epidemiology of the childhood acute leukemias. *Pediatric Clinics of North America*, 35, 675–92.

Pinkel, D. (1971). Five-year follow-up of 'total therapy' of childhood leukemia. *JAMA*, 216, 648–52.

Pui, C.H. (1995). Childhood leukemia. *New England Journal of Medicine*, 332,(24), 1618–30.

Ravindranath, Y., Yeager, M., Chang, M.N., Steuber, C.P., Krischer, J., Graham-Pole, J., *et al.* (1996). Autologous bone marrow transplantation versus intensive consolidation chemotherapy for acute myeloid leukemia in childhood. *New England Journal of Medicine*, 334, 1428–34.

Reiter, A., Schrappe, M., Ludwig, W.D., Hiddeman, W., Sauter, S., Henze, G., *et al.* (1994). Chemotherapy in 998 unselected childhood acute lymphoblastic leukemia patients. Results and conclusions of the multicenter trial ALL-BFM 86. *Blood*, 84(9): 3122–33.

Riehm, H., Gadner, H., Henze, G., Kornhuber, B., Lampert, F., Niethammer, D., *et al.* (1990). Results and significance of six randomized trials in four consecutive ALL-BFM studies. *Haematol Blood Transfus*, 33, 439.

Rivera, G.K., Pinkel, D., Simone, J.V., Hancock, M.L., and Crist, W.M. (1993). Treatment of acute lymphoblastic leukemia. 30 years experience at St. Jude Children's Research Hospital. *New England Journal of Medicine*, 329 (18): 1289–95.

Rohatiner, A. (1994). Myelodysplasia and acute myelogenous leukaemia after myeloablative therapy with autologous stem-cell transplantation. *Journal of Clinical Oncology*, 12, 2521–3.

Savitz, D.A. (1993). Overview of epidemiologic research on electric and magnetic fields and cancer. *Am Ind Hyg Assoc J*, 54, 197–204.

Sawyers, C.L. (1997). Molecular genetics of acute leukaemias. *Lancet*, 349, 196–200.

Schorin, M.A., Blattner, S., Gelber, R.D., Tarbell, N.J., Donnelly, M., Dalton, V., *et al.* (1994). Treatment of childhood acute lymphoblastic leukemia: results of Dana-Farber Cancer Institute/Children's Hospital Acute Lymphoblastic Leukemia Consortium Protocol 85–01. *Journal of Clinical Oncology*, 12:740.

Slørdahl, S.H., Smeland, E.B., Holte, H., Gronn, M., Lie, S.O., and Seip, M. (1993). Leukemic blasts with markers of four cell lineages in Down's syndrome (megakaryoblastic leukemia), *Medical and Pediatric Oncology*, 21(4), 254–8.

Smith, M.A., Rubinstein, L., and Ungerleider, R.S. (1994). Therapy-related acute myeloid leukaemia following treatment with epipodophyllotoxins: Estimating the risks. *Medical and Pediatric Oncology*, 23, 86–98.

Steenbergen, E.J., Verhagen, O.J.M.H., van Leeuwen, E.F., van den Berg, H., Behrendt, H., Slater, R.M., *et al.* (1995). Prolonged persistence of PCR-detectable minimal residual disease after diagnosis or first relapse predicts poor outcome in childhood B-precursor acute lymphoblastic leukaemia. *Leukemia*, 9, 1726–1734

Steinhertz, P., Gaynon, P., Breneman, J., Cherlow, J.M., Grossman, N.J., Kersey., Johnstone, H.S., *et al.* (1996). Cytoreduction and prognosis in acute lymphoblastic leukemia–the importance of early marrow response. Report from the Children's Cancer Group. *Journal of Clinical Oncology*, 14(2), 389–398.

Trueworthy, R., Shuster, J., Look, T., Crist, W., Borowitz, M., Carroll, A., *et al.* (1992). Ploidy of lymphoblasts is the strongest predictor of treatment outcome in B-progenitor cell acute lymphoblastic leukemia of childhood: A Pediatric Oncology Group Study. *Journal of Clinical Oncology*, 10(4), 606–13.

Veerman, A.J.P., Hählen, K., Kamps, W.A., Van Leeuwen, E.F., De Vaan, G.A.M., Solbu, G., *et al.* (1996). High cure rate with a moderately intensive treatment regimen in non-high-risk childhood acute lymphoblastic leukemia: Results of protocol ALL VI from the Dutch Childhood Leukemia Study Group. *Journal of Clinical Oncology*, 14, (3), 911–8.

Vormoor, J., Boos, J., Stahnke, K., Jurgens, H., Ritter, J., and Creutzig, U. (1996), Therapy of childhood acute myelogenous leukemias. *Annals of Haematology*, 73, 11–24.

Warrell Jr, R.P., Maslak, P., Eardley, A., Heller, G., Miller Jr, W.H., and Frankel, S.R. (1993). Treatment of acute promyelocytic leukaemia with all-trans retinoic acid: an update of the New York experience. *Leukemia*, 8 (6), 929–33.

Winick, N.J., McKenna, R.W., Shuster, J.J., Schneider, N.R., Borowitz, M.J., Bowman, W.P., *et al.* (1993), Secondary acute myeloid leukaemia in children with acute lymphoblastic leukaemia treated with etoposide. *Journal of Clinical Oncology*, 11, 209–17.

Woods, W.G., Kobrinsky, N., Buckley, J.D., Lee, J.W., Sanders, J., Neudorf, S., *et al.* (1996). Timed-sequential induction therapy improves postremission outcome in acute myeloid leukemia: A report from the Children's Cancer Group. *Blood*, 87, 4979–89.

9 Non-Hodgkin's lymphomas

M. Büyükpamukçu

Lymphomas are the third most common malignancies in children and adolescents, accounting in most developed countries for 10–13% of newly diagnosed cancers in this age group. But in developing countries, especially in Africa and some of the East Mediterranean countries, they are the most common malignancy in childhood (Ries *et al.* 1994; Shad and Magrath 1997). The lymphomas are a heterogeneous group of diseases with two main types: Hodgkin's disease (HD) and non-Hodgkin's lymphomas (NHL). Non-Hodgkin's lymphomas comprise approximately 60%.

Epidemiology

Non-Hodgkin's lymphomas are 1.5 times commoner than HD in children under 15 years. Unlike Hodgkin's disease, which has a bimodal age distribution with peaks in early and late adulthood, the incidence of NHL increases steadily throughout life. For reasons that remain unclear, the average annual incidence of paediatric NHL rose by almost 30% in the US between 1973 and 1991 (Ries *et al.* 1994). The average annual incidence is approximately 9 cases per million White children younger than 15 years, and 5 cases per million Black children. There is a male predominance, with a male to female ratio of 3:1. The peak incidence occurs between the ages of 5–7 years. Involvement before the age of three is uncommon.

It is clear that the disease results from genetic changes, probably influenced by environmental factors. Patients at increased risk of NHL include those with congenital immunodeficiency syndromes (ataxia-telangiectasia, Wiskott-Aldrich syndrome, common variable immunodeficiency disease, severe combined immunodeficiency disease, and the X-linked lymphoproliferative syndrome), acquired immunodeficiency syndrome, and those who have received immunosuppressive therapy (Taylor *et al.* 1996). In some of these immunodeficiency states, the genetic instability associated with the chromosomal abnormality contributes to the increased risk of lymphoid malignancy; for example translocations involving the long arm of chromosome 14q32 are frequently encountered in ataxia-telangiectasia. In neoplasms of B-cell origin, translocational involvement of the immunoglobulin heavy chain locus is common, and the activity of the enzyme system that mediates immunoglobulin gene rearrangement in ataxia-telangiectasia probably accounts for the increase in NHL-associated chromosomal translocation. In X-linked lymphoproliferative syndrome, Epstein-Barr Virus (EBV) can cause fatal infectious mononucleosis and B-cell malignancies, and EBV genomes are frequently found in tumour cells. Long-term immunosuppressive therapy for organ recipients may increase the risk of lymphoproliferative syndromes that are almost all EBV associated. In patients with HIV (Human Immunodeficiency Virus) infection, CNS lymphomas, which are commoner than in the immunocompetent person, appear to be invariably associated with EBV (Ziegler 1991).

There are striking geographical differences in both the incidence rates and the distribution of histological subtypes of NHL. Non-Hodgkin's lymphoma is relatively rare in Japan, whereas Burkitt's lymphoma accounts for almost half of all childhood cancers in equatorial Africa. Similarly, a striking predominance of the Burkitt's subtype has been reported among cases of NHL diagnosed in North-Eastern Brazil (Pedrosa *et al.* 1993). Razzouk *et al.* (1996) showed that viral DNA in some tumours indicates greater involvement of virus in sporadic Burkitt's lymphoma than previously documented, and suggested that the process of viral DNA rearrangement and loss during malignant progression is consistent with an initiating role for EBV in tumourogenesis. All these findings suggest that EBV has a widespread role in the pathogenesis of NHL.

Chronic treatment with hydantoin drugs like phenytoin has been associated with the development of pseudolymphomas and malignant lymphomas. NHL may develop as a second malignancy in patients treated with chemotherapy for Hodgkin's disease, particularly in combination with radiation therapy. This risk of developing NHL and other solid tumours increases steadily after 10 years follow-up, and the incidence of second NHL at 15 years goes up to 17% after combined modality treatment (Prosper *et al.* 1994).

Histopathology, molecular biology, and immunophenotyping

Over the past few years, spectacular progress has been made in understanding the biology of NHL in children, making these tumours a model of oncogenic processes in human malignancy.

Recent biological and immunological studies have greatly contributed to a better understanding and classification of NHL, although the superimposition of immunological, cytogenetic, and molecular classifications can still be confusing. Childhood lymphoma is mainly divided into three histological and immunological subtypes:

(1) B-cell origin (small noncleaved, undifferentiated);

(2) T-cell origin (majority of lymphoblastic lymphomas express T-cell markers);

(3) large-cell lymphomas (B- and T-cell origin, also Ki-1 positive cells in anaplastic large-cell lymphomas).

At a histological level, childhood non-Hodgkin's lymphomas are all diffuse lymphomas of high grade, except for some large-cell lymphomas (large non-cleaved or large cleaved cells) which are intermediate grade.

Paediatric NHL can be divided into three major histopathological categories, according to the most widely accepted different classification schemes (see Table 9.1).

B-cell lymphomas

Undifferentiated small non-cleaved lymphoma, B-cell lymphomas (Burkitt's and non-Burkitt's) comprise 40–50% of childhood NHL.

Table 9.1   Histopathological classification of childhood NHL

Scheme	LBL	BCL	LCL
Rappaport	lymphoblastic lymphoma	Burkitt's non-Burkitt's	histiocytic lymphoma
Kiel	lymphoblastic convoluted and unclassified types	lymphoblastic, Burkitt's type, and other B-cell	immunoblastic, centroblastic
Working formulation	lymphoblastic	small, non-cleaved cell	Diffuse large cell, immunoblastic
REAL	T lymphoblastic	high-grade B-cell lymphoma Burkitt's	large cell anaplastic large cell

LBL, lymphoblastic lymphoma; BCL, B-cell lymphoma; LCL, large-cell lymphoma; REAL, revised European-American lymphoma.

In 1958, Burkitt described a lymphoid tumour occurring in Black African children, with a distinctive clinical presentation, histological features, and geographical distribution. Later, in other parts of the world, lymphoma in childhood with the same characteristic histopathological pattern was described. However, the clinical presentation was quite different with abdominal involvement, in contrast to the jaw involvement characteristic of African endemic tumours.

Small, non-cleaved cell lymphomas are either histologically indistinguishable from African Burkitt's lymphoma or differ only in the degree of pleomorphism or the number of large, single nucleoli. This group of lymphomas can be subdivided into Burkitt's and non-Burkitt's lymphomas based on the degree of pleomorphism, but there are no known clinical, phenotypic, karyotypic, or nuclear features in children that correspond to this histological subdivision. Small, non-cleaved cells have a high nuclear-cytoplasmic ratio, the nucleus is round or oval, has an open, nuclear chromatin pattern, and contains multiple, (usually 2–5), readily discernable nucleoli. Some cells may only have a single central nucleolus. If such cells are frequent, pathologists would diagnose non-Burkitt's lymphoma. The cytoplasm usually contains lipid vacuoles and its rim is very basophilic. The cells are frequently interspersed with macrophages in which nuclear debris is discernable, giving rise to the starry sky appearance.

Small, non-cleaved lymphomas show B-cell phenotype, express mostly IgM class surface immunoglobulins with either kappa or lambda light chains, and B-cell antigen presented by the monoclonal antibodies CD19 and CD20. HLA-DR antigens and common ALL antigen (CD10) are also present, and terminal deoxyribonucleotide transferase (TdT) enzyme is absent. American- (sporadic) type Burkitt's lymphoma expresses surface IgM, whereas African (endemic) Burkitt's lymphoma cells appear not to secrete this immunoglobulin.

Malignant cells from endemic and sporadic Burkitt's lymphomas have the same morphology and differentiation patterns, even in the presence of EBV in most cases. In 75% of cases, the malignant cells display a reciprocal translocation of the distal end of the long arm of chromosome 8 to the long arm of chromosome 14 (t(8;14) (q24;q32)). Other translocations occur in 16% of cases; the same small segment of chromosome 8 translocates to the long arm of chromosome 22 (t(8;22) (q24;q11)), or to the short arm of chromosome 2 (t(2;8) (q24;p12)).

The oncogene, c-*myc*, a gene involved in the control of cellular proliferation (through the G1 phase into the S phase of the cell cycle), is present on chromosome 8q24 precisely where the break points of chromosomal translocation occur. The genes for immunoglobulin heavy and light chain lambda and kappa are located on chromosomes 14, 22, and 2, respectively. In these translocations, the oncogene c-*myc* moves from its normal position and is juxtaposed to one of the immunoglobulin receptor subunit genes on chromosome 14, 22, or 2. This leads to altered expression of c-*myc* oncogene with consequently inappropriate cellular proliferation. Normally, the expression of c-*myc* is closely regulated, with rapid induction of transcription after mitogenic stimulation. Molecular studies have shown heterogeneity of break points on both translocated chromosomes. Sporadic and endemic lymphomas can be differentiated at the molecular level, according to whether the breakpoint on chromosome 8 is some distance away from the gene (endemic) or within the gene itself (sporadic).

C-Myc forms heterodimers with a related protein, MAX, which can bind to DNA, itself, or other proteins. After EBV-induced immortalization of B cells, and proliferation of these cells, facilitated by suppression of T cells by co-existing malaria, translocation-induced, dysregulated expression of c-*myc* probably increases the proportion of transcription-activating Myc-MAX complexes, leading to the progression of the cell cycle and lymphoproliferation (Ayer *et al.* 1993).

The blocking of the function of c-Myc as an inducer of apoptosis in B-cell lymphoma suggests that additional molecular changes might be involved in the formation of the tumour (Croce 1993). The introduction of the c-*myc* oncogene, driven by immunoglobulin, induces lymphoid malignancy in transgenic mice (Adams *et al.* 1985).

Lymphoblastic lymphoma

Lymphoblastic lymphomas (convoluted and nonconvoluted) comprise 30–40% of childhood NHL. More than 90% of lymphoblastic lymphomas are derived from immature T cells and express the immunophenotypic markers of intrathymic T-cell differentiation. The thymocytes can be classified as early (T10 and/or T9), intermediate (T6, T10, T4, T8), or mature (T4, T8, T3) in the differentiation process. Although childhood T-cell acute lymphoblastic leukaemia and NHL show specific clinical features, it is difficult to conclude that ALL is derived from earlier precursor T cells than lymphoblastic lymphoma, because there is considerable overlap between the immunological markers of both disorders. Separation of the entities according to the percentage of blast cells in the bone marrow is unsatisfactory and reported differences in response to treatment are more a reflection of stage than of real biological differences. A small percentage of cases have a B-cell progenitor immunophenotype in lymphoblastic lymphoma cells.

The chromosomal translocation identified in T-cell leukaemias and lymphomas, like those in Burkitt's lymphoma, inappropriately activates proto-oncogenes by placing them near the regulatory sequences of immunologically important genes (in this case, T-cell-antigen receptor genes on chromosome 7 or 14). These T-cell-antigen receptor gene (*TCR*) rearrangements involve transcription factor genes (*TAL1*) that participate in developmental processes not usually operative in T cells (Bash *et al.* 1993). Very few studies have focused on lymphomas, but submicroscopic deletion of *TAL1* can be detected in T-cell leukaemias (25%), suggesting that this deletion may also be the common molecular defect in lymphoblastic lymphoma. Precise explanation of how *TAL1* and other translocated transcription factor genes contribute to the malignant transformation of T cells is currently under investigation. Some of the translocations described in lymphoblastic lymphomas are: t(1:14) (p32;q11), t(10:14) (p24;q11), t(7:14) (q35;p11), t(8:14) (q24;q11), and t(1:7) (p34;q34).

Lymphoblastic lymphomas are indistinguishable histologically and cytologically from the acute lymphoblastic leukaemias (ALL). The cells are usually quite uniform in appearance but some of them may have irregular nuclear margins, caused by nuclear convolution and multiple nucleoli. There is usually a thin rim of pale cytoplasm with a high nuclear-cytoplasmic ratio. The distinction from ALL is arbitrary and can only be made on the basis of clinical features. The extent of bone marrow involvement has been used to separate lymphoma, where less than 25% of nucleated cells are lymphoblasts, from leukaemia (more than 25%). Such a distinction is of questionable biological significance, because it depends on adequate sampling of the bone marrow.

Large-cell lymphomas

Large-cell lymphomas are of two main types: large-cell, non-cleaved (B-cell origin) and cleaved lymphomas (immunoblastic). The recently described Ki-1 lymphoma is classified as immuno-blastic or anaplastic large-cell lymphoma (Stein *et al.* 1985). A small number of large-cell lym-phomas are truly histiocytic and can be separated by specific monoclonal antibodies.

Large-cell lymphomas (10% of childhood NHL) are immunoblastic lymphomas, including Ki-1 positive or anaplastic large-cell lymphomas (ALCL) (Harris *et al.* 1994).

Large-cell, non-Hodgkin's lymphoma is a heterogeneous group of tumours that can have T-cell, B-cell, or indeterminate immunophenotype. In children, these immunotypes occur with equal frequency, whereas in adults approximately 80% of large-cell lymphomas are B-cell tumours. Anaplastic large-cell lymphomas, which usually express CD30 (recognized by Ki-1 and Bcr-H_2 monoclonal antibodies), are of T-cell lineage, and have a t(2;5) (p23;q35) chromosomal translocation in about 50% of cases (Sandlund *et al.* 1994*a*,*b*). The t(2;5) translocation results in the fusion of the involved genes in the amino-terminal portion of the nucleophosmin gene, *NPM*, on chromosome 5 with the catalytic domain of anaplastic lymphoma kinase gene, *ALK*, on chro-mosome 2. The resulting chimeric NPM-ALK protein product engages in activities that are not characteristic of its components (Morris *et al.* 1994). When rearranged, NPM, a nonribosomal nuclear phosphoprotein, loses its nuclear localization signal, and the NPM-ALK chimera becomes primarily localized in the cytoplasm. Under these circumstances, the truncated ALK component can inappropriately phosphorylate the substrates involved in normal cell growth and differentiation. Molecular characterization of the t(2;5) translocation has led to the development of a reverse-transcriptase polymerase chain reaction (RT-PCR) assay that reliably detects NPM-ALK fusion transcripts. This RNA marker has been found in some non-anaplastic lymphomas, some CD30 positive anaplastic lymphomas, and some lymphomas that lacked the t(2;5) translo-cation on routine cytogenetic analysis. Thus, the RT-PCR assay provides an important diagnostic tool and should also expand our understanding of the subgroup of tumours characterized by t(2;5) translocation, expression of CD30, and anaplastic features.

Presentation and clinical features

The clinical presentation of non-Hodgkin's lymphomas in children is varied and depends on histological subtype, the extent of the disease, and primary site of the tumour. Children with NHL typically have extranodal disease. The disease often grows rapidly and spreads by blood-borne dissemination. Almost two-thirds of children and adolescents with NHL have locally advanced or metastatic disease at the time of diagnosis. Patients with lymphoma which has spread to the central nervous system (CNS) have malignant pleocytosis or cranial nerve palsies. The presence of pancytopaenia suggests bone marrow involvement.

Primary site of disease is mostly correlated to the histological subtype. Sporadic cases of Burkitt's lymphoma (small, non-cleaved cell lymphoma) present with abdominal tumour, with or without ascites, in approximately 90% of cases. Abdominal tumours are often associated with pain or swelling, nausea, and vomiting, resulting from intestinal obstruction caused by direct compression of the bowel lumen, or intussusception. Presentation with a right iliac fossa mass is common and can be confused with appendicitis or an inflammatory appendiceal mass. 50% of patients with endemic Burkitt's lymphoma present with a jaw mass (Fig. 9.1). Jaw involvement is usually age dependent, occurring particularly in young children under 5 years. Primary abdominal tumours are also common, and occasionally the orbit and paraspinal areas are involved. Bone marrow involvement is more common in sporadic than endemic cases, and *vice versa* for CNS involvement. Patients with large abdominal masses, mostly with ascites, are at risk for tumour lysis syndrome, especially when chemotherapy is started (Fig. 9.2). Spinal cord compression in children with epidural masses also requires immediate attention. Prompt administration of chemotherapy is crucial once the diagnosis has been established. If the patient does not

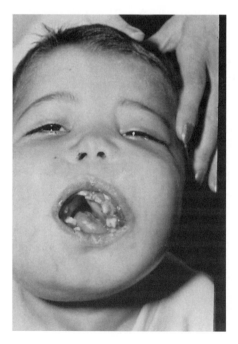

Fig. 9.1 A child with Burkitt's lymphoma of the jaw with extension to the oral cavity.

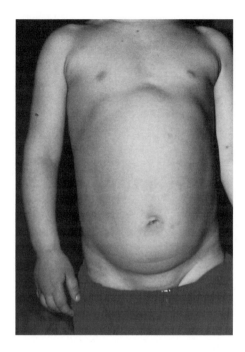

Fig. 9.2 A child with abdominal Burkitt's lymphoma with bilateral involvement of axillary and cervical lymphatic nodes.

have a rapid response, or if a diagnostic tissue-biopsy specimen is unavailable, low-dose radiation therapy or laminectomy may be necessary.

Lymphoblastic lymphoma most commonly presents as a mediastinal tumour, often with an associated pleural effusion (Fig. 9.3). Children present with severe respiratory distress from airway compression, or swelling of neck, face, and arms from obstruction of the superior vena cava. If there is marked tracheal compression, sedation must be avoided. The liver and spleen may also be involved in patients with lymphoblastic lymphoma, although isolated, primary, abdominal disease is rare. Other sites, such as bone, skin, and testis are not usually associated with a large mediastinal mass. The CNS, including cranial nerve involvement, is rarely involved at diagnosis, and in the presence of widespread (more than 25%) bone marrow involvement, leukaemia is usually diagnosed.

Patients with large-cell lymphoma can present with an anterior mediastinal mass and symptomas similar to those of lymphoblastic disease, or with abdominal disease causing intestinal obstruction, as in sporadic Burkitt's lymphoma. Sites of extranodal disease include skin, bone, lung, and soft tissue (Ki-1 positive anaplastic large-cell lymphoma). Dissemination to the bone marrow is somewhat less frequent in patients with large-cell lymphomas than in those with other histological subtypes, and CNS disease is relatively rare.

Diagnosis, staging, and prognosis

Non-Hodgkin's lymphoma grows very rapidly in children; therefore, expeditious diagnosis is essential. The diagnosis is mostly established by examining tumour tissue obtained by open

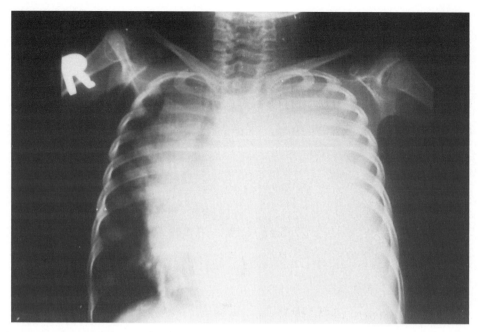

Fig. 9.3 Very large mediastinal tumour due to lymphoma with left pleural fluid. There is tumoural extension to the right, and cardiac and tracheal shift to the right.

biopsy, which should be sufficient to permit morphological, immunophenotypic, cytogenetic, and molecular studies. If the patient's clinical condition is unstable, or if there is large abdominal or mediastinal mass with fluid, the diagnosis can often be made by less invasive procedures (percutaneous fine-needle biopsy, aspiration of a peripheral lymph node, or examination of cerebrospinal, pleural, peritoneal fluid, and bone marrow). Determination of the histological subtype and immunophenotypic and cytogenetic examinations are very important to decide treatment. The material used for these special studies should contain minimal amounts of normal tissue unless molecular or combined morphological/phenotyping studies are to be performed. Clonal populations can be detected by PCR, even if they represent only a small percentage of the total number of cells. Since immunophenotyping can be done on cytocentrifuged preparations, imprints, or smears requiring little material, it is rare that leukocyte common antigen (LCA) will be the only antigen that can be examined. LCA is not present on non-haematological malignancies, and provides adequate confirmation of a lymphoid cell population, as opposed to another type of 'small, round, blue cell tumour'. Distinction between lymphomas and other 'small, round, blue cell tumours', including neuroblastoma, rhabdomyosarcoma, and Ewing's sarcoma, is usually not difficult on histological grounds alone, but immunophenotyping and molecular studies will resolve any diagnostic problems.

The minimal and optimal studies needed to establish the diagnosis and staging are given in Table 9.2.

Serum studies do not aid the specific diagnosis of lymphomas, but may help to exclude nonlymphoid tumours (for example, high level of catecholamines in neuroblastomas and

Table 9.2   Initial staging studies for the diagnosis of histological subtypes of NHL

Complete blood count (with differential)
Test for Human Immunodeficiency Virus (HIV) and Epstein-Barr Virus (EBV)
Blood chemistry
     electrolytes, uric acid, calcium, phosphorus,
     lactic dehydrogenase, BUN (blood urea nitrogen), creatinine
Examination of cerebrospinal fluid
Bone marrow aspiration (bilateral) and bone marrow biopsy
     peritoneal and/or pleural fluid examination
Bilateral chest X-ray
Abdominal ultrasonography
CT scan
MRI (CNS and paraspinal disease)
Bone scintigraphy (optional, depending on clinical features)
Adequate biopsy and/or cytological studies (histology and immunophenotype)

alpha-fetoprotein in germ-cell and liver tumours). Raised lactate dehyrogenase and high serum levels of soluble interleukin-2 receptors (SIL-2R) and B_2-microglobulin provide prognostic information.

In children with non-Hodgkin's lymphoma, staging systems predominantly reflect the tumour volume. The most widely used staging is the St Jude system, which is modified from the system proposed at Ann Arbor for Hodgkin's disease (see Table 9.3) (Murphy 1980).

Certain problems are not taken into account with this staging system, such as the predominance of extranodal primaries, the unpredictable pattern of spread, the size and the number of tumours, and immunohistological characteristics. But this system has the advantages of clarity, simplicity, and prognostic usefulness. It is applicable to all histological types of childhood NHL and separates patients with localized stage disease (stage I and II) from those with advanced, intrathoracic and intra-abdominal (stage III) disease. Patients with bone marrow infiltration with less than 25% tumour cells and involvement of the CNS are separated into the advanced group with the worst prognosis (stage IV).

Accurate staging is essential because of the marked differences in intensity and duration of therapy, as well as the differences in prognosis for patients with localized and advanced disease. Prognostic distinction is made between apparently localized, gastrointestinal tract lymphoma *versus* more extensive, intra-abdominal disease because of the different patterns of survival after appropriate therapy. Stage II disease is typically limited to a segment of the gut, with or without associated mesenteric lymph nodes, and the primary tumour can be completely excised. Stage III disease has frequently spread to para-aortic and retroperitoneal areas, ascites may be present, and complete resection of all gross tumour is not possible.

One of the main determinants of treatment outcome is the tumour burden at presentation. Tumour burden is reflected in the clinical stage and the presence of elevated serum levels of molecules, either secreted or shed by tumour cells or which accumulate as a consequence of tumour cell breakdown. These include lactic dehydrogenase (LDH), SIL-2R, B_2-microglobulin, uric acid,

Table 9.3 St Jude's staging for childhood non-Hodgkin's lymphoma

Stage I	A single tumour (extranodal) or single anatomical area (nodal) with the exclusion of the mediastinum or abdomen.
Stage II	A single tumour (extranodal) with regional node involvement.
	Two or more nodal areas on the same side of the diaphragm.
	Two single (extranodal) tumours with or without regional node involvement on the same side of the diaphragm.
	A primary gastrointestinal tract tumour, usually in the ileocaecal area, with or without involvement of associated mesenteric nodes only, grossly completely resected.
Stage III	Two single tumours (extranodal) on opposite sides of the diaphragm.
	Two or more nodal areas above or below the diaphragm.
	All the primary intrathoracic tumours (mediastinal, pleural, thymic).
	All extensive primary intra-abdominal disease, unresectable.
	All paraspinal or epidural tumours, regardless of other tumour site(s).
Stage IV	Any of the above with initial CNS and/or bone marrow involvement.

and lactic acid. In patients with Burkitt's lymphoma, CNS disease at the time of diagnosis is associated with greatest risk of treatment failure. In patients with large-cell lymphoma, bone marrow involvement and a T-cell or indeterminate immunophenotype appear to be associated with a poorer prognosis. The expression of CD30 may be a favourable prognostic feature in patients with anaplastic, large-cell lymphoma, although this finding is controversial.

Finally, every effort must be made to avoid delays in therapy and to initiate successive cycles as soon as there has been sufficient bone marrow recovery.

Treatment

There has been remarkable improvement in the response and long-term prognosis for non-Hodgkins lymphoma in childhood over the past decade. These advances can be attributed mainly to the introduction of intensive combination chemotherapy given as primary treatment. The advances have been validated with randomized, multicentre trials chosen according to the stage and histological subtype of disease.

Principles of therapy and pretreatment considerations

Before the 1970s, the overall survival of children with NHL was poor, few patients survived 5 years after diagnosis, and most of those had localized disease. Surgery and radiation therapy were effective in patients with stage I and II disease, but more than two-thirds of the patients experienced relapse. Chemotherapy is now the main treatment modality for all histologies and stages of childhood non-Hodgkin's lymphomas. Children with localized NHL can be cured by a chemotherapy regimen of reduced intensity and duration, and radiotherapy can be safely omitted without substantially jeopardizing the excellent chance of cure. Advanced childhood abdominal

NHL can be cured with intensive multidrug therapy without irradiation to the primary tumour (Patte *et al.* 1991). There is no good evidence that irradiation adds therapeutic benefit to children with NHL, but it does increase both short-term and long-term toxicity (Link *et al.* 1990). A few indications for radiotherapy still remain, such as emergency treatment for superior vena caval and ureteric obstruction, and intraparenchymal involvement of the central nervous system (CNS). In these conditions, chemotherapy is usually as effective as radiotherapy. Localized residual tumour may, however, benefit from radiotherapy.

There are very few indications for surgery in the treatment of childhood NHL. Laparatomy is frequently performed at the time of presentation to make the diagnosis in patients who present as an abdominal emergency or have tumour confined to the abdomen. There is no indication for partial reduction of tumour bulk by surgery. Surgery may be needed in certain special situations, such as intussusception, intestinal perforation, suspected appendicitis, and serious gastrointestinal bleeding. If these complications occur during the neutropaenic state, the mortality rate is very high. At the time of remission evaluation, a residual mass can be removed or widely biopsied for careful, pathological examination to decide whether complete or partial remission has been obtained. In the French experience, less than one-third of residual masses contain viable malignant cells (Helardot *et al.* 1989).

At the time of presentation, some tumour-associated problems will require immediate attention. A large mediastinal mass may cause life-threatening respiratory problems, superior vena caval (SVC) obstruction, cardiac irregularities or tamponade, paraplegia, or acute gastrointestinal complications. Patients with a large mediastinal mass are also at increased risk of complications during anaesthesia; cardiac arrest and bleeding from enlarged mediastinal vessels may occur. If the tumour is limited to the mediastinum, biopsy is performed by mediastinoscopy or by a small parasternal incision. When anaesthesia is considered too hazardous and needle biopsy is not feasible, the only way to reduce the mediastinal mass is limited radiation or corticosteroid therapy until it is sufficiently small for safe biopsy to be performed.

If there is a high tumour burden, the patient with NHL may develop uric acid nephropathy before or immediately after chemotherapy, when the biochemical abnormalities of the acute tumour lysis syndrome may lead to renal failure. Before therapy starts, it is essential to ensure the serum uric acid level is not elevated, the patient is well hydrated, and is able to maintain a high urine flow (250 ml/m^2/hr). Serum uric acid can be reduced to normal levels by alkaline diuresis and allopurinol administration in all patients except those with additional renal compromise from ureteric obstruction, or, less commonly, tumour involvement of the kidneys. In these circumstances, the only option may be haemodialysis before chemotherapy.

Lymphoblastic lymphoma (LBL)

The most widely used chemotherapy protocols for LBL are based upon protocols designed for acute lymphoblastic leukaemia (ALL). Most successful protocols are LSA$_2$L$_2$ from Memorial Sloan Kettering and German BFM protocols. Almost all effective regimens have included either adriamycin or daunorubicin. LSA$_2$L$_2$ protocols have been used with similar success in several countries, 60–80% long-term, disease-free survival (DFS) for patients with extensive disease, and around 90% for patients with limited, localized disease (Anderson *et al.* 1983). Patients with localized LBL do not benefit from specific CNS preventive treatment unless they present with involvement of parameningeal sites.

The LSA$_2$L$_2$ schedule contained 10 drugs in an intensive regimen (Wollner *et al.* 1979). At the Institut Gustav Roussy, the original protocol was modified by the addition of HDMTX (high dose methotrexate) (3 g/m^2 in 3 hours infusion), and the French investigators took a more aggressive initial approach, treating localized LBL with the same intensive and prolonged regimen used for advanced disease. The EFS was 79% and 72% in stage III and IV patients, respectively, with one CNS relapse (Patte *et al.* 1992). In 1993, Schrappe *et al.* (1993) reported results of three, consecutive, multicentric BFM trials in non-B-cell NHL in which methotrexate dosage was increased, induction therapy intensified, and the dose of cranial radiation reduced from 18 to 12 Gy. BFM 81, 83, and 86 trials showed EFS of 69%, 76%, and 77%, respectively.

Subsequent refinements included intensification of the regimen of high-dose methotrexate, the addition of a reinduction phase, and the inclusion of newly identified active agents.

Updated results of BFM 86 showed 78% EFS with a follow-up duration of 3.6–7 years (median 5 years) (Reiter *et al.* 1995). In this protocol, eight-drug induction was followed by a consolidation phase in stage I and II patients, whereas stage III and IV patients received an additional reinduction protocol and cranial irradiation in the second phase of reinduction, followed by maintenance therapy. The radiation dose was 12 Gy for all patients without CNS disease, 18 Gy for those older than 3 years with overt disease, and 24 Gy in older children. Children under 1 year with CNS disease did not receive cranial radiotherapy. The total duration of treatment was 18–24 months. The long-term, event-free survival rate for this group of patients has remained 65–78% in the last decade.

Current studies are investigating the potential benefit of incorporating epipodophyllotoxins, high-dose asparaginase, and cytarabine into treatment regimens.

B-cell lymphomas

Because localized B-cell lymphoma (stage I and II) has an excellent prognosis with a cure rate of about 90%, all centres tend to treat patients with localized disease with less intensive regimens. The primary therapeutic question is how little treatment can be given without reducing the excellent survival rates. The CCSG study indicates that the COMP and LSA$_2$L$_2$ regimens were equally effective in patients with localized disease, regardless of histology (Anderson *et al.* 1983). Another CCSG trial showed 6 months to be as effective as 18 months treatment in patients with non-lymphoblastic lymphoma of limited extent (Meadows *et al.* 1989). In the NCI 77–04 protocol, even 6 months' treatment appears to be longer than necessary, and currently, successful chemotherapy can be given over a period of only 9 weeks (Link *et al.* 1990).

In Europe, treatment of localized NHL, as of advanced stage NHL, is adapted according to histology and immunophenotype. In the BFM protocols of 1981, 83, and 1986, patients with limited disease received only 8 and 6 weeks of therapy, respectively, with a survival rate of over 90%. In the SFOP (the Society of French Paediatric Oncology) LMB protocol, only two cycles of therapy (COPAD) are given for patients with stage I disease, or those with abdominal disease with complete resection. In all these studies, radiation has been shown to be of no benefit to the patients with localized disease.

Disseminated B-cell lymphomas

In this group of patients, abdominal, bone marrow (BM), and central nervous system (CNS) involvement occurs separately or together. Patients with abdominal disease without BM and CNS involvement have a cure expectancy of 60–90% with all major protocols. In the last 10 years, well organized, multicentre studies in Europe (BFM and LMB) and in North America (NCI, CCG, St Jude and POG) showed considerable improvement in childhood NHL.

In SFOP's LMB-081 protocol, 75% of patients with bone marrow involvement achieved long-term survival. There was no difference between survival of patients with less or more than 25% of tumour cells in the bone marrow, although patients with CNS disease had a poor prognosis (19% DFS at 2 years).

The general scheme of the LMB protocols, which can be given over a relatively short period (2–8 months), is a cytoreductive phase, with low dose of cyclophosphamide (CPM), vincristine (VCR), and prednisone (COP) given a week before an intensive induction based on HDMTX, fractionated CPM, and adriamycin. This is followed by a consolidation phase based on continuously infused Ara-C. CNS-directed therapy is given with HDMTX and intrathecal (ITMTX) (Helardot *et al.* 1989; Patte *et al.* 1996*b*). The most recent protocol (LMB 89) for patients with BCL, including large-cell lymphoma with B-cell markers, adapts treatment intensity to three risk groups. Group A (resected stage I and stage II) patients receive two polychemotherapy (COPAD) courses without any CNS prophylaxis. In group B (other stage I and II, stage III and IV and ALL with bone marrow involvement <70%) patients received initial COP, 2 COPADM, and then CPM and continuous ara-C, followed by a further COPADM. In group C (patients with >70 % blasts in bone marrow and/or CNS involvement) treatment lasts for 7 months. After COP and 2 COPADM (MTX $8gm/m^2$), consolidation with HD ara-C ($3 gm/m^2$) and VP16 ($200 mg/m^2$ for 5 days) and CNS treatment with HDMTX, HD ara-C and triple intrathecal is given; 24 Gy cranial irradiation is given to patients with CNS involvement. These protocols are shown in Fig. 9.4. Conclusions from consecutive LMB studies are: 1. Stage III and IV CNS-negative NHL have reached an 85–93% EFS. 2. Bone marrow involvement is not a poor prognostic factor. 3. CNS therapy with HDMTX and ITMTX is effective (CNS relapse rate is less than 3%). 4. Treatment intensification and high-dose therapy with bone marrow transplantation can convert partial remission to cure. 5. Residual tumour must be confirmed histologically since two-thirds of abdominal masses are necrotic. 6. No tumour reduction after cytoreductive therapy indicates a poor prognosis. Short intensive chemotherapy regimen results in high cure rates in B-cell NHL, even in patients with known poor prognostic factors such as high LDH or CNS involvement (EFS is 83%).

Similar results are obtained in the German and Austrian cooperative studies with BFM protocols (Reiter *et al.* 1995).

Other groups in North America, Italy, and Great Britain have adopted similar, intensive, combined chemotherapy for childhood NHL, with similar results (Pinkerton *et al.* 1993).

Today, in undifferentiated and B-cell NHL, there is good evidence that intensive therapy need not be prolonged beyond a few months, even in patients with the most advanced disease, and these short protocols also reduce short- and long-term toxicity and are more convenient.

Large-cell lymphomas

Because of the biological heterogeneity of large-cell lymphomas, their optimal treatment and data on long-term outcome are not yet established. Most centres treat all large-cell lymphomas with the same protocols used for B-cell lymphomas or lymphoblastic lymphomas. 50 out of 62 Ki-1 ALCL patients treated with the BFM B-cell protocol were in continuous, complete remission for a median of 2.5 years with short-pulse chemotherapy (EFS 83%) (Reiter *et al.* 1995). In this study, skin

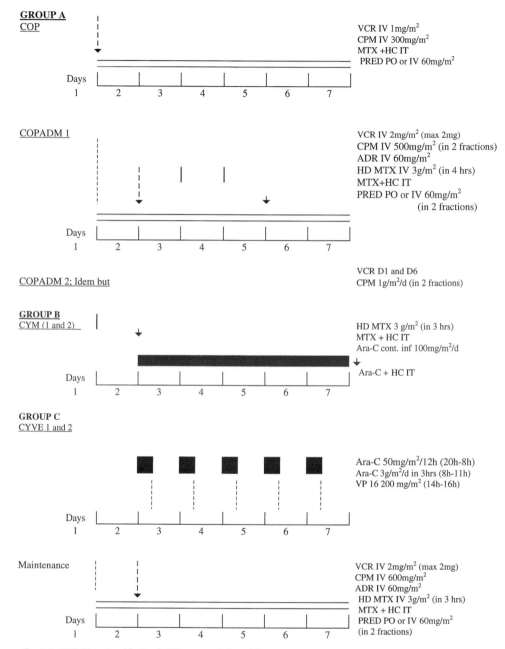

Fig. 9.4 LMB 89 protocol for B-cell NHL, groups A, B, and C.

involvement was the only negative prognostic parameter. In St Jude's Children's Hospital, 13 children with advanced, diffuse, large-cell non-Hodgkin's lymphoma were treated with a 12-week MACOP-B protocol. One patient had a partial response and 12 (92%) achieved complete response, and 2-years' EFS was only 52($\pm$15[S.E.])% (Santana *et al.* 1993). APO regimen and LSA$_2$L$_2$

regimen give similar results. The French SFOP group treated large-cell lymphoma with the same risk-adapted polychemotherapy regimen as Burkitt's lymphoma, with similar outcome (Patte *et al.* 1996*a*).

The most recent data suggest that immunophenotype-directed treatment may be more effective in improving survival. B-cell tumours and Ki-1 ALCL respond well to short-term, intensive chemotherapy used for Burkitt's lymphoma (Reiter *et al.* 1995). Tumours of T-cell origin probably require more intensive and prolonged therapy.

Relapse

The prognosis of relapsed NHL in children is very poor, especially for those who initially received intensive chemotherapy. Recent studies have attempted to prolong survival with various high-dose protocols, with or without bone marrow transplantation. Chemotherapy that includes etoposide, iphosphamide, and cytarabine can induce second remission in some patients with relapsed B-cell lymphomas, and the combination of dexamethasone, cytarabine, and cis-platin often induces second remission in patients with relapsed, large-cell lymphoma. Patients who remit are considered candidates for bone marrow transplantation. Very intensive protocols, such as the BACT regimen (BCNU, CPM, Ara-C, and 6-thioguanine), have some success with autologous bone marrow transplantation (ABMT) (Philip *et al.* 1988). In an NCI study, half of the patients received the above protocol, with ABMT previously cryopreserved after intensive chemotherapy. Four of 19 patients achieved long-term survival. Similar results have been obtained in Lyon, France. A problem in interpreting such studies is that patients are invariably selected, and it is not clear whether ABMT and high-dose therapy are necessary. This issue is currently under study in an international trial. Preliminary results do not show a clear advantage for ABMT, and it always carries the risk of reinfusion of malignant cells. Overall results for allogeneic BMT are quite similar to the ABMT experience. Patients with progressive disease at the time of transplant do poorly.

Long-term sequelae of therapy

The long-term complications and the quality of life after treatment of non-Hodgkin's lymphoma of childhood have become very important, as results have shown excellent outcomes. The potentially serious consequences of radiation therapy have almost ceased to exist, as this therapy modality has a smaller and smaller role in the overall therapeutic strategy, including CNS-directed therapy. The trend towards shorter chemotherapy duration in the B-cell lymphomas will reduce the likelihood and severity of late effects. Potential complications of chemotherapy, especially impaired reproductive function from alkylating agents, late cardiac failure due to anthracyclines, secondary malignancies, and psychological consequences must be seriously considered, and patients should be followed up for the duration of their lives. The development of therapies that are equally or more effective, but less toxic, remains an important challenge. Because most cases of limited-stage disease are curable with relatively non-toxic therapy, future efforts should focus on the two-thirds of patients who have advanced disease at the time of diagnosis.

References

Adams J.M., Harris A.W., Pinkert CA., Corcoran, L.M., Alexander, W.S., Cory, S. *et al.*, (1985). The c-*Myc* Oncogene driven by immunoglobulin enhances induced lymphoid malignancy in transgenic mice. *Nature* 318: 533–8.

Anderson, J.R., Wilson, J.F., Jenkin, D.T., Meadows, A.T., Kersey, J., Chilcote, R.R. *et al.*, (1983). Childhood non-Hodgkin's lymphoma: results of a randomized therapeutic trial comparing a 4 drug regimen (COMP) to a 10 drug regimen (LSA$_2$L$_2$). *New England Journal of Medicine.*, 308, 559–65.

Ayer D.E., Kretzner L., and Eisenman R.N. (1993). Mad: a heterodimeric partner for Max that antagonizes Myc transcriptional activity. *Cell*, 72, 211–22.

Bash R.O., Crist W.M., Shuster J.J., Link, M.P., Amylon, M., Pullen, J., *et al.* (1993). Clinical features and outcome of T-cell acute lymphoblastic leukaemia in childhood with respect to alterations at the TAL-I locus: a Paediatric Oncology Group Study. *Blood*, 81, 2110–7.

Croce, C.M. (1993). Molecular biology of lymphomas. *Seminars in Oncology*, 20, (suppl 5), 31–46.

Harris, N.L., Jaffe, E.S., Stein, H., Banks, P.M., Chan, J.K., Cleary, M.L., *et al.* (1994). A revised European-American Classification of lymphoid neoplasms: A proposal from the International Lymphoma Study Group. *Blood*, 84, 1361–92.

Helardot, P.G., Wakim, A., Kalifa, L., Leclere, J., Lacombe, M.J., and Patte, C. (1989). The place of surgery in the remission assessment of childhood abdominal malignant non-Hodgkin's lymphoma (NHL). *Medical and Paediatric Oncology*, 17, 322, Abstract.

Link, M.P., Donaldson, S.S., Bernard, C.W., Shuster, J.J., and Murphy, S.B. (1990). Result of treatment of childhood localized non-Hodgkin's lymphoma with combination chemotherapy with or without radiotherapy. *New England Journal of Medicine*, 322, 1769–74.

Meadows, A.T., Sposto, R., Jenkins, R.D.T., Kersey, J.H., Chilcote, R.R., Siegel, S.E., *et al.* (1989). Similar efficiency of 6 and 18 months of therapy with four drugs (COMP) for localized non-Hodgkin's lymphoma of children: A report from the Children's Cancer Study Group. *Journal of Clinical Oncology*, 7, 92–9.

Morris, S.W., Kirstein, M.N., Valentine, M.B., Dittmer, K., Shapiro, D.N., Look, A.T., *et al.* (1994). Fusion of a kinase gene, ALK to a nuclear protein gen, NPM in non-Hodgkin's lymphoma. *Science*, 263, 1281–4.

Murphy, S.B. (1980). Classification, staging and results of treatment of childhood non-Hodgkin's lymphomas in adults. *Seminars in Oncology*, 7, 332–9.

Patte C., Philip T., Rodary C., Zucker, J.M., Behrendt, H., Gentet, J.C., *et al.* (1991). High survival rate in advanced stage B cell lymphomas and leukaemias without CNS involvement with a short intensive polychemotherapy. Results of a non randomized trial from French Paediatric Oncology Society (SFOP) on 216 children, *Journal of Clinical Oncology*, 9, 123–32.

Patte, C., Kalifa, C., Flamant, F., Hartmann, O., Brugieres, L., Valteau Couanet, D., *et al.* (1992). Results of the LMT81 protocol, a modified LSA$_2$L$_2$ protocol with high dose methotrexate, on 84 children with non B-cell lymphoma, *Medical and Paediatric Oncology*, 20, 105–13.

Patte, C., Michon, J., Behrendt, H., Bergeron, C., Lutz, P., Leverger, G., *et al.* (1996*a*). B-cell large cell lymphoma in children, description and outcome when treated with the same regimen as Burkitt's. SFOP experience with the LMB 89 protocol. Annals of Oncology. 7 (Suppl 3): 29 A.

Patte, C., Michon J., Behrendt, H., Leverger, G., Frappaz, D., Robert, A. *et al.* (1996*b*). Updated results of the LMB 89 protocol of the SFOP (French Paediatric Oncology Society) for childhood B cell lymphoma and leukaemia ALL. Annals of Oncology, 7, 30 A.

Pedrosa, F., Fonseca, T., Leimig, T., Verissimo, I., Ribeiro, R.C., and Sandlund, J. (1993). Clinical and biological characteristics of childhood non-Hodgkin's lymphoma (NHL) in northeast Brazil. *Medical Pediatric Oncology*, 21, 532 abstract.

Philip, T., Hartmann, Q., Biron, P., Cahn, J.Y., Pein, F., Bordigoni, P., *et al.* (1988). High dose therapy and autologous bone marrow transplantation in partial remission after first line induction therapy for diffuse non-Hodgkin's lymphoma *Journal of Clinical Oncology*, 6, 1118–24.

Pinkerton, C.R., Gerrard, M., Hann, I., Eden, O.B., and Carter, R. (1993). United Kingdom Children's Cancer Study Group (UKCCSG) experience with the French SFOP intensive regimen for advanced B cell lymphoblastic lymphoma. *Medical and Paediatric Oncology*, 21, 532, Abstract.

Prosper, F., Robledo, C., Cuesta, B., Rifon, J., Barbolla, J.R., Parolo J., *et al.* (1994). Incidence of non-Hodgkin's lymphoma in patients treated for Hodgkin's disease, *Lymphoma*, 12, 457–462.

Razzouk, BI., Srinivas, S., Sample, C.E., Singh, V., and Sixbey, J.W. (1996). Epstein-Barr virus DNA recombination and loss in sporadic Burkitt's lymphoma *Journal of Infectious Diseases*, 173:529–35.

Reiter, A., Schrappe, M., Parwaresch, R., Henze, G., Muller-Weihrich, S., Sauter, S., *et al.* (1995). Non-Hodgkin's lymphoma of childhood and adolescence: results of a treatment stratified for biologic subtypes and stage-a report of the Berlin-Frankfurt-Münster Group. *Journal of Clinical Oncology*, 13, 359–72.

Ries LAG, Miller, B.A., Hankey, B.F., Kosary, C.L., Harras, A., Edward's B.K eds (1994). SEER cancer statistics review, 1973–1991: tables and graphs. Bethesda. Md: *National Cancer Institute*. (NIH publication no:94–2789.)

Sandlund, J.T., Pui, C.H., and Roberts, W.M. (1994*a*). Clinicopathologic features and treatment outcome of children with large cell lymphoma and the t(2:5) (p23, q35). *Blood*, 84, 467–71.

Sandlund, J.T., Pui, C.H., Santana, V., Mahmoud, H., Roberts, W.M., Morris, S., *et al.*, (1994*b*). Clinical features and treatment outcome for children with CD30 + large cell non-Hodgkin's lymphoma, *Journal of Clinical Oncology*, 12, 895–8.

Santana, V.M., Abromowitch, M., Sandlund, J.T., Behm, F.G., Ayers, G.D., Robertson, P.K., *et al.* (1993). MACOP-B treatment in children and adolescents with advanced diffuse large-cell non-Hodgkin's lymphoma. *Leukaemia*, 7, (2), 187–191.

Schrappe, M., Reiter, A., Brandt, A., Gadner, H., Muller-Weihrich, S., Genze, G., *et al.* (1993). Childhood Non-Hodgkin's lymphoma of the non-B cell type: Treatment results of three BFM trials. *Medical and Paediatric Oncology*, 21(8):531 A.

Shad, A. and Magrath, I.T. (1997). Malignant non-Hodgkin's lymphomas in children, In Pizzo, P.A., Poplack, D.G eds: Principles and practice of paediatric oncology. 3rd ed. Philadelphia, J.B. Lippincott, pp. 545–587.

Stein, H., Mason, D.Y., Gerdes, J., O'Connor, N., Wainscoat, J., Pallesen, G., *et al.* (1985). The expression of the Hodgkin's disease associated antigen Ki–1 in reactive and neoplastic lymphoid tissue: Evidence that Reed-Sternberg cells and histiocytic malignancies are derived from activated lymphoid cells. *Blood*, 66, 848–58.

Taylor, A.M.R., Metcalfe, J.A., Thick, J., and Mak, Y.F. (1996). Leukaemia and lymphoma in ataxia-telangiectasia, *Blood*, 87, 423–38.

Wollner, N., Exelby, P.R., and Lieberman, P.H. (1979). Non-Hodgkin's lymphoma in children. A progress report on the original patients treated with LSA_2L_2 protocol. *Cancer*, 44, 1990–9.

Ziegler, J.L. (1991). Biologic differences in acquired immune deficiency syndrome-associated non-Hodgkin's lymphoma. *Journal of Clinical Oncology*, 9, 1329–1331.

10 Hodgkin's disease

O. Oberlin

Aetiology, biology, epidemiology, and incidence

Hodgkin, in his first description of the disease subsequently named after him, called it lympho granuloma malignum—a name which remains appropriate (Wallhauser 1933). While the aetiology of Hodgkin's disease remains unknown, the biology of the disease confirms neoplastic behaviour. Cytogenetic studies suggest that the Reed-Sternberg cells represent the malignant cells in Hodgkin's disease. Most authorities believe that this cell comes from activated lymphocytes. With present technical progress in the generation of single cell analysis of Hodgkin/Reed-Sternberg cells, it appears that the majority of these cells may represent a B-cell-derived, monoclonal population (Wolf *et al.* 1996). There are many possible sources of transformation in Hodgkin's cells, including cytogenetic abnormalities, evidence for proto-oncogene involvement, and Epstein-Barr virus (EBV) infection and/or activation. There is now strong evidence linking Hodgkin's disease with Epstein-Barr virus genomes, and gene products can be detected in Reed-Sternberg cells in a proportion of cases. This is approximately 40% in developed countries but much higher in countries such as China, Brazil, Costa Rica, or Kenya (Jarrett *et al.* 1996; Weinreb *et al.* 1996). The heterogeneity of the clinical and histological appearances of Hodgkin's disease and the multitude of different and controversial cellular markers might be explained by the theory that Hodgkin's disease is a group of aetiopathophysiologically associated, but not identical, disease entities. The origin could be the same target cell transformed at different stages of maturation, or, alternatively, several biologically related diseases, each with a different aetiopathogenesis.

The disease has been reported to occur more frequently among young children from developing countries than among those from countries of advanced socioeconomic status. No clear relation exists between Hodgkin's disease and specific HLA histocompatibility antigens; however, there are data demonstrating increased risk of disease among parents and siblings, which may relate to an environmental or genetic influence (Gutensohn and Cole 1981; Grufferman and Delzell 1984).

Age-specific incidence rates reveal a characteristically bimodal curve, with the first peak in the 15–30-year age-range followed by a distinct trough, and a second peak in the 45–55-year group. Thus, children under 15 years of age represent the minority. There is a slight overall male predominance, which decreases with progressive age. Among teenagers and young adults, incidence rates are consistent with secular changes in sociodemographic conditions, suggesting that exposure to infectious agents is involved in the pathogenesis (Glaser and Schwartz 1990).

Diagnosis and pathology

Accurate diagnosis of Hodgkin's disease can be made only by microscopic examination of one or more tissue specimens. It is best to perform an excisional biopsy of an enlarged lymph node. Definitive diagnosis from extranodal tissue, such as lung or bone marrow, is much more difficult. Needle-aspiration biopsy and frozen section material are not optimal for examining the architecture and stromal cellular pattern of a lymph node. Identification of the characteristic Reed-Sternberg cell, a large, multinucleated giant cell with inclusion-like nucleoli, facilitates the diagnosis of Hodgkin's disease. However, the presence of these cells alone does not confirm the histological diagnosis, since cells of similar appearance have been found in reactive processes including infectious mononucleosis, phenytoin-induced pseudolymphoma, rubeola, graft-versus-host disease, and also non-Hodgkin's lymphoma.

The Rye modification of the Lukes-Butler classification divides Hodgkin's disease into four categories: lymphocyte predominance, nodular sclerosis, mixed cellularity, and lymphocyte depletion (Lukes *et al.* 1966). Using this classification, histological subcategorization is age related. The lymphocyte-predominance subtype is seen more commonly in children in the earlier decades, whereas lymphocyte depletion is rare. The majority of children present with nodular-sclerosing or mixed-cellularity subtype, the nodular-sclerosing subtype being most common in the adolescent age-group, and the mixed-cellularity subtype in the prepubertal age-group (Parker *et al.* 1976). Histological subtypes also correlate with certain patterns of disease. The lymphocyte-predominant type is often associated with localized cervical or inguinal-femoral disease, while the nodular-sclerosing subtype commonly presents in the mediastinum. The mixed-cellularity and lymphocyte-depletion subtypes often present with advanced stage of disease.

Clinical presentation and staging

Painless cervical lymphadenopathy is the most common presenting sign in children with Hodgkin's disease, often with a fluctuating course leading to a delay in diagnosis. While 80% of children present with neck disease, only 60% have mediastinal involvement (Donaldson and Kaplan, 1982). Fewer than 5% present with disease limited to the upper cervical lymph nodes, above the level of the hyoid bone (Pao and Kun 1989). The majority of patients presents with supradiaphragmatic disease, although subdiaphragmatic presentation does not indicate an unfavourable prognosis. Some 20–30% of children present with systemic B symptoms, as defined by the Ann Arbor staging criteria of fever over 38°C, drenching night sweats, and an unexplained weight loss of over 10% of body weight at the time of presentation (Carbone *et al.* 1971). The frequency of these symptoms increases with advanced stage of disease. The Ann Arbor staging system is shown in Table 10.1.

Clinical staging involves a careful history and physical examination with special attention to the lymphatic system. If an enlarged lymph node is palpable at a site where involvement would influence staging or treatment, it is a wise policy to biopsy the node to assess involvement. Any suspicious lymph nodes should also be biopsied or treated as if involved. Characteristically, involved lymph nodes are not painful or tender but have a 'rubbery' firmness to palpation, often

Table 10.1   Ann Arbor staging for Hodgkin's disease

Stage I	Involvement of a single lymph-node region (I) or a single extralymphatic organ or site (I_E).
Stage II	Involvement of two or more lymph-node regions on the same side of diaphragm (II) or solitary involvement of an extralymphatic organ or side, and of one or more lymph-node regions on the same side of diaphragm (II_E).
Stage III	Involvement of lymph-node regions on both sides of the diaphragm (III), which may also be accompanied by involvement of spleen (III_S or by solitary involvement of an extralymphatic organ or site (III_E) or both (III_{SE}).
Stage IV	Diffuse or disseminated involvement of one or more extralymphatic organs or tissues, with or without associated lymph node involvement.

The absence or presence of fever over 38°C for 3 consecutive days, drenching night sweats, and unexplained loss of more than 10% of body weight in last 6 months are to be denoted in all cases by the suffix letters A or B, respectively.

with a variable growth rate. Although Waldeyer's ring involvement is infrequent, it may present as asymmetric tonsillar enlargement; thus, examination of the nasopharynx, oropharynx, and hypopharynx is important.

Routine laboratory studies involved in the staging of children should include a complete blood count, erythrocyte sedimentation rate, and liver function studies including alkaline phosphatase. Eosinophilia occurs in approximately 15% of patients, while lymphopaenia, often a sign of advanced disease, is less common. An elevated erythrocyte sedimentation rate is related both to stage and systemic symptoms, and is an important prognostic indicator as well as a useful marker of disease activity (Tubiana *et al.* 1984). The alkaline phosphatase level is a nonspecific indicator of disease activity and is less useful in children than in adults, since it is characteristically elevated as a function of active growth. However, unusually elevated alkaline phosphatase, with or without symptoms of bone pain, is a signal to evaluate the skeletal system by bone scan. Serum copper, also a nonspecific marker of disease activity, is useful as an indicator of relapse (Hrgovic *et al.* 1973), but may also reflect normal hormonal activity in young patients. False-positive evaluations of serum copper have been observed in children with Hodgkin's disease, secondary to inflammatory disease (and in pregnancy or with oral contraceptive medication). Elevated serum levels of interleukin-2 receptor and CD8 antigen correlate with advanced disease, B symptoms, and a poor prognosis (Pui *et al.* 1989).

A chest radiograph (posteroanterior and lateral) is essential in all cases. In addition, thoracic computed tomography (CT) or thoracic magnetic resonance imaging is indicated. A mediastinal mass ratio of greater than one-third the intrathoracic diameter, as evaluated by the plain chest X-ray, is generally considered to represent advanced disease, which is optimally treated more aggressively than is limited disease. The major value of CT is in the detection of subtle mediastinal adenopathy in the child with an apparently normal chest X-ray; it is also of value in the child with obvious intrathoracic disease. In approximately 50% of previously untreated patients, disease including pericardial or chest wall invasion, retrocardiac masses, and pulmonary parenchymal involvement was discovered on thoracic CT after having been previously missed on plain film. (Rostock *et al.* 1983). The value of magnetic resonance imaging in the staging of the chest is being evaluated. It appears to be complementary to CT but of less value in assessing the pulmonary parenchyma than is the thoracic CT. Although mediastinal adenopathy is common, hilar adenopathy is less so and almost never appears in the absence of mediastinal adenopathy. Pulmonary and pleural involvement are also uncommon and almost never occur without mediastinal/hilar disease. Pleural effusions may be commonly seen but are usually secondary to lymphatic obstruction from large, central disease and are rarely cytologically positive for Hodgkin's disease. Children present the unique problem of differentiating the normal thymus gland from thymic infiltration with Hodgkin's disease. Thymic involution secondary to immunosuppressive chemotherapy with subsequent thymic enlargement, following cessation of chemotherapy, has been observed, and may be mistaken for disease progression.

Optimal imaging studies for subdiaphragmatic and retroperitoneal areas have been a matter of controversy for a long time. Lymphography was useful to detect involved retroperitoneal lymph nodes, visualising both size and architecture of these nodes. However, this procedure is technically difficult, requires general anaesthesia in young children, and cannot be performed in patients with massive mediastinal and lung involvement. Abdominopelvic CT scan and ultrasound are easier and less invasive procedures than a lymphogram. At first they appeared complementary to the lymphogram, since they enabled visualization of upper abdominal disease in the coeliac axis-porta hepatis area, which is not well demonstrated by lymphography. The accuracy of current CT scans and ultrasound has progressively improved, and their accuracy has become better than the lymphogram, providing information not only on all the abdominal nodes, but also on the echogenicity of the spleen and of the liver.

Radionuclide studies have limited usefulness in Hodgkin's disease. Routine liver and spleen scans are not useful (Silverman *et al.* 1972). Although gallium scanning is often employed, it has limited accuracy in subdiaphragmatic sites, with true-positive findings (sensitivity) in only approximately 40% of patients (Hagemeister *et al.* 1990). Technetium-99 m bone scanning is helpful in symptomatic children with bone complaints and in those with an unexplained elevation of serum alkaline phosphatase.

Bone marrow biopsies should be performed in all children with systemic symptoms and in those with clinical stage III or IV disease. The bone marrow needle biopsy has a low yield of involvement in children with supradiaphragmatic clinical stage IA and IIA disease. Bone marrow aspiration is not adequate for the staging of Hodgkin's disease and is not an alternative to percutaneous needle or open bone marrow biopsy.

The role of staging laparotomy in children is controversial, largely because of concerns about morbidity or mortality related to an elective, operative procedure and removal of the spleen. Staging laparotomy has been shown to be of value in the accurate staging of the disease (Donaldson *et al.* 1976). Complete clinical staging is accurate in approximately two-thirds of children, while the clinical stage in at least one-third is altered by the findings of surgical staging at laparotomy with splenectomy, most frequently by the findings of occult, splenic disease in the setting of a normal lymphogram, normal abdominal CT scan, and a normal physical examination. The most common sites of subdiaphragmatic disease are the spleen (39%), splenic hilar lymph nodes (28%), coeliac lymph nodes (17%), periportal lymph nodes (15%), and para-aortic lymph nodes (15%) (Green *et al.* 1983).

When staging laparotomy was performed, it included splenectomy, liver biopsy, biopsy of selected nodes of the coeliac axis, porta hepatis, and para-aortic nodes, as well as any lymph nodes that were suspicious, and open bone marrow biopsy. However, this procedure was associated with a risk of short-, medium-, and long-term morbidity. The major short-term problems are wound infections. The major medium-term problems are intestinal obstruction related to adhesions that may require surgical correction. The major long-term problems are overwhelming postsplenectomy infections. The incidence of serious bacterial infection in children with Hodgkin's disease has ranged from 10–13%, with a mortality of up to 5% (Chilcote *et al.* 1976; Donaldson *et al.* 1978). The use of pneumococcal vaccine and prophylactic antibiotics is not sufficient to prevent these infections.

This procedure was the gold standard when radiotherapy was used as a single modality therapy; it was indicated to delineate the radiotherapy volumes. However, this procedure is questionable when other treatment options are chosen. When one considers treatment with chemotherapy alone, accurate evaluation and extent of subdiaphragmatic disease may not be needed. Most investigators now recommend combined modality therapy. In the past, such programmes used chemotherapy with radiotherapy to involved fields as defined by surgical staging (Donaldson and Link 1987; Donaldson *et al.* 1990; Jenkin *et al* 1990). In other series, therapy consisted of multiagent chemotherapy, with radiotherapy limited to areas of known disease at the time of initial staging (Andrieu *et al.* 1981; Oberlin *et al.* 1992). These studies demonstrated that chemotherapy can control radiologically inapparent disease in the vast majority of patients. German investigators have studied the value of pathological staging and laparotomy in a stepwise procedure, routinely using pathological staging in their earlier studies, then restricting splenectomy on the basis of intraoperative findings, before omitting laparotomy and splenectomy in their most recent studies (Schellong *et al.* 1986; Brämswig *et al.* 1990; Schellong *et al.* 1994*b*).

Therapy

Treatment for children with Hodgkin's disease may involve radiotherapy, chemotherapy, or combined modality therapy. Many of the guidelines determined from studies in adults may be applied to children, since young age is a favourable prognostic indicator, and children fare as well as or better than adults. However, when planning treatment programmes for the paediatric population who are undergoing active growth and development at the time of diagnosis and treatment, practical consideration must be given to tissue development and organ function.

Late consequences of treatment

High-dose, large-volume radiotherapy administered to young and prepubescent children is recognized to result in impairment of soft-tissue and bone growth. The growth disturbance is related largely to the age of the child at the time of treatment and the dose of radiation administered. The most marked impairment is observed when radiation doses in excess of 35 Gy are given to children under the age of 13 years (Donaldson and Kaplan 1982). It appears that doses less than 25 Gy do not cause the disproportionate standing- and sitting-height abnormalities seen with higher doses. Thus, a dose of 25 Gy, in fractions of 1.8–2 Gy, may be a threshold beyond which growth retardation is more likely to occur.

Gonadal toxicity in both boys and girls remains a major problem. Pelvic lymph node irradiation is known to carry a high likelihood of ablating ovarian function. The probability of maintaining ovarian function following radiotherapy is directly related to pelvic dose and age at the time of treatment. The younger the girl at the time of treatment, the higher the probability of maintaining regular menses following therapy. Oophoropexy with appropriate shielding at the time of radiotherapy has allowed the preservation of ovarian function, and normal pregnancies after such procedures have been reported. The pregnancies have been uncomplicated, the offspring normal, and there has been no increased fetal wastage or spontaneous abortion.

In contrast to girls, the issue of sterility in boys is of much greater severity and requires longer periods of follow-up for accurate assessment. High doses of irradiation to the pelvis, in a standard inverted-Y field, may be associated with transient oligospermia or azoospermia; however, recovery of function is common (Pedrick and Hoppe 1986). Testicular shields should be routinely used during pelvic radiotherapy, although they are anatomically difficult to use effectively in prepubertal boys. Testicular injury following combination chemotherapy, specifically MOPP, is more complete than that observed following radiotherapy. There are no data to suggest that the prepubertal testis is in any way protected from the testicular injury that is observed among pubertal boys receiving six cycles of MOPP chemotherapy. However, data now suggest potential recovery of spermatogenesis 12–15 years following six cycles of MOPP (mustine, oncovin, prednisone, procarbazine). Recovery is more likely following three or fewer cycles of MOPP as compared with the standard six cycles (Sy Ortin *et al.* 1990). The ABVD (adriamycin, bleomycin, vinblastine, DTIC) combination appears to carry a lower risk of sterility (Santoro *et al.* 1987).

Hypothyroidism, as judged by an elevated level of thyroid-stimulating hormone, is common following mantle irradiation. The incidence of elevated thyroid-stimulating hormone in children with Hodgkin's disease is higher than in adults, suggesting a greater sensitivity of the thyroid among the rapidly growing pre-adolescent or adolescent age-group (Green *et al.* 1980). The risk of hypothyroidism appears related to radiation dose. Among children who receive neck irradiation of up to 26 Gy, the incidence of hypothyrodism is only 17%, as compared to 78% incidence among children who receive doses over 26 Gy. Approximately 36% of children show normalization in biochemical studies and a spontaneous reversal of their thyroid dysfunction (Constine *et al.* 1984). Children who are chemically or clinically hypothyroid are candidates for thyroid replacement therapy, as the long-term effect of unopposed stimulation of the thyroid gland is unknown, and both thyroid adenomas and thyroid carcinomas have been reported among long-term survivors.

Cardiopulmonary complications may be related both to radiotherapy and chemotherapy. Pneumonitis and fibrosis may result from radiation and/or bleomycin, and are dose and volume dependent. While most children are asymptomatic following radiotherapy, echocardiography and pulmonary function or exercise tests reveal that approximately three-quarters have some abnormalities in pulmonary function (Kadota *et al.* 1988). In combined modality programmes, pulmonary dysfunction appears to be related more to the doses of chemotherapy than to radiotherapy (Fryer *et al.* 1990). In the Stanford series of children, who received 15–25 Gy and six cycles of ABVD/MOPP, alterations in pulmonary function were observed in as many as 40% of cases, with abnormalities in diffusing capacity in 55% (Mefferd *et al.* 1989). The Children's Cancer Study Group reported that 9% of children who received 12 courses of ABVD followed by 21 Gy regional radiation developed grade 3 or 4 pulmonary toxicity, largely abnormalities in carbon monoxide diffusing capacity, and that one child died of pulmonary toxicity (Fryer *et al.* 1990). The incidence of pericarditis and pancarditis was reported to be as high as 13% in children during the era when high-dose, large-volume mantle radiotherapy was used (Schellong *et al.* 1994*b*).

However, with the more recent use of low doses of mantle radiation to smaller volumes, radiation-related cardiac injury is much reduced. On the other hand, the addition of adriamycin in the ABVD combination may well enhance cardiac injury. In the Stanford series of children receiving only three cycles of ABVD and low-dose radiation, 14% of asymptomatic children had cardiac abnormalities, demonstrated by cardiac nuclear-gated angiogram testing, at short-term follow-up (Mefferd *et al.* 1989). Longer follow-up is certainly necessary, as premature coronary artery disease with coronary fibrosis and accelerated atherogenesis has been observed in long-term survivors of Hodgkin's disease. The true risk of cardiac and pulmonary injury following current therapy remains unknown.

The second malignant tumours represent a major concern for those who treat children with Hodgkin's disease, most of whom will be successfully treated and will have a very long life span. Large studies on survivors of childhood Hodgkin's disease show that the incidence of any second neoplasm 15 years after the diagnosis is 7–8% (Bhatia *et al.* 1996). The Late Effects Study Group (LESG) followed a cohort of 1380 patients treated for HD between 1955 and 1986, and reported that the risk of leukaemia reaches a plateau at 2.8% at 15 years, while the incidence of solid second tumours continues to rise even 25 years after diagnosis. It also demonstrated that the incidence of leukaemias is related to the doses of alkylating-agent chemotherapy given. All these studies underscore the high risk of developing breast cancer. In the LESG study, the estimated, cumulative probability approached 35% at 40 years of age. Older age (10–16 *vs* < 10 years) and a higher dose of radiation (20–40 Gy *vs* < 20 Gy) were associated with increased risk of breast cancer (Bhatia *et al.* 1996). This calls for adequate surveillance and screening of this very high-risk population.

Psychosocial problems among children with Hodgkin's disease include a decline in energy and sexual activity, perception of impaired body image, work-related problems, and difficulties obtaining health insurance. These problems have received little attention and are extremely important issues to the child who is cured of his/her disease.

Because of the known late effects of both chemotherapy and radiotherapy in children, arguments for the last 15 years have been in favour of single modality treatments to minimize the toxicity of the therapy. The different approaches available are summarized and the advantages of combined modality treatment discussed.

Radiation therapy alone

Even for adults, for whom late effects linked to growth do not occur, the choice between radiation therapy alone or combined with chemotherapy in favourable cases continues to be a point of controversy. Several criteria have been defined as indications for combined modality treatment in adults: massive mediastinal mass, B symptoms, the dissemination of Hodgkin's lymphoma to three or more lymph-node areas, infra-diaphragmatic disease, an elevated erythrocyte sedimentation rate, and mixed cellularity or lymphocyte-depleted subtype. Radiation therapy alone is therefore applicable to only 10–15% of patients. Yet, in this subgroup of patients, laparotomy and splenectomy, in spite of their inherent risks, should be included in the staging procedure to delineate the radiation fields; high doses (40–44 Gy) and extended fields are required. Such factors are the matter for long debate, even with respect to adults and, so far, 22 randomized trials of radiotherapy *versus* radiotherapy plus combination chemotherapy have been conducted worldwide without compellingly establishing the superiority of one approach over another (Specht *et al.* 1992).

Chemotherapy alone

As soon as chemotherapy was shown to be effective, the next question was whether children could be cured without the use of radiation. The rationale for most protocols using chemotherapy alone was always based on the experience of Olweny in Uganda where radiation machines were not available. Actuarial survival rates of 75% and 60% were achieved in stages I and II and in stages III and IV disease, respectively, in a series of 48 children who received six cycles of MOPP alone, without radiation therapy (Olweny *et al.* 1971).

Against this background, several teams opted for chemotherapy alone. In Australia, children with stage I and II received six courses of MOPP, and children with more advanced disease received from 6–12 courses (Ekert *et al.* 1988). In the United Kingdom and in Amsterdam, patients without large mediastinal mass or bulky lymph nodes (< 4 cm) received six cycles of MOPP or ChlVPP (chlorambucil, vinblastine, prednisone, procarbazine) without additional radiotherapy (Behrendt *et al.* 1987; Martin and Radford 1989).

In all these studies, children received at least four and mostly six cycles or more of chemotherapy containing alkylating agents and procarbazine. In both our paediatric and adult experience, six cycles of MOPP induces sterility in more than 90% of the boys, as well as an increased risk of secondary leukaemia that we consider unjustifiable. The Paediatric Oncology Group addressed the question of the efficacy of chemotherapy alone *versus* chemotherapy combined with radiation therapy in a randomized study in advanced stages. Four cycles of MOPP and four cycles of ABVD, with or without 21 Gy total or subtotal nodal irradiation, were given to children with stages IIB, IIIA2, IIIB, and IV. The difference between the event-free free survival of the two schedules was not statistically significant (78.4% without additional radiation therapy and 78.2% with radiation therapy). Survival was comparable in the two groups (94% and 88%, respectively) (Weiner *et al.* 1995).

A randomized study was conducted in stages III and IV disease by the Children's Cancer Study Group. It compared MOPP alternating with ABVD for 12 months to ABVD for 6 months followed by 21 Gy. The event-free survival in the two schedules was similar at 2 years (84.8% and 88.5%) (Fryer *et al.* 1990). The addition of radiotherapy did not seem to offer a significant advantage over chemotherapy alone. However, it is noteworthy that the children treated without radiation therapy in these studies received six, eight, and 12 cycles of chemotherapy alternating MOPP and ABVD which are toxic combinations. The risks of six cycles of MOPP have already been mentioned. Six cycles of ABVD lead to high cumulative doses of adriamycin, (300 mg/m^2) and bleomycin, (120 mg/m^2). These doses account for the very high pulmonary toxicity, with one death reported in the CCSG experience. These results should dissuade physicians from administering so many courses of ABVD in combination with radiation therapy to the mediastinum (Fryer *et al.* 1990). The same remark applies to potential late toxicity of the six cycles of ABVD given in the Dutch study attempting to treat patients with chemotherapy alone in stage I–IV patients (Behrendt *et al.* 1996).

The known late effects of splenectomy, of high-dose radiation therapy, and of high cumulative doses of chemotherapy argue in favour of the wide use of combined modality therapy to treat childhood Hodgkin's disease. Such an approach would enable a gradual decrease of both radiation therapy and chemotherapy.

Combined modality treatment

Using chemotherapy allowed a reduction in the fields and doses of radiation therapy, while the use of radiation therapy made it possible to reduce the duration of chemotherapy and the use of combinations other than MOPP.

Reduced radiation fields

The Hodgkin's Disease Intergroup for Childhood Hodgkin's Disease performed a randomized three arm study in pathologically staged disease. It compared involved-field radiotherapy alone, extended-field radiotherapy, and involved-field radiation given with six cycles of MOPP. The overall survival did not differ significantly between arms, but disease-free survival in the MOPP arm was excellent (93%) and in striking contrast to the results of the other two arms (41% and 67%, respectively). This result showed that with combined radiation therapy and chemotherapy, radiation therapy fields can be limited to involved areas (Gehan *et al.* 1990).

The first paediatric study conducted at Institute Gustav Roussy included 60 children with clinically staged disease. Treatment included involved-field radiation after chemotherapy by MOPP. The disease-free survival rate was 86% and only two relapses occurred outside an irradiated area (Oberlin *et al.* 1992). The Polish paediatric group obtained similar good results for patients treated with involved field radiotherapy after MOPP or B-DOPA (bleomycin, doxorubicin, adriamycin, vincristine, prednisone) (Balwierz *et al.* 1991).

The term 'involved fields' should be clearly defined in each study since this definition may differ from one institution to another or from one group to another. Some investigators give preference to the anatomical definition of separate lymph-node regions adopted for staging purposes at the Rye symposium. Some groups recommend exclusively irradiating the clinically involved nodal areas, ignoring staging definitions.

Reduced radiation doses

The Stanford group pioneered this strategy. Fifty five children were given six MOPP cycles after systematic splenectomy. Radiation doses (ranging from 15–25 Gy) were determined according to the age of the child and response to treatment, and were often supplemented by boosts (Donaldson and Link 1987). Extended-field radiation was given with six MOPP cycles of chemotherapy in the Toronto study. Both series achieved the same excellent results as the previous studies using high-dose radiotherapy, with survival exceeding 90% (Jenkin *et al.* 1990).

Other national studies confirmed the efficacy of such doses on larger groups of patients. The first French study tailored the radiation according to response to primary chemotherapy. At the end of chemotherapy, patients who had achieved a good response (at least 70% regression of initially measurable disease) received 20 Gy. Only 5% of the patients who did not achieve this good response were given 40 Gy. The updated results show that overall survival and disease-free survival rates are, respectively, 93% and 86% at 5 years (Oberlin *et al.* 1992). In the first Italian study, the radiation dose was 20 or 25 Gy (according to the age of the patient) (Vecchi *et al.* 1993). In the German studies, the radiation doses were dependent on the duration of prior chemotherapy: 35 Gy in stages I–IIA after two cycles, 30 Gy in stages IIB–IIIA after four cycles and 25 Gy after six cycles (Schellong *et al.* 1992). These good results demonstrate clearly that a dose of 20 Gy of radiotherapy can be safely used to cure patients after efficient primary chemotherapy.

The follow-up of most of the patient cohorts is not long enough to evaluate the definitive effects of such low-dose radiation. However, our experience of children given 20 Gy at a younger age for a malignancy other than Hodgkin's disease (for instance for a Wilms' tumour) suggests that patients with Hodgkin's disease who have received such a dose will sustain no or mild late effects, and these mild, adverse effects are not comparable to those observed after 40 Gy.

Reducing the duration of chemotherapy

To limit the risk of sterility and secondary acute leukaemias induced by alkylating agents and procarbazine, the next goal was to reduce exposure to MOPP. First, the number of cycles was reduced. Adult patients with stage I and II were randomized to receive three or six cycles of MOPP in a French trial. The results of laparotomy for restaging after MOPP and the disease-free survival were similar in both arms (Fermé *et al.* 1984). The study conducted in children in Villejuif confirmed that six cycles of MOPP were no more effective than three, with a reduction in the cumulative doses of mustine and procarbazine (Oberlin *et al.* 1985).

Chemotherapy other than MOPP

The second strategy for reducing the toxicity of chemotherapy was to use less toxic drugs than those of the MOPP regimen. The ABVD combination was tested as an alternative to MOPP. Once this combination was firmly demonstrated to be effective in patients who had failed with MOPP, alternating cycles of these two regimens (MOPP and ABVD) proved to be the most effective option in advanced disease, and clearly superior to MOPP alone (Bonadonna *et al.* 1989). The Milan team, then the Cancer and Leukaemia Group B, and the EORTC group tested the efficacy of ABVD alone *versus* alternating courses of MOPP and ABVD in advanced stages in adults. They concluded that ABVD was as effective as the alternating regimen (Bonadonna *et al.* 1989; Canellos *et al.* 1992). The only randomized study to be conducted in children was the first French national study that showed that four cycles of ABVD were equivalent to two MOPP plus two ABVD cycles in localized-stage disease (Oberlin *et al.* 1992).

Several other paediatric teams corroborated the efficacy of ABVD alone combined with low-dose radiation therapy in non-randomized studies (The National Italian Group, the Milan paediatric team, and the Children's Cancer Study Group) (Fryer *et al.* 1990, Fossati-Bellani *et al.* 1993, Vecchi *et al.* 1993).

ABVD became an interesting alternative to MOPP since it contains no alkylating agents or procarbazine. However, it consists of drugs known to be potential inducers of lung damage or cardiomyopathy (Mefferd *et al.* 1989).

For this reason, some groups have preferred combinations other than MOPP or AVBD, striving to eliminate both mustine and adriamycin from the chemotherapy regimen.

Up to 1985, the German paediatric group opted for OPPA (vincristine, prednisone, and procarbazine at MOPP doses, combined with adriamycin, 40 mg/m^2 twice) and COPP (cycles comparable to MOPP but with cyclophosphamide replacing mustine). In 1985, this group initiated a study to eliminate procarbazine from the chemotherapy. OPPA became OPA, and methotrexate replaced procarbazine in the COPP combination giving rise to the COMP regimen. Progressions and relapses were significantly higher in advanced stages than in the preceding protocol, so the study was stopped prematurely, on the grounds that a more effective drug was needed to replace procarbazine (Schellong *et al.* 1994*a*).

Active drugs which are non-toxic or have acceptable toxicity are few and far between in Hodgkin's disease. Preliminary data indicated etoposide (VP16) as a potential alternative, and this drug has been included in paediatric studies. For instance, OPPA became OEPA in the German HD90 (Schellong *et al.* 1994*a*), and the Memphis team added VP16 to vinblastine and adriamycin for advanced stages (Hudson *et al.* 1993).

In 1990, the French national group based its new study in stage I and II disease on the 'VBVP' combination consisting of etoposide (100 mg/m^2 for 5 days), bleomycin (10 mg/m^2 day 1), vinblastine (6 mg/m^2 days 1 and 8), and prednisone (40 mg/m^2 for 7 days). All patients with clinical stages I and II are given four cycles of VBVP at 3-weekly intervals, and the subsequent treatment is tailored to fit response to chemotherapy. Additional radiation therapy (20 Gy) is given to good responders after four cycles. Patients not achieving such a good response are given two cycles of OPPA chemotherapy described above. Response to these further two cycles determines the dose of radiation therapy, namely 20 Gy for good responders and 40 Gy for poor responders (Landman-Parker *et al.* 1995). To date, 177 patients have completed their four VBVP cycles; only 29 patients have received additional cycles of OPPA chemotherapy, and seven a 40 Gy dose. The projected 3-year, disease-free and overall survivals are 94% and 97%, respectively. Pending longer follow-up, these results imply that a strategy based on primary response to treatment permits a safe decrease in therapy, and that the majority of the patients can be cured with low-dose radiation therapy after chemotherapy without mustine, procarbazine, and anthracyclines.

We should, however, not underestimate the concern regarding the risk of secondary leukaemias attributed to etoposide. This risk seems to be dose related, and all the reported leukaemias but two have occurred after cumulative doses of more than 4 g/m^2. This dose has never been recommended. The NCI report is not convincing regarding the leukaemogenic effects of VP16 (Smith *et al.* 1993) and, furthermore, this drug has been given in favourable cases to avoid alkylating agents whose leukaemogenic risk is well established. When administered for poor risk disease, VP16 is given in combination with alkylating agents to improve the initial efficacy of chemotherapy.

Poor prognosis Hodgkin's disease in childhood

Stage IV disease has the most dismal outcome. As only 8–16% of children have stage IV disease, the absolute number in published series is often small. The results of several studies demonstrate that these patients fare worse than those with less advanced disease. For instance, the event-free survival of such cases was only 61% in the first French study (Oberlin *et al.* 1992) and 65% in the Toronto study (Jenkin *et al.* 1990). The German group obtained the best results in two consecutive, multicentric studies. They were based on surgical staging and chemotherapy, with two cycles of OPPA and four cycles of COPP, as previously described. Radiation therapy was given to involved nodes (25 Gy) and involved extra lymphatic organs (12–15 Gy).

An SIOP study was initiated in 1987 for stage IV, to attempt to reproduce the good German results internationally, and to limit the radiation dose to 20 Gy after a good response to chemotherapy (Oberlin *et al.* 1993). By December 1994, 97 patients from six countries had been included in the study, and their median follow-up exceeded 4 years. The projected 4-year survival was 95%, and the disease-free survival was 79%, similar to the 81% observed in the previous German studies. These results confirm that OPPA-COPP chemotherapy followed by 20 Gy is a valid therapeutic approach for stage IV in children.

Refractory or relapsed disease is the second group with a poor prognosis. Attempts have been made to improve the efficacy of chemotherapy by incorporating new drugs in standard regimens or dose intensification with stem-cell rescue.

Few cytotoxic drugs offer promising results in advanced Hodgkin's disease. Etoposide, already mentioned, has been included by several teams in third-line therapy after MOPP and anthracycline-containing regimens, with combinations such as MIME (methyl GAG, iphosphamide, methotrexate, and etoposide), MINE (derived from MIME but with an increased dose of iphosphamide and VP16), and vinorelbine (navelbine). Such combinations in disease refractory to standard chemotherapy have yielded response rates of 66% and 75%, respectively (Hagemeister *et al.* 1987, Fermé *et al.* 1995).

Tumour cell relative resistance to cytotoxics can be overcome by administering very high doses of drugs with bone marrow or peripheral stem-cell support. Encouraging results have been obtained in adults with prolonged responses in refractory disease. Experience in children is limited, as the number who enter this high-risk group is small. However, as their outcome is comparable with that of adults, they ought to be treated in the same way (Bessa *et al.* 1993; Williams *et al.* 1993).

In conclusion, the results of recent studies suggest that the cure rate, whose curve was constantly rising between 1960 and 1980, has practically plateaued. Since 1980, efforts have been directed towards curing the disease with minimal morbidity. Combined modality therapy is clearly a strategy allowing the administration of less toxic, shorter chemotherapy and low-dose, limited-field radiation therapy. It will be difficult to drastically improve upon the present situation. The efforts currently deployed to cure patients with chemotherapy without recourse to procarbazine and adriamycin are encouraging in favourable cases.

We hope that during the next decade, progress in the field of biology will help us to understand the aetiology and pathogenesis of Hodgkin's disease and its apparent heterogeneity, and to continue refining therapy for the benefit of each individual patient.

References

Andrieu, J.M. Asselain, B., Bayle, C., Teillet, F., Clot, P., Dana, M., *et al.* (1981). La séquence polychimiothérapie MOPP-Irradiation ganglionnaire sélective dans le traitement de la maladie de Hodgkin, stades cliniques IA-IIIB. *Bull Cancer (Paris)*, 68, 190–199.

Balwierz, W., Armata, J., Moryl-Bujakowska, A., Depowska, T., Najbar, A., Radwanska, U., *et al.* (1991). Chemotherapy combined with involved field radiotherapy for 177 children with Hodgkin's disease treated in 1983–1987. *Acta Paediatr Jpn*, 33, 703–8.

Behrendt, H., van Bunningen, B., and van Leeuwen, E.F. (1987). Treatment of HD in children without radiotherapy. *Cancer*, 59, 1870–1873.

Behrendt, H., Brinkhuis, M., and Van Leeuwen, E.F. (1996). Treatment of childhood Hodgkin's disease with ABVD without radiotherapy. *Medical and Paediatric Oncology*, 26, 244–247.

Bessa, E., Pacquement, H., Hartmann, O., Poulvier, E., Bordigoni, P., Bertrand, Y., *et al.*, (1993). Long term survival of refractory or relapsed Hodgkin's disease treated by high dose chemotherapy with hematopoietic support. *Medical and Paediatric Oncology*, 21, 84.

Bhatia, S., Robison, L.L., Oberlin, O., Greenberg, M., Bunin, G., Fossati-Bellani, F., *et al.* (1996). Breast cancer and other second neoplasms after childhood Hodgkin's disease. *New England Journal of Medicine*, 21.334, 745–751.

Bonadonna, G., Valagussa, P., Santoro, A., Viviani, S., Bonfante, V., and Banfi, A. (1989). Hodgkin's disease: the Milan Cancer Institute experience with MOPP and AVBD. *Recent Results Cancer Research*, 117, 169–174.

Brämswig, J.H., Hornig-Franz, I., Riepenhausen, M., and Schellong, G. (1990). The challenge of paediatric Hodgkin's disease-where is the balance between cure and long-term toxicity? *Leukaemia and Lymphoma*, 3, 183–193.

Canellos, P.G., Anderson, J.R., Katheleen, J.P. Propert, K.J., Nissen, N., Cooper, M.R., *et al.* (1992). Chemotherapy of advanced Hodgkin's disease with MOPP, ABVD or MOPP alternating with ABVD. *New England Journal of Medicine*, 327, 1478–1484.

Carbone, P., Kaplan, H.S., Musshoff, K., Smithers, D.W., and Tubiana, M. (1971). Report of the Committee on Hodgkin's Disease Staging Classification. *Cancer Research*, 31, 1860–1861.

Chilcote, R.R., Baehner, R.L., and Hammond, D. Children's Cancer Study Group (1976). Septicemia and meningitis in children splenectomized for Hodgkin's disease. *New England Journal of Medicine*, 295, 798–800.

Constine, L.S., Donaldson, S.S., McDougall, I.R., Cox, R.S., Link, M.P., and Kaplan, H.S. (1984). Thyroid dysfunction after radiotherapy in children with Hodgkin's disease. *Cancer*, 53, 878–883.

Donaldson, S.S. and Kaplan, H.S. (1982). Complications of treatment of Hodgkin's disease in children. *Cancer Treatment Reports*, 66, 977–989.

Donaldson, S.S., and Link, M.P. (1987). Combined modality treatment with low-dose radiation and MOPP chemotherapy for children with Hodgkin's disease. *Journal of Clinical Oncology*, 5, 742–749.

Donaldson, S.S., Glatstein, E., Rosenberg, S.A., and Kaplan, H.S. (1976). Paediatric Hodgkin's disease. II. Results of therapy. *Cancer*, 37, 2436–2447.

Donaldson, S.S., Glatstein, E., and Vosti, K.L. (1978). Bacterial infections in paediatric Hodgkin's disease: relationship to radiotherapy, chemotherapy, and splenectomy. *Cancer*, 41, 1949–1958.

Donaldson, S.S., Whitaker, S.J., Plowman, P.N., Link, M.P., and Malpas, J.S. (1990). Stage I-II paediatric Hodgkin's disease: long-term follow-up demonstrates equivalent survival rates following different management schemes. *Journal of Clinical Oncology*, 8, 1128–1137.

Ekert, H., Waters, K.D., Smith, P.F., Toogood, I., and Mauger, D. (1988). Treatment with MOPP or CHIVPP chemotherapy only for all stages of childhood Hodgkin's disease. *Journal of Clinical Oncology*, 6, 1845–1850.

Fermé, C., Teillet, F., d'Agay, M.F., Gisselbrecht, C., Marty, M., and Boiron, M. (1984). Combined modality in Hodgkin's disease. Comparison of six versus three courses of MOPP with clinical and surgical restaging. *Cancer*, 54, 2324–2329.

Fermé, C., Bastion, Y., Lepage, E., Berger, F., Brice, P., Morel, P., *et al.* (1995). The MINE regimen as intensive salvage chemotherapy for relapsed and refractory Hodgkin's disease. *Annals of Oncology*, 6, 543–549.

Fossati-Bellani, F., Gasparini, M., Ballerini, E., Cefalo, G., Giadani, R., Pizzeti, P., *et al.* (1993). ABVD and limited field radiotherapy in 85 consecutive children with stage I-III Hodgkin's disease. Abstract, *Medical and Paediatric Oncology*, 21, 543.

Fryer, C.J., Hutchinson, R.J., Krailo, M., Collins, R.D., Constine, L.S., Hays, D.M., *et al.* (1990). Efficacy and toxicity of 12 courses of ABVD chemotherapy followed by low-dose regional radiation in advanced Hodgkin's disease in children: a report from the Children's Cancer Study Group. *Journal of Clinical Oncology*, 8, 1971–1980.

Gehan, E.A., Sullivan, M.P., Fuller, L.M., Johnston, B.A., Kennedy, P., Fryer, C., *et al.* (1990). The Intergroup Hodgkin's Disease in Children. A study of stages I and II. *Cancer*, 65, 1429–1437.

Glaser, S.L. and Schwartz, W.G. (1990). Time trends in Hodgkin's disease incidence. The role of diagnostic accuracy. *Cancer*, 66, 2196–2204.

Green, D.M., Brecher, M.L., Yakar, D., Blumenson, L.E., Lindsay, A.N., Voorhess, M.L., *et al.* (1980). Thyroid function in paediatric patients after neck irradiation for Hodgkin's disease. *Medical Paediatric Oncology*, 8, 127–136.

Green, D.M., Ghoorah, J., Douglass, H.O., Allen, J.E., Berjian, R.J., Jewett, T.C., *et al.* (1983). Staging laparotomy with splenectomy in children and adolescents with Hodgkin's disease. *Cancer Treatment Review*, 10, 23–38.

Grufferman, S.L. and Delzell, E. (1984). Epidemiology of Hodgkin's disease. *Epidemiology Review*, 6, 76–106.

Gutensohn, N. and Cole, P. (1981). Childhood social environment and Hodgkin's disease. *New England Journal of Medicine*, 304, 135–140.

Hagemeister, F.B., Tannir, N., McLaughlin, P., Salvador, P., Riggs, S., Velasquez, W.S., *et al.* (1987). MIME (Methyl GAG, iphosphamide, methotrexate, etoposide) chemotherapy as treatment for recurrent Hodgkin's disease. *Journal of Clinical Oncology*, 5, 556–561.

Hagemeister, F.B., Fesus, S.M., Lamki, L.M., and Haynie, T.P. (1990). Role of the gallium scan in Hodgkin's disease. *Cancer*, 65, 1090–1096.

Hrgovic, M., Tessmer, C.F., Thomas, F.B., Fuller, L.M., Gamble, J.F., and Shullenberger, C.C. (1973). Significance of serum copper in adult patients with Hodgkin's disease. *Cancer*, 31, 1337–1345.

Hudson, M.M., Weinstein, H.J., Donaldson, S.S., Greenwald, C., Kun, L., Tarbell, N.J., *et al.* (1993). Acute hypersensitivity reactions to etoposide in a VEPA regimen for Hodgkin's disease. *Journal of Clinical Oncology*, 11, 1080–1084.

Jarrett, A.F., Armstrong, A.A., and Alexander, E. (1996). Epidemiology of EBV and Hodgkin's lymphoma. *Annals of Oncology*, 7, (suppl. 4) 5–10.

Jenkin, D., Doyle, J., Berry, M., Blanchette, V., Chan, H., Doherty, M., *et al.* (1990). Hodgkin's disease in children: treatment with MOPP and low-dose, extended field irradiation without laparotomy. Late results and toxicity. *Medical Paediatric Oncology*, 18, 265–272.

Kadota, R.P., Burgert, E.O., Driscoll, D.J., Evans, R.G., and Gilchrist, G.S. (1988). Cardiopulmonary function in long-term survivors of childhood Hodgkin's lymphoma: a pilot study. Mayo *Clin Proc*, 63, 362–367.

Landman-Parker, J., Oberlin, O., Pacquement, H., Robert, A., Coze, C., Thuret, I., *et al.* (1995). Localized Hodgkin's disease: chemotherapy regimen with VP16, Bleomycin, Vinblastine and Prednisone before Low-dose radiation therapy. Results of the study by the French Society of Paediatric Oncology. Abstract Third International Symposium on Hodgkin's lymphoma. Cologne, 188.

Lukes, R.J., Craver, L.F., Hall, T.C., Rappaport, H., and Rubin, P. (1966). Report of the Nomenclature Committee. *Cancer Research*, 26, 1311.

Martin, J. and Radford, M. (1989). Current practice in Hodgkin's disease. The United Kingdom Children's Cancer Study Group. In: Kamps WA, Humphrey GB, Poppema S (eds) Hodgkin's disease in children: controversies and current practice. Kluwer, Boston, pp 263–275.

Mefferd, J., Donaldson, S.S., and Link, M.P. (1989), Paediatric Hodgkin's disease: pulmonary, cardiac, and thyroid function following combined modality therapy. *International Journal of Radiation Oncology, Biology and Physics*, 16, 679–685.

Oberlin, O., Boilletot, A., Leverger, G., Sarrazin, D., and Lemerle, J. (1985). Clinical staging, primary chemotherapy and involved field radiotherapy in childhood Hodgkin's disease. *European Paediatric Hematology and Oncology*, 2, 65–70.

Oberlin, O., Leverger, G., Pacquement, H., Raquin, M.A., Chompret, A., Habrand, J.L., *et al.* (1992). Low-dose radiation therapy and reduced chemotherapy in childhood Hodgkin's disease. The experience of the French Society of Paediatric Oncology. *Journal of Clinical Oncology*, 10, 1602–8.

Oberlin, O., Hörnig-Franz, I., Pacquement, H., Vecchi, V., Lacombe, M.J., Wagner, H.P., *et al.* for the SIOP Hodgkin's Disease Study Group. (1993). Stage IV Hodgkin's disease: results of the study of the International Society of Paediatric Oncology. Abstract Fifth International conference on malignant lymphoma, Lugano: 71.

Olweny, C.L., Katongole-Mbidde, E., and Kilre, C. (1971). Childhood Hodgkin's disease in Uganda. *Cancer*, 27, 1295–1301.

Pao, W.J. and Kun, L.E. (1989). Hodgkin's disease in children. *Hematol Oncol Clin North Am*, 3, 345–365.

Parker, B.R., Castellino, R.A., and Kaplan, H.S. (1976). Paediatric Hodgkin's disease. I. Radiographic evaluation. *Cancer*, 37, 2430–2435.

Pedrick, T.J. and Hoppe, R.T. (1986). Recovery of spermatogenesis following pelvic irradiation for Hodgkin's disease. *International Journal of Radiation Oncology, Biology and Physics*, 12, 117–121.

Pui, C.H., Ip, S.H., Thompson, E., Dodge, R.K., Brown, M., Wilimas, J., *et al.* (1989). Increased serum CD8 antigen level in childhood Hodgkin's disease relates to advanced stage and poor treatment outcome. *Blood*, 73, 209–213.

Rostock, R.A., Siegelman, S.S., Lenhard, R.E., Wharam, M.D., and Order, S.E. (1983), Thoracic CT scanning for mediastinal Hodgkin's disease; results and therapeutic implications. *International Journal of Radiation Oncology, Biology and Physics*, 9, 1451–1457.

Santoro, A., Bonadonna, G., Valagussa, P., Zucali, R., Viviani, S., Villani, F., *et al.* (1987). Long term results of combined chemotherapy-radiotherapy approach in Hodgkin's disease. Superiority of ABVD plus radiotherapy versus MOPP plus radiotherapy. *Journal of Clinical Oncology*, 5, 27–37.

Schellong, G., Waubke-Landwehr, A.K., Langermann, H.J., Riehm, H.J., Brämswig, J. and Ritter, J. (1986). Prediction of splenic involvement in children with Hodgkin's disease: significance of clinical and intraoperative findings–a retrospective statistical analysis of 154 patients in the German therapy study DAL-HD-78. *Cancer*, 57, 2049–2056.

Schellong, G., Brämswig, J.H., and Hörnig-Franz, I. (1992). Treatment of children with Hodgkin's disease. Results of the German Paediatric Oncology Group. *Annals of Oncology*, 3, 73–76.

Schellong, G., Hörnig-Franz, I., and Rath, B. OEPA versus OPPA in combined modality treatment of Hodgkin's disease. Preliminary results of the German-Austrian multicentric trial DAL HD 90 (1994*a*). *Medical and Paediatric Oncology*, 23, 61.

Schellong, G., Hornig-Franz, I., Rath, B., Ritter, J., Riepenhausen, M., Kabisch, H., *et al.* (1994*b*). Reducing radiation dosage to 20–30 Gy in combined chemo-/radiotherapy of Hodgkin's disease in childhood. A report of the cooperative DAL-HD-87 therapy study. *Klin Padiatr*, 206, 253–262.

Schellong, G., Brämswig, J.H., Hörnig-Franz, I., Schwarze, E.W., Potter, R., and Wannenmacher, M. (1994*c*). Hodgkin's disease in children: combined modality treatment for stages IA, IB and IIA. Results in 356 patients of the German/Austrian Paediatric Study Group. *Annals of Oncology*, 5, 113–115.

Silverman, S., DeNardo, G.L., Glatstein, E., and Lipton, M.J. (1972). Evaluation of the liver and spleen in Hodgkin's disease. II. The value of splenic scintigraphy. *American Journal of Medicine*, 52, 362–366.

Smith, M.A., Rubinstein, L., Cazenave, R.S., Cazenave, L., Ungerleider, R.S., Maurer, H.M., *et al.* (1993). Report of the Cancer Therapy Evaluation Program monitoring plan for secondary acute myeloid leukemia following treatment with epipodophyllotoxins. *Journal of the National Cancer Institute*, 85, 554–558.

Specht, L., Carde, P., Mauch, P., and Magrini, S.T. (1992). Radiotherapy versus combined modality in early stages. *Annals of Oncology*, 3, 77–81.

Sy Ortin, T.T., Shostak, C.A., and Donaldson, S.S. (1990). Gonadal status and reproductive function following treatment for Hodgkin's disease in childhood: the Stanford experience. *International Journal of Radiation Oncology, Biology and Physics*, 19, 873–880.

Tubiana, M., Henry-Amar, M., Burgers, M.V., Van Der Werf-Messing, B., and Hayat, M. (1984). Prognostic significance of ESR in clinical stages I and II Hodgkin's disease. *Journal of Clinical Oncology*, 2, 194–200.

Vecchi, V., Pileri, S., Burneli, R., Bontemri, N., Comelli, A., Testi, A.M., *et al.*, (1993). Treatment of paediatric Hodgkin's disease tailored to stage, mediastinal mass and age. *Cancer*, 72, 2049–57.

Wallhauser, A. (1933). Hodgkin's disease. *Arch Path*, 16, 522–562; 672–712.

Weiner, M., Leventhal, B., Brecher, M., Marcus, R., Cantor, A., Ternberg, J., *et al.* (1995). A randomized study of intensive MOPP-ABVD ± low dose total nodal irradiation therapy in the treatment of stages IIB, IIIA2, IIIB, IV Hodgkin's disease: a Paediatric Oncology Group Study. *Proc Am Soc Clin Oncol*, 14, 40.

Weinreb, M., Day, P.J., Niggli, F., Powell, J.E., Raafat, F., Hesseling, P.B., *et al.* (1996). The role of Epstein-Barr virus in Hodgkin's disease from different geographical areas. *Arch Dis Child*, 74, 27–31.

Williams, C.D., Goldstone, A.H., Pearce, R., Green, S., Armitage, J.O., Carella, A., *et al.* (1993). Autologous bone marrow transplantation for paediatric Hodgkin's disease: a case-matched comparison with adult patients by the European Bone Marrow Transplant Group Lymphoma Registry. *Journal of Clinical Oncology*, 11, 2243–2249.

Wolf, J., Bohlen, H., and Diehl, V. (1996). Report on the workshop on biology in the third international symposium on Hodgkin's lymphoma in Cologne 1995. *Annals of Oncology*, 7, (suppl.4), 45–47.

11 Langerhans cell histiocytosis

H. Gadner and N. Grois

Langerhans cell histiocytosis (LCH) is a proliferative process characterized by an accumulation of dendritic cells with epidermal Langerhans cell (LC) phenotype in various tissues and organs. The disease may involve a variety of clinical entities ranging from a spontaneously regressing solitary bone lesion to a widespread, life-threatening disorder. In the literature, a broad spectrum of synonyms has been used, including 'histiocytosis X', 'eosinophilic granuloma', Hand-Schueller-Christian disease', 'Abt-Letterer-Siwe disease', 'self-healing reticulohistiocytosis', etc. Since it became evident that the lesional cells are LCs, the disease has been called LCH (see Table 11.1) (Writing Group of the Histiocyte Society 1987).

Incidence and epidemiology

LCH can present at any age ranging from birth to adulthood. Predominantly young children between 1–3 years are affected. The incidence is approximately 0.2–1.0 per 100 000 children per year (median 0.4 per 100 000) with males outnumbering females (Carstensen and Ornvold 1993). More than one-third of children—especially those under 2 years—are prone to 'multisystem' disease with 'organ dysfunction' (Lahey 1975).

The disease is essentially sporadic, and has been reported rarely in twins and certain kindreds. In adults, there is some evidence that cigarette smoking plays a key role in the development of pulmonary disease. Other data regarding epidemiological aspects are not conclusive.

Aetiology and pathogenesis

The aetiology of LCH is still unknown, and the pathogenesis not understood. The disease is widely accepted to be a reactive process rather than a malignancy, although a clonal origin of the lesional LC was found recently (Willman 1994). Pathophysiologically, a deficiency of the intercellular communication between T-cells and LCs is suspected. It has been postulated that either an atypical immunological response, a reactive process following viral infection, or a dysequilibrium of cytokines may be involved in the disease.

Table 11.1 Classification of histiocytosis syndromes

Class I	**Dendritic-cell-related**
	Langerhans cell histiocytosis
	Secondary dendritic cell processes
	Juvenile xanthogranuloma
	Solitary dendritic histiocytoma
Class II	**Macrophage-related**
	Haemophagocytic lymphohistiocytosis
	Primary: familial
	sporadic
	Secondary: infection-associated
	malignancy-associated
	other
	Rosai–Dorfman disease (Sinus histiocytosis with massive lymphadenopathy)
	Multicentric reticulohistiocytosis, often arthritis-associated
Class III	**Malignant disorders**

(Source: Farera *et al.* 1997)

Pathology

The LCH lesions consist of an aggregation of dendritic cells of Langerhans type with a variable admixture of other cells (eosinophils, neutrophils, lymphocytes, fibroblasts, and multinucleated giant cells) forming granulomas with proliferative and locally destructive behaviour. These granulomas initially have a high cellular content, which decreases gradually resulting in a xanthomatous and fibrotic pattern. The typical LC is a 'histiocytic' cell with abundant, homogeneous, pink cytoplasm in haematoxylin-eosin stained sections, and a lobulated, 'coffee-bean'-like nucleus. These cells express a number of phenotypic markers, which can be demonstrated by immunohistochemistry and electron microscopy (Chu and Jaffe 1994; Favara and Jaffe 1994). The most important are class II MHC (mixed histocompatibility complex) molecules and the CD1a complex. In addition, the Birbeck granule, detectable in the cytoplasm by electron microscopy, is specific for LCs. LCH cells also produce a wide variety of cytokines. Many of them may be implicated in the organ damage seen in this disease (e.g. fibrosis in the lungs and liver, gliosis in the brain).

To avoid difficulties in distinguishing LCH from other histiocytosis syndromes, the histopathological diagnosis of LCH is based on different confidence levels (see Table 11.2) (Writing Group of the Histiocyte Society 1987). The definitive diagnosis can be proven only by conventional light microscopy with the addition of immunohistochemical detection of CD1a epitopes on the cell surface and/or demonstration of Birbeck granules in the cytoplasm by electron microscopy.

Table 11.2 Histopathological diagnosis of LCH

Level of confidence	Based on
Presumptive diagnosis	Conventional histology
Designated diagnosis	Conventional histology plus positive staining for two or more: ATPase, S100 protein, alpha-D-mannosidase, Peanut agglutinin
Definitive diagnosis	Conventional histology plus Birbeck granules (ELM) or CD1a staining

(Source: Writing Group of the Histiocyte Society 1987)

Clinical presentation

The clinical presentation of LCH is highly variable. Almost every organ in the body can be affected. According to the number of organs and systems involved, we discriminate between 'single' and 'multisystem' disease (see Table 11.3). Symptoms and signs vary considerably and depend on the localization and extent of the disease (Gadner and Grois 1993; Broadbent *et al.* 1994; Egeler and Nesbit 1995). In older children, 'single system' disease, characterized by local swelling, pain, and functional impairment and usually affecting bone, is commonly found. Infants most frequently present with 'multisystem' disease, often with 'organ dysfunction' (see Table 11.4) and very pronounced general symptoms like pain, irritability, skin rash, weight loss, failure to thrive, and fever. Various combinations of involvement of bone, soft tissue, skin, liver, spleen, lungs, bone marrow, lymph nodes, and central nervous system are seen.

Bone and soft tissue involvement

The organ most frequently involved in 'single' and 'multisystem' disease is the skeleton (see Table 11.5). The skull is most commonly affected, followed by lesions in the mastoid or petrous

Table 11.3 Stratification of LCH

Single system disease
    Single site: single bone lesion
                    isolated skin disease
                    solitary lymph-node involvement
    Multiple site: multiple bone lesions
                    multiple lymph-node involvement
Multisystem disease
    Multiple organ involvement (with or without organ dysfunction)

(Source: Consensus of the Histiocyte Society 1991)

Table 11.4   Organ dysfunction criteria

Liver dysfunction
 hypoproteinaemia (total protein < 5.5 g dl^{-1}) and/or
 hypoalbuminaemia (< 2.5 g dl^{-1})
 oedema, ascites
 hyperbilirubinaemia (> 1.5 g dl^{-1})
 coagulopathy (PT < 50%)

Lung dysfunction
 tachypnoea and/or dyspnoea, cyanosis, cough
 pneumothorax, pleural effusion

Haemopoietic dysfunction
 anaemia (Hb < 10 g dl^{-1}, not caused by iron deficiency or infection)
 leukopaenia (< 4.0 × 10^9 l^{-1}), granulocytopaenia (< 1.5 × 10^9 l^{-1}),
  thrombocytopaenia (< 100 × 10^9 l^{-1})

(Source: modified according to Lahey 1975; PT, thromboplastin time)

Table 11.5   Organ involvement in LCH (275 patients)

Organ	Involvement (%)
Bone	79
Skin	25
Liver	11
Spleen	9
Ears	8
Lungs	6
Diabetes insipidus	6
Gastrointestinal mucosa	5
Endocrinopathies	3
Eyes	2

(Source: DAL HX-83/90 studies)

bone, and in the periorbital region (leading to proptosis due to adjacent soft tissue swelling). Jaw lesions may provoke premature eruption and loss of 'floating' milk teeth. Frequently, long bones, pelvic bones, and ribs are affected. Spinal cord compression may be a rare complication of vertebral destruction.

Bone lesions present on X-ray as typical, well defined osteolytic areas, surrounded by a 'halo' of sclerosis if the healing process has started, and sometimes excessive periostial reaction. For the detection of bone lesions, a skeletal survey is better than a bone scan (Parker *et al.* 1980). Soft tissue swelling adjacent to a bone lesion, caused by extension of the granuloma or by local oedema, is a common finding and is usually not considered as a separate organ involvement. An isolated granuloma in the soft tissue is found only rarely.

Skin lesions

The cutaneous eruptions largely resemble seborrhoeic or atopic dematitis. Skin rash may be the only manifestation in infants or can occur as part of a 'multisystem' disease. Areas of predilection are the trunk, abdomen, and scalp, showing scattered pinkish-brown papules, often covered by a scale. Especially in the intertriginous regions, the eruptions tend to become erosive and crusted, sometimes forming ulcers and granulomas, e.g. groin, perianal, axillary or neck folds, and retroauricular (Gadner and Grois 1993). Skin rash in the aural canal may cause otitis externa. This aural discharge may be difficult to distinguish from the secretion related to a bone lesion with tissue extension into the ear canal. A particular form of a purely cutaneous manifestation in neonates is the 'congenital self-healing reticulohistiocytosis', with numerous firm skin nodules of a brownish-red colour scattered over the trunk, head, palms, and soles with spontaneous regression within 6 months (Hashimoto and Pritzker 1973).

Lymphohaematopoietic system

Lymph node involvement is seen frequently in LCH, either adjacent to bone or skin manifestations, or as part of 'multisystem' disease. Most commonly, cervical lymph nodes and nodes in the mediastinum and abdomen are affected, sometimes reaching considerable size. Waldeyer's ring involvement and obstruction of the superior vena cava by lymph nodes have been reported. Thymic enlargement may occasionally be seen on chest X-ray. Morphological changes in the thymic tissue without organ enlargement are also reported, especially in those patients who died of disease. Various immunological changes, including reversal of the CD4/CD8 ratio, have been described in patients with LCH (Osband *et al.* 1981).

LCs do not normally appear in bone marrow. In 'multisystem' disease, however, diffuse infiltration and clustering of LCH cells (together with haemophagocytic macrophages) may be detected. Severe pancytopaenia, frequently observed in young infants, is usually associated with huge hepatosplenomegaly, and is related to bone marrow 'dysfunction' rather than infiltration (McClain *et al.* 1983). In contrast, in cases with mild anaemia, the differential diagnoses of iron deficiency or malabsorption related to occult gut disease have to be considered.

Liver and spleen

Hepatosplenomegaly is common in 'multisystem' disease, often associated with functional impairment. Ascites and oedema due to hypoalbuminaemia, which may be associated with hypocoagulopathy (prolonged prothrombin time/partial thromboplastin time) or hyperbilirubinaemia, are typical signs of liver 'dysfunction' (Lahey 1975) (see Table 11.4). Due to the LCH cell infiltration in the periportal area, the disease can progress from mild cholestasis to severe liver failure with fibrosis or even biliary cirrhosis. The histological picture can resemble sclerosing cholangitis resulting from Kupffer-cell hypertrophy, and hyperplasia due to an activation of the cellular immune system, caused by cytokine release (Favara and Jaffe 1994). Enlargement of the spleen is a typical sign of 'multisystem' disease in very young children, and may be an additional factor responsible for pancytopaenia.

Pulmonary disease

Lung involvement in LCH is usually part of 'multisystem' disease and can occur at any age. Often the diagnosis is suspected when a chest X-ray shows a typical, micronodular, interstitial shadowing. On CT scanning, there may be nodules and cystic lesions. With time, these cysts increase in number and size and form 'honeycomb lungs'. A rupture of such a bulla may result in a pneumothorax (Favara and Jaffe 1987). The prominent clinical sign is tachypnoea with sub-costal retraction. Respiratory function tests typically show a decreased total lung volume and compliance. For confirmation of the diagnosis, the finding of LCH cells on biopsy or in the alve-olar fluid obtained by bronchoalveolar lavage (more than 5% CD1a positive cells) is required (Auerswald *et al.* 1991).

Mucous membranes and gastrointestinal tract

Mucous membrane lesions may affect the buccal mucosa, gingiva, and palate, as well as the anal and perianal area, or the vulvar and vaginal region. The localized or disseminated lesions present as whitish, granulomatous plaques with a tendency to transform into ulcers and to bleed.

The frequency of gastrointestinal involvement is often underestimated, because it does not lead to specific clinical symptoms. The most prominent sign is chronic diarrhoea or failure to thrive due to malabsorption caused by LCH infiltration of the mucosa and submucosa, most often occurring in the colon (Egeler *et al.* 1990). The diagnosis should be proven by endoscopic biopsy.

Endocrine system

Diabetes insipidus (DI) is the most common endocrinopathy in LCH. It may appear before, at the same time, or after the disease presents in other organs. Often, DI can be found in patients with bone disease affecting the skull, and in patients with 'multisystem' disease. The diagnosis must be confirmed by an appropriate water deprivation test and, if available, measurement of urinary arginine vasopressin levels (Dunger *et al.* 1989). Gadolinium-enhanced magnetic resonance imaging (MRI) is the method of choice to demonstrate the typical morphological changes. These are thickening of the pituitary stalk (> 2.5 mm) and loss of the posterior, pituitary 'bright' signal in T1-weighted images (Rosenfield *et al.* 1990).

Growth failure in children with LCH is commonly reported, and its cause appears to be multi-factorial (Braunstein and Kohler 1981; Dean *et al.* 1986). Compromised, anterior pituitary func-tion with growth hormone deficiency, hypogonadism, and hyperprolactinaemia is described in only a few cases. Panhypopituitarism may occur in cases with a hypothalamic mass. Occult gut involvement with malabsorption, vertebral collapse, prolonged steroid therapy, and persistent cytokine release in chronic, 'multisystem' disease may also have some importance.

Central nervous system

CNS problems in patients with LCH, other than DI and anterior pituitary disease, are enigmatic and rare. Symptoms may occur in all age-groups, particularly in patients with multiple organ involvement. They may occur years before, but more often years after, the initial diagnosis of LCH. In order of frequency the following localizations have been observed: cerebellum, pons, cerebral hemispheres, choroid plexus, basal ganglia, spinal cord, optic tract, and nerves. A classification system describing several subtypes of changes seen by MRI techniques distinguishes between white matter and grey matter lesions, with and without gadolinium enhancement and choroid plexus or dural-based lesions. Biopsy of the affected areas may show histiocytic infiltrate, with a xanthomatous character, or degenerative changes with gliosis (Grois *et al.* 1994).

Neurological symptoms range from discrete intellectual and behavioural changes, or subtle hypo- or hyperreflexia, to severe ataxia, tremor, dysarthria, nystagmus, blurred vision, and cranial nerve deficits, eventually leading to fatal CNS degeneration despite various treatment approaches (Grois *et al.* 1993).

Permanent consequences

Permanent consequences are disease-linked, long-term disabilities in patients with LCH (Gadner *et al.* 1994). In 'single system' disease, with its excellent prognosis, long-term effects are usually minimal. In contrast, patients with 'multisystem' disease, particularly if the disease course is undulating and refractory, show an overall incidence of late sequelae in more than 50% of survivors (Komp *et al.* 1980). In more than half of these patients, permanent consequences linked to the initial presentation of LCH are present at diagnosis, and in the majority of patients they are clearly related to the disease location and activity (Gadner *et al.* 1994). Most common permanent consequences are: small stature, growth hormone deficiency, diabetes insipidus, partial deafness, cerebellar ataxia, loss of dentition, orthopaedic problems, pulmonary fibrosis, and biliary cirrhosis with portal hypertension (see Table 11.6). Furthermore, in 5% of long-term survivors, the development of a malignancy is reported (Greenberger *et al.* 1981). The recognition of a high

Table 11.6 Permanent consequences in 35/106 patients with disseminated disease

	Present at diagnosis n = 19 (18%)	Developing after diagnosis n = 22 (21%)	Total n = 35 (33%)
Diabetes insipidus	6	10	16
Orthopaedic disabilities	8	4	12
Growth failure	4	4	8
Anterior pituitary dysfunction	3	5	8
Hearing impairment	4	1	5
Liver fibrosis	0	3	3
Lung fibrosis	0	2	2
Tooth loss	1	1	2
Goitre	0	1	1
Psychomotor retardation	0	1	1

(Source: Gadner *et al.* 1994)

association of malignancy and LCH, even without any treatment and frequently preceding the diagnosis of LCH (Egeler *et al.* 1993), makes the interpretation of this data difficult, and the concern regarding the prolonged use of high doses of potentially carcinogenic drugs is warranted (Gadner *et al.* 1994).

Diagnostic procedures

A biopsy is essential to obtain a definitive diagnosis of LCH. The Writing Group of the Histiocyte Society outlined a classification of histiocytosis syndromes and standards for histopathological diagnosis which have been widely accepted (Writing Group of the Histiocyte Society 1987). According to this proposal, morphological, immunohistochemical, and clinical criteria are required for the definitive diagnosis (see Tables 11.1 and 11.2).

In a rare disease like LCH, with a highly variable clinical presentation, it is crucial to use uniform guidelines for clinical evaluation and assessment of disease extent. Based on an accurate history and meticulous clinical examination, mandatory, baseline investigations should be performed uniformly in every newly diagnosed patient (see Table 11.7a) and, in selected cases, other specific diagnostic procedures are required (see Table 11.7b) (Writing Group of the Histiocyte Society 1989).

Differential diagnosis

To ensure a correct diagnosis of LCH, it is important to consider it in the context of a wide range of possible clinical presentations. Skin disease may mimic seborrhoeic or atopic dermatitis, juvenile xanthogranuloma, or unusual infection. Solitary subcutaneous nodules may resemble malignant lymphoma or metastatic tumour. In the case of massive cervical lymphadenopathy, histology may exclude lymphoma or 'sinus histiocytosis with massive lymphadenopathy' (Rosai Dorfman disease). Localized bone lesions must be distinguished from osteomyelitis or other bone tumours. In 'multisystem' disease without a prominent skin rash or bone involvement, distinction from familial or sporadic haemophagocytic lymphohistiocytosis (HLH) and infection-associated haemophagocytic syndrome should be easy, especially if typical HLH-associated laboratory abnormalities are lacking, e.g. raised serum triglycerides, decreased plasma fibrinogen, CSF pleocytosis, and marked haemophagocytosis in the bone marrow. Malignant histiocytosis, extremely rare in children, can be ruled out by histopathological findings.

Current management

Background

The lack of knowledge of the pathogenesis of LCH and the failure to establish generally accepted diagnostic criteria have inhibited not only the understanding of the disease but also the development of a rational treatment policy. Empirically, it has been shown that the treatment of LCH should depend on the extent of the disease (Ladisch and Gadner 1994). Patients are stratified as having 'single' or 'multisystem' disease (see Table 11.3).

Table 11.7a Diagnostic guidelines

CLINICAL

Complete history:

fever, pain irritability, failure to thrive, nutritional status, loss of appetite, diarrhoea, polydipsia, polyuria, activity level, behavioural changes, neurological changes

Complete physical examination:

measurement of temperature, height, weight, head circumference, pubertal status, skin and scalp rashes, purpura, bleeding, and aural discharge, orbital abnormalities, lymphadenopathy, gum and palatal lesions, dentition, soft tissue swelling, dyspnoea, tachypnoea, intercostal retraction, liver and spleen size, ascites, oedema, jaundice, neurological examination, papilloedema, cranial nerve abnormalities, cerebellar dysfunction

	Follow-up evaluations		
	+ organ involvement	– organ involvement	isolated bone
LABORATORY			
Haemoglobin and/or haematocrit	monthly	6-monthly	none
White blood count and differential	monthly	6-monthly	none
Platelet count	monthly	6-monthly	none
Liver enzymes and function tests (SGOT, SGPT, alkaline phosphatase, bilirubin, total protein, albumin)	monthly	6-monthly	none
Coagulation studies (PT, PTT, fibrinogen)	monthly	6-monthly	none
Urine osmolality (measurement after overnight water deprivation)	6-monthly	6-monthly	none
RADIOGRAPHIC			
Chest radiograph, p.a., and lateral	monthly	6-monthly	none
Skeletal radiograph survey	6-monthly	none	6-monthly

(Source: Writing Group of the Histiocyte Society 1989)

The disease may follow different courses, ranging from spontaneous regression to an often chronic or undulating course. Therefore, a new definition and assessment of response to a given treatment had to be established. Response has been defined as a measurable resolution of symptoms and signs, and prevention of permanent consequences (see Fig. 11.1).

'Single system' disease

The clinical course of LCH in patients with 'single system' disease (usually bone, lymph node, or skin) is generally benign, with a high chance of spontaneous remission and favourable outcome over a period of months to years (McLelland *et al.* 1990). Some therapeutic principles have emerged from clinical experience. Bone lesions usually do not require any treatment, other than biopsy or curettage at the time of diagnosis, for confirmation of diagnosis. Only if weight-bearing

Table 11.7b   Evaluations required upon specific indication

Test	Indication
Bone marrow aspirate and trephine biopsy	Anaemia, leukopaenia, or thrombocytopaenia
Pulmonary function tests	Abnormal chest radiograph, tachypnoea, intercostal retraction
Lung biopsy, preceded by bronchoalveolar lavage, when available; when diagnostic lung biopsy not needed	Patients with abnormal chest radiograph in whom chemotherapy is being considered, to exclude opportunistic infection
Small bowel series and biopsy	Unexplained chronic diarrhoea or failure to thrive, evidence of malabsorption
Liver biopsy	Liver dysfunction, including hypoproteinaemia not due to protein-losing enteropathy, to differentiate active LCH of the liver from cirrhosis
MRI of brain/hypothalamic-pituitary axis, with iv gadolinium-DTPA	Hormonal, visual, or neurological abnormalities
Panoramic dental radiograph of mandible and maxilla; oral surgery consultation	Oral involvement
Endocrine evaluation	Short stature, growth failure, diabetes insipidus, hypothalamic syndromes, galactorrhoea, precocious or delayed puberty; CT or MRI abnormality of hypothalamus/pituitary
Otolaryngology consultation and audiogram	Aural discharge, deafness

(Source: Writing Group of the Histiocyte Society 1989)
CT, computed tomography; MRI, magnetic resonance imaging

bones are involved, with the risk of spontaneous fracture, or locations causing pain or unacceptable deformity, is further local therapy needed. Intralesional infiltration of steroids (75–150 mg methylprednisolone) has been shown to be an effective and safe treatment (Egeler *et al.* 1993). The use of radiation therapy in the management of localized bone or soft tissue disease has decreased considerably with experience of late sequelae and secondary malignancy (Greenberger *et al.* 1981). However, under particular circumstances, when the disease is threatening the function of a critical organ (e.g. optic nerve or spinal cord), and local infiltration of steroids is not recommended, urgent treatment with low-dose radiotherapy (6–10 Gy) is warranted. A huge, localized tumour mass, which is difficult to excise surgically, or polyostotic bone disease may require a short course of systemic steroid therapy. Indomethacin may be a useful alternative approach for bone disease due to its analgesic effect and prostaglandin properties (McLean and Pritchard 1996).

For isolated lymph node involvement or nodular skin lesions, surgical excision is undoubtedly the therapy of choice. Rarely, systemic steroid therapy may be needed to treat regional lymph-node involvement.

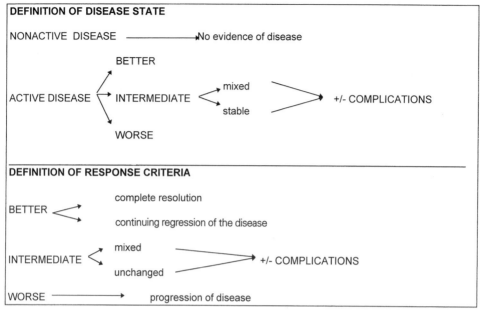

(Source: Consensus of the Histiocyte Society 1991)

Fig. 11.1   Definition of disease state and criteria for treatment response.

Correct treatment of patients with isolated skin disease is critical. Whereas mild skin disease may respond to topical steroids, in severe symptomatic skin involvement with widespread areas of crusting and excoriation, topical application of a 20% solution of nitrogen mustard is useful (Sheehan *et al.* 1991). Generalized skin lesions may also be controlled by PUVA photo-chemotherapy (a combination of psoralen and long-wave ultraviolet radiation). Both of these treatment approaches, however, can be recommended only for short-term therapy. With chronic application, the possibility of carcinogenicity must be considered. Resistant skin manifestations, particularly those with ulceration, do clearly benefit from systemic steroid therapy, with or without vinca alkaloids.

'Multisystem' disease

Chemotherapy, including cytostatic agents, has been shown to be beneficial. No single drug or regimen, however, has been unequivocally demonstrated to influence the unpredictable course associated with a high mortality rate in severely affected children. There has been a continuing search for systematic, therapeutic approaches using new agents in addition to the currently widely used, reasonably effective drugs (Ladisch and Gadner 1994).

For the treatment of 'multisystem' disease in LCH throughout the last decade, two major strategies were common: a conservative approach with treatment used only during disease exacerbation, and an aggressive polychemotherapy plan for rapid initiation of treatment immediately after diagnosis with prolonged maintenance therapy, aiming for a rapid decrease of disease activity, reduction of mortality, and prevention of recurrences and chronic disease.

Conservative approach

Based upon the observations of spontaneous remission, a conservative approach has been followed in several institutions for many years. In one large, single institution series, only cases with evidence of general symptoms (fever, pain, immobility, failure to thrive) or progressive disease in vital organs were treated initially with prednisolone, followed by the addition of either vincristine, vinblastine, or etoposide (VP16). Overall mortality rate was 14%, and 36% in children with 'organ dysfunction'. The majority of survivors (67%) had permanent consequences. DI occurred in 36% (McLelland *et al.* 1990).

Intensive chemotherapy

There has been uniform agreement that the best prognostic parameters available at diagnosis are age, extent of disease, and presence of 'organ dysfunction' as defined by Lahey (1975). In 1983, two large, prospective, multicentre trials were started, the AIEOP-CNR-HX 83 study in Italy (Ceci *et al.* 1993) and the DAL-HX 83 study in Austria/Germany (Gadner *et al.* 1994). In both trials, patients were stratified according to the extent of disease and the presence of 'organ dysfunction' at diagnosis. Patients with 'multisystem' disease were treated with risk-adapted chemotherapy. In the Italian study, 9 months initial treatment with sequential vinblastine, adriamycin, and VP 16 was followed by 9 months of continuation therapy including vincristine, cyclophosphamide, adriamycin, and prednisolone. In the DAL-HX 83 series, a 6-weeks initial treatment consisted of prednisone, vinblastine, and VP 16 followed by 12 months continuation therapy including 6-mercaptopurine, vinblastine, and prednisone for all patients, with the addition of VP 16 and methotrexate in more severely affected subgroups of patients.

The overall mortality in both of these series was low (8% and 9%, respectively), but increased in the poorest prognostic groups, and was 54% in the Italian study and 38% in the DAL study. The low incidence of disease reactivations seen in the DAL-HX study (overall 23%) provides evidence that effective treatment may beneficially influence the natural course of the disease. Disease-related, permanent consequences were encountered in 48% of patients in the Italian series and in 33% of the DAL group. Strikingly, DI occurred only in 20% and 10%, respectively. In contrast to these data, the overall incidence of permanent consequences reported in the literature is higher than 50%, and the incidence of DI, in particular after conservative management, is estimated to be 36% (Komp 1981; McLelland *et al.* 1990; Gadner *et al.* 1994).

The foundation of the Histiocyte Society in 1985 was followed by general agreement on uniform criteria for diagnostic and clinical evaluation in LCH (Writing Group of the Histiocyte Society 1987), and led to the first randomized chemotherapy trial, LCH-1, initiated by the Histiocyte Society in 1991. In this prospective international study, all patients with 'multisystem' disease were randomized between two treatment arms consisting of monochemotherapy with either VP 16 (150 mg/m^2 iv for 3 days every 3 weeks) or vinblastine (6 mg/m^2 as a bolus iv weekly) for 6 months (Ladisch *et al.* 1994).

The trial endpoints were response, mortality, disease reactivation, toxicity, and late sequelae.

The findings were:

(1) results with vinblastine or VP 16 given as monotherapy do not differ with respect to response, mortality, and reactivation frequency;

(2) the evaluation of response at 6 weeks discriminates between responders (50% of patients) and non-responders (19%), and non-response at 6 weeks is the most important prognostic discriminator predicting outcome;

(3) patients with severe disease who fail to respond initially rarely benefit from changing to alternative chemotherapy, and are at high risk of a fatal outcome (34% mortality);

(4) for non-responders, therefore, an early switch to an experimental salvage therapy is indicated;

(5) there is no statistical difference between responders and non-responders in terms of age or number of organs involved, nor can they be stratified by type or 'dysfunction' of organs involved.

These results of the LCH-1 study compare unfavourably with the DAL-HX 83 study. In this series the response rate was even higher (79% *vs* 50% in the LCH-1 study), indicating that patients with severe 'multisystem' disease appear to benefit from a more aggressive chemotherapy. These results formed the basis of the LCH-2 protocol, opened in 1996, in which the strategy of the DAL concept is compared with a milder treatment in a randomized way.

Other therapies

Only preliminary data exist on the efficacy of alternative treatment approaches in 'multisystem' disease (Ladisch and Gadner 1994). In some patients, a positive clinical response after administration of thymic hormones or extracts was seen, associated with an improvement or correction of immunological abnormalities (Osband *et al.* 1981). Monoclonal antibody therapy directed against the CD1a antigen on LCs may be of interest in future studies (Kelly *et al.* 1994). Alpha-interferon (IFN-alpha) is another drug used occasionally in recurrent LCH, but without consistent success (Jakobson *et al.* 1987). Recent studies suggest that cyclosporin A (CSA) may be a potent immune-modulator, especially in young children with advanced chemotherapy-resistant 'multisystem' disease. Persistent response, however, was obtained only by adding conventionally used drugs, e.g. steroids, vinblastine, etc. (Mahmoud *et al.* 1991). The successful use of 2-chlorodeoxyadenosine or 2′-deoxycoformycin in refractory LCH has only been reported anecdotally (Saven *et al.* 1993; McCowage *et al.* 1996). Little data is available regarding the role of bone marrow transplantation (BMT) in recurrent 'multisystem' disease (Greinix *et al.* 1992). Certainly, all these approaches urgently need to be evaluated in a prospective manner.

References

Auerswald, U., Barth, J., and Magnussen, H. (1991). Value of CD-1-positive cells in bronchoalveolar lavage fluid for the diagnosis of pulmonary histiocytosis X. *Lung*, 169, 305–309.

Braunstein, G. and Kohler, P. (1981). Endocrine manifestations of histiocytosis. *American Journal of Pediatric Hematology and Oncology*, 3, 67–75.

Broadbent, V., Egeler, R.M., and Nesbit, M.E. (1994). Langerhans cell histiocytosis- clinical and epidemiological aspects. *British Journal of Cancer*, 70(Suppl XXIII), SII-6.

Carstensen, H. and Ornvold, K.(1993). Langerhans-cell histiocytosis (histiocytosis X) in children. *Ugeskr Laeger*, 155, 1779–83,

Ceci, A., de Terlizzi, M., Colella, R., Loiacono, G., Bladucci, D., Surico, G., *et al.* (1993). Langerhans cell histiocytosis in childhood: results from the Italian Cooperative AIEOP-CNR-HX83 Study. *Medical and Pediatric Oncology*, 21, 259–64.

Chu, T. and Jaffe, R. (1994) The normal Langerhans cell and the LCH cell. *British Journal of Cancer*, 70, (suppl XXIII), S4-S10.

Dean, H.J., Bishop, A., and Winter, J.S. (1986), Growth hormone deficiency in patients with Histiocytosis X. *Journal of Pediatrics*, 109, 615–18.

Dunger, D.B., Broadbent, V., Yeoman, E., Seckl, J.R., Lightman, S.L., Grant, D.B., *et al.*, (1989), The frequency and natural history of diabetes insipidus in children with Langerhans cell histiocytosis. *New England Journal of Medicine*, 321, 1157–62.

Egeler, R.M. and Nesbit, M.E. (1995). Langerhans cell histiocytosis and other disorders of monocyte-histiocyte lineage. *Crit Rev Oncol Hematol*, 18, 9–35.

Egeler, R.M., Schipper, M.E., and Heymans, H.S (1990). Gastrointestinal involvement in Langerhans cell histiocytosis (Histiocytosis X): a clinical report of three cases. *European Journal of Pediatrics*, 149, 325–9.

Egeler, R.M., Neglia, J.P., Puccetti, D.M., Brennan, C.A., and Nesbit, M.E. (1993). Association of Langerhans cell histiocytosis with malignant neoplasms. *Cancer*, 71, 865–73.

Favara, B.E. and Jaffe, R. (1987). Pathology of Langerhans cell histiocytosis. *Hematology/Oncology Clinics of North America*, 1, 75–97.

Favara, B.E. and Jaffe, R. (1994). The histopathology of Langerhans cell histiocytosis. *British Journal of Cancer*, 70 (Suppl XXIII), S17–S23.

Favara, B.E., Feller, A.C., Pauli, M., Jaffe, E.S., Weiss, L.M., Arico, M., *et al.* (1997). Contemporary classification of histiocytic disorders. *Med. Pediatr. Oncol.* 29:3, 157–66.

Gadner, H. and Grois, N. (1993). The Histiocytosis Syndromes. *Dermatology in general medicine*, (ed. T.B. Fitzpatrick et al), vol II, pp. 2003–23. McGraw-Hill Inc.

Gadner, H., Heitger, A., Grois, N., Gatterer-Menz, I., and Ladisch, S. (1994). Treatment strategy for disseminated Langerhans cell histiocytosis. DAL HX-83 Study Group. *Medical and Pediatric Oncology*, 23, 72–80.

Greenberger, J.S., Crocker, A.C., Vawter, G., Jaffe, N., and Cassady, J.R. (1981). Results of treatment of 127 patients with systemic histiocytosis (Letterer-Siwe Syndrome, Schuller- Christian Syndrome and multifocal eosinophilic granuloma). *Medicine*, 60, 311–38.

Greinix, H.T., Storb, R., Sanders, J.E., and Petersen, F.B. (1992). Marrow transplantation for treatment of multisystem progressive Langerhans cell histiocytosis. *Bone Marrow Transplantation*, 10, 39–44.

Grois, N., Barkovich, A.J., Rosenau, W., and Ablin, A.R. (1993), Central nervous system disease associated with Langerhans cell histiocytosis. *American Journal of Pediatric Hematology and Oncology*, 15, 245–54.

Grois, N., Tsunematsu, Y., Barkovich, A.J., and Favara, B.E. (1994). Central nervous system disease in Langerhans cell histiocytosis. *British Journal of Cancer*, 70, (Suppl XXIII), S24–S28.

Hashimoto, K. and Pritzker, M.S. (1973). Electron microscopic study of reticulohistiocytoma. An unusual case of congenital self-healing reticulohistiocytosis. *Archives of Dermatology*, 107, 263–70.

Jakobson, A.M., Kreuger, A., Hagberg, H., and Sundstrom, C. (1987). Treatment of Langerhans cell histiocytosis with alpha-interferon. *Lancet*, 2, 1520–21.

Kelly, K.M., Beverley, P.C., Chu, A.C., Davenport, V., Gordon, I., Smith, M., *et al.* (1994). Successful *in vivo* immunolocalization of Langerhans cell histiocytosis with use of monoclonal antibody, NA1/34. *Journal of Pediatrics*, 125, 717–22.

Komp, D.M. (1981). Long-term sequelae of histiocytosis X. *American Journal of Pediatric Hematology and Oncology*, 3, 163–8.

Komp, D.M., El Mahdi, A., Starling, K.A., Easley, J., Vietti, T.J., Berry, D.H., *et al.* (1980). Quality of survival in histiocytosis X: a Southwest Oncology Group Study. *Medical and Pediatric Oncology*, 8, 35–40.

Ladisch, S. and Gadner, H. (1994). Treatment of Langerhans cell histiocytosis—evolution and current approaches. *British Journal of Cancer*, 70,(Suppl XXIII), S41–S46.

Ladisch, S., Gadner, H., Arico, M., Broadbent, V., Grois, N., Jacobson, A., *et al.* (1994). LCH-I: a randomized trial of etoposide vs. vinblastine in disseminated Langerhans cell histiocytosis. The Histiocyte Society. *Medical and Pediatric Oncology*, 23, 107–10.

Lahey, M.E. (1975). Histiocytosis X—an analysis of prognostic factors. *Journal of Pediatrics*, 87, 184–89.

Mahmoud, H.H., Wang, W.C., and Murphy, S.B. (1991). Cyclosporine therapy for advanced Langerhans cell histiocytosis. *Blood*, 77, 721–5.

McClain, K., Ramsay, N.K., Robison, L., Sundberg, R.D., and Nesbit, M. Jr. (1983). Bone marrow involvement in histiocytosis X. *Medical and Pediatric Oncology*, 11, 167–71.

McCowage, G.B., Frush, D.P., and Kurtzberg, J. (1996). Successful treatment of two children with Langerhans cell histiocytosis with 2′-deoxyocoformycin. *Journal of Pediatric Hematology and Oncology*, 18, 154–58.

McLean, T.W. and Pritchard, J. (1996). Langerhans cell histiocytosis and hypercalcemia: clinical response to indomethacin. *Journal of Pediatric Hematology and Oncology*, 18, 318–20.

McLelland, J., Broadbent, V., Yeoman, E., Malone, M., and Pritchard, J. (1990), Langerhans cell histiocytosis: the case for conservative treatment. *Archives of Diseases in Childhood*, 65, 301–3.

Osband, M.E., Lipton, J.M., Lavin, P., Levey, R., Vawter, G., Greenberger, J.S., *et al.* (1981). Histiocytosis X: Demonstration of abnormal immunity, T-cell histamine H2-receptor deficiency and successful treatment with thymic extract. *New England Journal of Medicine*, 304, 146–53.

Parker, B.R., Pinckney, L., and Etcubanas, E. (1980). Relative efficacy of radiographic and radionuclide bone surveys in the detection of the skeletal lesions of histiocytosis X. *Radiology*, 134, 377–80.

Rosenfield, N.S., Abrahams, J., and Komp, D. (1990). Brain MRI in patients with Langerhans cell histiocytosis findings and enhancement with Gd-DTPA. *Pediatric Radiology*, 20, 433–36.

Saven, A., Figueroa, M.L., Piro, L.D., and Rosenblatt, J.D (1993). 2-Chlorodeoxyadenosine to treat refractory histiocytosis. *Lancet*, 329, 734–5.

Sheehan, M.P., Atherton, D.J., Broadbent, V., and Pritchard, J. (1991) Topical nitrogen mustard: an effective treatment for cutaneous Langerhans cell histiocytosis. *Journal of Pediatrics*, 119, 317–322.

Willman, C.L. (1994). Detection of clonal histiocytes in Langerhans cell histiocytosis: biology and clinical significance. *British Journal of Cancer*, 70(Suppl XXIII), S29–S33.

Writing Group of the Histiocyte Society (1987). Histiocytosis syndrome in children. *Lancet*, 1, 208–9.

Writing Group of the Histiocyte Society (1989). Histiocytosis syndromes in children: II. Approach to the clinical and laboratory evaluation of children with Langerhans Cell Histiocytosis. *Medical and Pediatric Oncology*, 17, 492–5.

12 Tumours of the central nervous system

R. Pötter, Th. Czech, K. Dieckmann, I. Slavc, D. Wimberger-Prayer, and H. Budka

Introduction

Tumours of the central nervous system constitute the most common solid tumour in children (2.7 cases per 100 000 children per year), and therefore contribute to a major part of daily practice in paediatric oncology. Brain tumours are very heterogeneous with regard to tissue, location, pattern of spread, clinical picture, natural history, and age of occurrence (from the neonatal period to adolescence). As significant progress has been achieved and is evolving in the different areas of diagnosis and treatment, adequate clinical management and follow-up nowadays brings a challenge to the interdisciplinary paediatric neuro-oncology team: neuropaediatrician, paediatric oncologist, neurosurgeon, radiotherapist, neuropathologist, neuroradiologist, and psychologist. Management decisions for childhood brain tumours should be based exclusively on such a team approach, in which the different members must be familiar with all available knowledge, experience, and developments in their respective fields (Cohen and Duffner 1994). The goal of brain tumour therapy is to achieve cure while avoiding unacceptable long-term sequelae.

Modern neurosurgery remains the mainstay of treatment for most brain tumours, followed by modern brain radiotherapy as the most important adjuvant procedure in a large number of patients (Thomas and Graham 1995). The role for adjuvant or neoadjuvant chemotherapy remains unsettled, although response rates for different regimens are encouraging.

Tumour classification and histological diagnosis

Progress in our understanding of the molecular basis of neoplastic development may lead to molecular tumour diagnosis in the future. At present, however, descriptive classification by histological examination remains pivotal for the appropriate management of CNS tumours. Since location and cellular differentiation are the basis of this diagnostic system, tumour classification has remained 'histogenetic'. The second edition of the WHO *Histological typing of tumours of the CNS* (Kleihues *et al.* 1993) lists 127 entities, reflecting the remarkable variety of cellular constituents of the CNS. Theoretically, all types might develop in children. However, the number of tumour types which are of special importance in children is significantly smaller (Table 12.1); the large majority of paediatric CNS tumours encompasses only five entities: medulloblastoma, pilocytic astrocytoma, diffuse astrocytoma, ependymoma, and craniopharyngioma.

As with their counterparts in adults, CNS tumours in childhood have important properties which deviate from those of tumours at other sites, but profoundly influence their behaviour:

(1) many are highly invasive, even when histologically of low malignancy;

(2) many are heterogeneous in composition with areas of mixed tumour types and differing malignancy (special attention is necessary in stereotactic biopsies);

(3) many are notorious for spreading to CSF pathways, thus enabling CSF seeding even in low-grade tumours;

(4) tumour progression may occur, leading from low- to high-grade tumours, most prominently in diffuse astrocytomas.

Most CNS tumour types occur preferentially in specific age-groups and specific sites (Table 12.1). Nevertheless, exceptions to these rules must be kept in mind. In comparison with tumours in adults, the posterior fossa site is overrepresented (about half of all paediatric CNS tumours). However, the distribution depends upon age: during the first year of life and in adolescence, supratentorial tumours are more frequent than those in infratentorial sites, which predominate during childhood. Spinal cord tumours are rare in children. Many CNS tumours in young age occur near the midline, suggesting a developmental aspect to their origin.

Histological grading of malignancy according to the WHO (Table 12.1) gives an idea how a given tumour type usually behaves on a four-point scale. Again, exceptions may occur. In general, histological malignancy is judged according to cellularity, pleomorphism, nuclear atypia, mitotic activity, invasiveness and metastasis, anaplasia (cellular differentiation), and secondary features such as necrosis and neovascularity; however, some of these items do not have the same meaning in all tumour types. It is important to separate the pilocytic astrocytoma, which is the most frequent glioma of childhood and has a usually excellent prognosis, from the much less favourable diffuse astrocytomas.

The impact of modern morphological techniques, with immunocytochemistry as an indispensable tool, on a refined histogenetic classification of CNS tumours cannot be overemphasized. Information on biological tumour properties, such as proliferation, can also be obtained. While CNS tumour proliferation indices in general reflect the malignancy scale of the present classification system, proliferation on its own has not yet been shown to be of decisive prognostic importance. Thus, it is the combined consideration of distinct features of the histological examination (tumour type, grade of malignancy, growth pattern, proliferative activity, etc.), which will provide the maximum relevant information for further management and therapy of an individual tumour.

The concept of the primitive neuroectodermal tumour (PNET)

In Bailey and Cushing's old histogenetic tumour classification, tumour morphology was considered to mirror specific stages of normal neural tissue development. Since then, highly undifferentiated neural neoplasms have been considered as 'embryonal', with the medulloblastoma as the most important clinicopathological entity. More recently, the unifying concept of the PNET was proposed to encompass all types of undifferentiated or primitive, small-celled, neural neoplasms, with a potential for multiple differentiation (neuronal, glial, ependymal, pineal ...), irrespective

Table 12.1 Histological CNS tumour types of special importance in children: preferential age and sites, WHO grade, and approximate percentage of all brain tumours in children*

Tumour type	WHO grade(s)	Preferential age(s)	Preferential site(s)	%*
Pilocytic astrocytoma	I	childhood and adolescence	cerebellum	12–18
			hypothalamus, optic pathways	4–8
Subependymal giant-cell astrocytoma (usually in tuberous sclerosis)	I	childhood, adolescence	Foramen of Monro region	
Diffuse astrocytoma (low grade)	II	adolescence, young adults	cerebral hemispheres	8–20
		childhood	brain stem	3–6
Pleomorphic xanthoastrocytoma	II	late childhood, adolescence	superficial cerebral hemispheres	
Anaplastic astrocytoma, glioblastoma	III, IV	all ages	cerebral hemispheres	6–12
		childhood	brain stem	3–9
Oligodendroglioma, mixed glioma, anaplastic oligodendroglioma	II, III	adolescence, young adults	cerebral hemispheres	2–7
Ependymoma, anaplastic ependymoma	II, III	childhood and adolescence	lateral and third ventricles	2–5
			fourth ventricle	4–8
Choroid plexus papilloma, choroid plexus carcinoma	I, IV	infancy, childhood	lateral and fourth ventricles	2–4
Gangliocytoma, ganglioglioma	I	childhood and adolescence	temporal lobe	1–5
Desmoplastic infantile ganglioglioma, desmoplastic cerebral astrocytoma of infancy	I	infancy	superficial cerebral hemispheres	
Dysembryoplastic neuroepithelial tumour	I	childhood to young adults	temporal lobe	
Central neurocytoma	I	adolescence, young adults	lateral ventricles	
Pineocytoma, pineoblastoma	II, IV	childhood to young adults	pineal region	0.5–2
Neuroblastoma	IV	infancy and childhood	cerebral hemispheres	
Ependymoblastoma	IV	infancy and childhood	lateral and fourth ventricles	

Table 12.1 *Continued*

Tumour type	WHO grade(s)	Preferential age(s)	Preferential site(s)	%*
Medulloblastoma	IV	infancy and childhood	cerebellum	20–25
Other primitive neuroectodermal tumours	IV	infancy and childhood	whole neuraxis	1–2
Germ-cell tumours, esp. germinoma and teratoma	I–IV	infancy and childhood	pineal region hypothalamus	0.5–2 1–2
Colloid cyst of third ventricle	I	adolescence, young adults	Foramen of Monro region	
Craniopharyngioma	I	adolescence	(supra)sellar	6–9
Meningioma	–	childhood, adolescence	supratentorial	1–2
Pituitary adenoma	I	adolescence	(supra)sellar	0.5–2.5

(Source: Pollack 1994)
* Percentages in children modified from Pollack (1994); some entities were not individually listed.

of their site of origin. The PNET concept has not been universally accepted, but has entered the present WHO classification in a somewhat hybrid format. The distinct clinicopathological tumour types, with traditional terminology such as the medulloblastoma, ependymoblastoma, and pineoblastoma, are retained in addition to PNETs with other presentations. Thus, PNET may be considered as a general term for all types of densely cellular ('blue-celled'), primitive, or 'embryonal' neural tumour. Whenever possible, however, further delineation as medulloblastoma, etc., should be given. To add to the terminological confusion, a 'PNET' (*peripheral* neuroectodermal tumour) is sometimes used to designate a peripheral nervous system tumour with similarities to Ewing's sarcoma.

'New' CNS tumour entities of childhood

In addition to PNETs and the long list of traditional tumour entities, the second edition of the WHO classification includes a number of recently recognized tumour types. The pleomorphic xanthoastrocytoma is a predominantly extracerebral growth with pleomorphic, lipidized astrocytes and a generally, but not universally, favourable prognosis. The desmoplastic infantile ganglioglioma and its variant, the desmoplastic cerebral astrocytoma of infancy, are usually very large tumours presenting during the first 2 years of life. The dysembryoplastic neuroepithelial tumour usually presents with long-standing complex partial seizures; it features a mixed glioneuronal population in a mucinous matrix, distributed in characteristic multiple cortical nodules. The central neurocytoma is almost invariably an intraventricular tumour of the lateral ventricle, and has been misdiagnosed for decades as oligodendroglioma or ependymoma; its prognosis is mostly, but not always, favourable (Kleihues *et al.* 1993).

Molecular biology

Cytogenetic and molecular techniques have resulted in the cloning of the neurofibromatosis type 1 (*NF-1*) and type 2 (*NF-2*) genes, and the characterization of the molecular physiology of the *p53* gene.

NF-1 occurs with a frequency of one in every 3500 live births and is the most common hereditary disease predisposing to neoplasia.

A role for the *NF-1* gene—hypothesized to be a tumour-suppressor gene—is suggested in the genesis of *NF-1*-associated, as well as of sporadic, pilocytic astrocytoma.

The most consistent abnormality seen in medulloblastoma is loss of genetic material on the distal arm of chromosome 17p, occuring in about 45% of tumours. Deletion of 17p has also been shown to have implications for clinical management, as the loss of DNA sequences located on this chromosome is strongly associated with a poor prognosis in some studies. The identification and cloning of a potential tumour-suppressor gene in this region will aid in better understanding the many, complex pathways that lead to medulloblastoma initiation and progression, as well as in guiding therapeutic strategies.

Work on paediatric astrocytomas suggests that the genes involved are different from those in adult gliomas. In contrast to adult astrocytic tumours, *p53* is rarely mutated in paediatric tumours, the epidermal growth factor receptor gene is rarely amplified or mutated, and chromosome 10 deletions are rare. Taken together, these observations imply that the pathways leading to the development of malignant astrocytomas in children may differ significantly from those involved in adults, which may, in part, account for the somewhat better prognosis of such tumours in children (Raffel 1996).

Epidemiology

Two peaks of incidence of brain tumours are noted, the first in the stage of younger life (approximately 2.5 per 100 000 per year) and the second occurring later in the third and subsequent decades. Embryonal tumours are commoner than gliomas. CNS tumours can be associated with several inherited syndromes including the phacomatoses, neurofibromatosis with visual pathway tumours, glial tumours, and meningiomas, tuberous sclerosis with glial tumours, subependymal giant cell astrocytoma, and ependymomas, von Hippel-Lindau syndrome with cerebellar haemangioblastoma. Patients with the Li Fraumeni syndrome may develop CNS tumours, commonly astrocytoma. Medulloblastoma may be seen in association with basal cell naevus syndrome (Gorlin's syndrome), as well as Turcot's and ataxia-telangectasia syndromes.

Clinical presentation

The signs and symptoms of neurological dysfunction in a child with a brain tumour are various and depend more on the age, premorbid developmental level, and site of origin than histology. Brain tumours may cause neurological impairment directly, by infiltrating or compressing normal CNS structures, or indirectly, by causing obstruction of cerebrospinal fluid flow and increased intracranial pressure (ICP). The latter is responsible for the 'classic' triad of ICP—morning headache, vomiting, and visual disturbances. When present, these symptoms strongly suggest a rapidly growing midline or posterior fossa tumour. More commonly, the initial signs of ICP are more subtle, subacute, non specific, and non-localizing. In school-age children, slowly developing ICP may be accompanied by declining academic performance, fatigue, changes in affect, energy level, motivation, personality, and behaviour, and complaints of vague, intermittent headaches. In the first few years of life, irritability, anorexia, developmental delay, and later, regression of intellectual and motor abilities, are frequently early signs of ICP.

Infratentorial tumours (brain stem and cerebellar) commonly present with deficits of balance or brain-stem function (truncal steadiness, extremity coordination and gait, cranial nerve function). Nystagmus and gaze palsy alone or, more likely, in combination with deficits of cranial nerves V, VII, and IX, strongly suggest invasion of the brain stem. Head tilt may be a presenting sign.

Supratentorial tumours may cause a variety of signs and symptoms, depending on the size and location of the tumour. The most common presenting complaint is headaches, followed secondly by seizures. Upper motor neurone signs, such as hemiparesis, hyperreflexia, and clonus, as well as associated sensory loss, may also be present.

Anorexia, bulimia, weight loss or gain, somnolence, mood swings, failure to thrive, diabetes insipidus, sexual precocity, or delayed puberty may be non-specific or suggest hypothalamic or pituitary dysfunction. Tumours of the region of the hypothalamus may also cause visual loss due to compression of the optic chiasm or the optic nerve.

Diagnosis and investigation

The advent of magnetic resonance imaging (MRI) has greatly altered the pre-operative and post-operative evaluation of children with brain tumours. Multiplanar imaging is extremely helpful in determining the exact extent of the tumour and its relationship to surrounding, normal structures. Using computerized tomography (CT), images have to be reformatted in coronal and sagittal planes, respectively, when information is needed about the relationship of the lesion to the tentorium, the foramen magnum (in case of posterior fossa tumours), or to midline structures (in case of lesions of the region of the pineal). However, reformatted images are of inferior quality, and abnormalities immediately adjacent to bony structures may be obscured by artefacts on CT scans. The administration of paramagnetic MR contrast agents, such as Gadolinium diethylene-triaminepentaacetic acid (DTPA), in MR studies, and iodinated contrast agents with CT, have been shown to identify tumours and metastatic disease in brain and spine more accurately (Barkovoch 1993).

In children with open fontanelles, sonography is the appropriate first investigation: children do not have to be sedated or transferred to an imaging centre, sections may be obtained in a multitude of orientations, and examinations can be repeated frequently. However, if a tumour is diagnosed by ultrasound, MRI or, if not available, CT is required for additional information.

Angiography is usually not needed unless a highly vascular lesion is suspected or a vascular malformation cannot be ruled out by non-invasive studies. In most cases, MR angiography is sufficient to answer these questions.

Spinal imaging

Leptomeningeal metastases may affect the entire neuraxis and necessitate evaluation of both the brain and the spinal cord. MRI has become the imaging method of choice as it has been shown to be clearly superior to myelography or CT myelography. When a brain tumour which is particularly prone to spinal seeding is diagnosed, MR imaging of the spine must be done before surgery of the primary tumour; otherwise postoperative, reactive, meningeal enhancement may mimic tumour involvement.

Postoperative imaging assessment

Surveillance imaging of the CNS at predetermined intervals is used to document the extent of tumour resection, to assess the tumour response to adjuvant treatment, to detect recurrence, and to evaluate the complications of treatment. The first contrast-enhanced, postoperative MR or CT scan should be scheduled within 72 hours of surgery: within this time, enhancing structures are due to residual disease and not to therapy-related, blood-brain-barrier disruption. Consecutive scans can then be reliably compared with this 'baseline' study.

Treatment modalities

Neurosurgical treatment

Surgical intervention remains the mainstay of the diagnostic and therapeutic management of primary brain tumours. The goals of surgery are

(1) to establish a tissue diagnosis;

(2) to excise or reduce the tumour volume and the mass effect;

(3) potentially to cure the disease.

Completeness of surgical excision is the most important prognostic factor. Accurate histological classification of a tumour is crucial for planning further therapy and determining prognosis. MRI- and CT-guided stereotactic biopsy is used as a first step in selected cases of thalamic and basal ganglia tumours, of multifocal lesions, and of radiologically diffusely infiltrating lesions without significant mass effect.

Most paediatric neurosurgeons prefer open craniotomy to stereotactic biopsy in the majority of children, even when only a subtotal resection is anticipated preoperatively. As the expanding mass or a resulting hydrocephalus leads to ICP, with the risk of herniation either through the tentorial notch or through the foramen magnum, prompt and effective cytoreduction can be life-saving, even when the tumour is only subtotally resected.

After acquisition of diagnostic imaging results, the child is prepared for surgery by first managing the most urgent symptomatic problems. This includes steroid administration to relieve accompanying brain oedema, and anticonvulsive treatment if indicated in supratentorial, hemispheric tumours. In patients who present with hydrocephalus, a preoperative shunt should be avoided if removal of the mass is anticipated. If necessary, external ventricular drainage is established before or at the time of tumour resection. This strategy allows the decision about permanent shunting to be made after surgery, as permanent hydrocephalus occurs in only 25–30% of all patients with posterior fossa tumours and hydrocephalus.

The safety and efficacy of surgery has improved because of advances in surgical techniques, progress in neuroimaging, and developments in neuroanesthesia and paediatric critical care.

Consideration of the anatomical location of the tumour as visualized by MRI (Fig. 12.1a), knowledge of the possibilities for postoperative adjuvant therapy depending on tumour type (determined by frozen section and smear), age of the patient, and, ultimately, the intraoperative findings will determine surgical aggressiveness. Surgery alone is increasingly able to cure, or keep in extended remission, some paediatric brain tumours. Tumours that invade deep grey nuclei, such as the hypothalamus, thalamus, or basal ganglia in the dominant hemisphere, tumours in eloquent cortical areas, and tumours that are intrinsic to the brain stem, can often not be totally resected without significant risk of devastating neurological sequelae. Technical adjuncts allowing for safer and more complete resection of radiologically well-defined tumours include intraoperative ultrasound, frameless stereotactic techniques allowing interactive 3-D-image-guided procedures (Fig. 12.1b), and neurophysiological monitoring of cortical, subcortical, and cranial nerve function (Berger 1996). The Cavitron ultrasonic aspirator (CUSA) enables the removal of firm tumours while minimizing injury to surrounding structures. The surgical laser is advocated by some as helpful, especially in dealing with intrinsic spinal cord tumours.

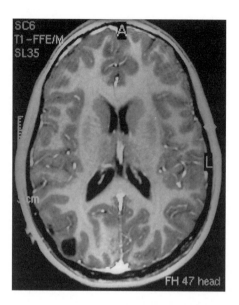

Fig. 12.1a MRI scan of a low grade glioma in the occipital lobe.

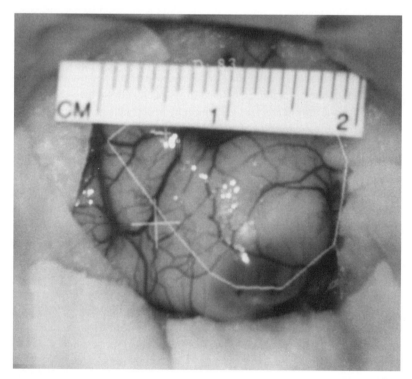

Fig. 12.1b The exposed cortex over the tumour with the contour of the lesion projected onto the operative site through a stereotactic surgical microscope.

Recent developments in endoscopical technology and instrumentation allow now for a third ventriculostomy to replace ventriculoperitoneal shunting in most patients with permanent hydrocephalus after posterior fossa tumour resection. Endoscopy may also assist the microsurgical procedure in evaluating the completeness of a resection, and offer alternatives for biopsy, and even resection, of intraventricular masses.

Radiotherapy

Radiotherapy has been proven to be an effective modality in the treatment of childhood brain tumours for decades. Nevertheless, local control and survival, in particular in aggressive and invasive tumours, still need to be significantly improved. On the other hand, late side-effects related to radiotherapy have been recognized more clearly with the increase in numbers and follow-up of long-term survivors (Halperin *et al.* 1994; Kun 1994 in Cohen and Duffner).

Current treatment policies, including radiotherapy, therefore aim at increasing the therapeutic ratio by different means: minimizing side-effects by limiting the indications for radiotherapy for good-prognosis tumours (e.g. low-grade astrocytoma accessible by modern neurosurgical techniques), postponing radiotherapy in very young children (e.g. medulloblastoma), by dose reduction in radiosensitive tumours (e.g. craniospinal irradiation in germ-cell tumours), by volume reduction through better adaptation of the treated volume to the target (e.g. circumscribed, low-grade tumours), improving local control by improving the quality of radiotherapy (e.g. medulloblastoma), or by dose escalation using modern radiotherapy techniques in the case of less radiosensitive tumours (e.g. high-grade glioma).

Radiation-related side-effects in CNS radiotherapy are generally related to total dose, fractionation of dose, radiation volume, area of CNS irradiated, and the age of the child at the time of treatment.

With advances in neuroimaging (MRI), target definition for radiotherapy has improved considerably in nearly all CNS tumours. With the integration of these sectional imaging tools into 3-D-treatment planning procedures and 'conformal radiotherapy' techniques (using multiple, individually shaped fields), the treated volume can now be more adequately tailored to the target volume. In conformal radiotherapy, the high-dose irradiation of normal brain tissue can thus be reduced, without jeopardizing treatment results, provided target definition has been correct. These 3-D-treatment planning-based conformal radiotherapy techniques have become more common in the last few years and will—in particular in brain tumours—most likely spread into general clinical practice within a short time-period.

A precondition for such precision radiotherapy is immobilization, which only permits minimal deviations throughout the planning procedure and the whole course of fractionated radiotherapy. Nowadays, different types of custom-made immobilization devices are available and should be in common use for the treatment of childhood brain tumours. One of the most difficult procedures is craniospinal irradiation (CSI), where children are treated in a prone position using a custom-made immobilization device for the head and the spinal axis. Detailed quality assurance procedures are necessary, and should be performed at regular intervals (e.g. weekly) during the treatment course to check the accuracy of the treatment set-up.

One of the most recent technical advances with much challenge for future developments has been the introduction of stereotactic radiotherapy. The advantage of this technique, using multiple radiation fields or arcs, is the extremely sharp fall-off of radiation dose (within millimeters to < 10–20%)

in all directions outside the treated volume. By this technique, small tumours (up to about 4 cm in diameter) directly adjacent to critical structures can be treated with high radiation doses without major radiation-related morbidity. Nevertheless, sufficient clinical data collected at various centers, with different techniques and fractionation schedules, will only be available after some years.

Image-guided, stereotactic, low-dose-rate interstitial and intracavitary brain radiotherapy with different isotopes (e.g. ^{125}I, ^{192}Ir, ^{90}Y, ^{32}P) has been in use in some specialist centres and may be indicated in specific situations in slowly proliferating, well-circumscribed lesions. However, great experience is necessary to handle these techniques adequately, and as the results reported so far are not clearly superior, these techniques should only be used in experienced hands and in prospective clinical protocols.

Chemotherapy

Progress in the chemotherapy of brain tumours has lagged behind that of other neoplasms of childhood. Reasons for this include

(1) problems related to the presence of the blood-brain barrier;

(2) tumour-cell heterogeneity;

(3) a low mitotic index of many brain tumours and thus a reduced susceptibility to cell-cycle-specific drugs. Nevertheless, chemotherapy is playing an ever increasing role in the treatment of paediatric brain tumours, and significant response rates have been reported for a number of chemotherapeutic agents. These include vincristine, procarbazine, the nitrosoureas BCNU and CCNU, etoposide, cisplatin, carboplatin, cyclophosphamide, iphosphamide, and methotrexate (Brecher 1994, in Cohen and Duffner, Heideman *et al.* 1997). Large cooperative trials are now using a variety of multidrug regimens as an adjuvant to surgery and radiotherapy. As a secondary consideration, chemotherapy is being used with reduced doses of radiotherapy to spare the cognitive side-effects of standard-dose craniospinal irradiation (CSI). However, it is not yet clear whether this reduction will detrimentally affect survival, improve cognition, or cause other sequelae. In an attempt to maximize the effect of chemotherapy, scheduling, dose intensity, and more effective drug-delivery strategies are being investigated. Cytokines and haematopoietic protectors such as amifostine may allow for further dose intensification of chemotherapy protocols, both by allowing dose escalation and decreasing the time interval between treatments. Another strategy to improve the response rate of poor-prognosis CNS tumours is high-dose chemotherapy with autologous stem-cell rescue. Early reports, in both newly diagnosed and recurrent CNS tumours, have shown some encouraging results, and new trials have begun in several centres.

As many brain tumours will spread throughout the cerebrospinal fluid (CSF) pathways, future design of brain tumour protocols may include administration of a drug directly into the CSF. The intrathecal route offers significant therapeutic advantages for molecules too large to pass the blood-brain barrier, and may avoid systemic toxicity. However, standard intrathecal agents such as methotrexate and cytarabine are not very effective in brain tumours.

The steep dose-response curve of bifunctional alkylating agents, coupled with their known activity against a variety of paediatric brain tumours, suggests the need for strategies to achieve high levels of these drugs in the CSF. Recent trials have demonstrated that agents such as maphosphamide, a preactivated cyclophosphamide derivative, can be safely administered into the CSF and may produce responses in leptomeningeal neoplasia.

Intratumoural administration of chemotherapeutic agents is also undergoing investigation as a new modality to improve drug delivery to the tumour.

Chemotherapy before surgery and/or radiotherapy may make local curative treatment more feasible and is currently under study.

Hopefully, better understanding of the molecular genetics and biology of brain tumours will translate into new treatments, including immunotherapy, gene therapy, and the use of antiangiogenesis factors and second messenger inhibitors.

Specific management

Low-grade glioma

Cerebellar astrocytoma

Cerebellar astrocytomas carry a more favourable prognosis than most other brain tumours (Campbell and Pollack 1996). The majority are histologically benign, slow growing, well circumscribed, often cystic lesions which involve the vermis and cerebellar hemispheres with approximately equal frequency. Invasion of the cerebellar peduncles or brain stem may occur. The goal in the treatment of these tumours is gross total resection. If achieved, a nearly 100% cure rate is expected. However, in some children, total removal may be impossible or hazardous due to brain-stem involvement or perioperative complications. Although subtotal resection may allow an extended period of disease control in these patients, a significant percentage of lesions ultimately progresses and requires additional therapy. At present, the role of radiotherapy after incomplete resection remains unclear. In the absence of convincing data favouring the routine use of radiotherapy, many groups defer radiotherapy until there is evidence of progressive disease that is surgically unresectable. Early experience at some institutions with radiosurgery and stereotactic radiotherapy for the treatment of focal areas of tumour recurrence suggests this modality is useful in managing small areas of unresectable disease in critical locations.

In contrast to the favourable results achieved with low-grade cerebellar astrocytomas, the prognosis for patients with high-grade lesions remains poor after conventional surgery, radiotherapy, and chemotherapy.

Gliomas of the optic pathway

Most gliomas of the optic pathways occur during the first 5 years of life and are low-grade, pilocytic astrocytoma. These tumours are associated in 15–20% with neurofibromatosis (NF-1). Clinical symptoms depend on the location along the optic pathway: exophthalmos, decrease in visual acuity, disc pallor, visual field changes, endocrine dysfunction, and the diencephalic syndrome.

The behaviour of these tumours is highly variable and unpredictable. Large tumours may remain stable for years, while initially small chiasmatic tumours may show rapid disease progression.

Management strategies for visual pathway gliomas include observation, chemotherapy, radiotherapy, surgery, and various combinations of these modalities.

The time for intervention and choice of treatment modality have to be considered carefully. The risks of treatment-related side-effects, such as optic nerve injury, vasculopathy, and endocrinopathy, have to be weighed against irreversible symptoms of tumour progression leading to deterioration of visual and endocrine function.

Children without evidence of tumour growth after diagnosis are followed by MR imaging and neurodevelopmental, ophthalmological, and endocrinological examinations. When tumour progression is diagnosed, therapeutic intervention should be considered.

Unilateral optic nerve gliomas without chiasmal involvement may be cured by resection of the affected optic nerve. An alternative optic-nerve-conserving approach is conformal or stereotactic radiotherapy.

Tumours involving the chiasm, and hypothalamic tumours, are treated by a combined approach including surgery, radiotherapy, and chemotherapy.

Neurosurgical intervention aims at tissue diagnosis, resection of exophytic tumour extensions, drainage of tumour cysts, and decompression of the optic nerve.

Local radiotherapy is performed, applying radiation doses of 40–50 Gy with conformal and stereotactic techniques (Kaye and Laws 1995).

New management strategies have been introduced for children younger than 5 years using chemotherapy (carboplatin/actinomycin D and vincristine) so that radiation therapy can be delayed till age five or later. If there is tumour progression during or after chemotherapy, local radiotherapy remains the treatment of choice.

Brain-stem glioma

Brain-stem gliomas have recently been classified into different entities based on MRI findings. Diffuse, intrinsic lesions in the pons account for about 80%. The remainder are small, focal tumours in the midbrain and medulla—often with a cystic component—dorsal exophytic tumours at the floor of the fourth ventricle, and cervicomedullary tumours. Except for diffuse, intrinsic tumours, most of the other tumour types are low-grade astrocytoma with a rather favourable prognosis.

Clinical symptoms depend on location and tumour size, and often consist of cranial nerve deficits (V-IX), long tract signs, and ataxia, whereas symptoms of hydrocephalus are rare except in tectal tumours. A short duration of symptoms (e.g. 1 month) and diffuse infiltration on MRI indicate a high grade of malignancy, and an unfavourable prognosis.

In tumours with favourable prognosis (focal, dorsal exophytic, cervicomedullary tumours; low-grade histology) overall survival rates approach 90%, if surgery leads to major removal. For these tumour types, neurosurgery, with improved techniques and perioperative care, has now become the method of choice and should result in as much tumour removal as feasible without introducing an unacceptable risk of morbidity. Stereotactic radiotherapy, as an interesting alternative to surgery, is under investigation in some centres.

Diffuse, intrinsic lesions mostly carry an unfavourable prognosis. As a rule, there is no need for histological confirmation by stereotactic biopsy, if the clinical presentation and the MR findings are characteristic, even though stereotactic procedures now carry a low risk of morbidity.

Radiotherapy thus remains the mainstay of treatment for the majority of brain-stem tumours. The target is the macroscopic lesion on MRI (T2-weighted) with a safety margin. The radio-responsiveness of these tumours may be marked, with response rates of about 70%. Nevertheless, most of these tumours recur at the site of the primary, resulting in a poor outcome (2-year survival < 20%). These findings have led to dose-escalation studies with hyperfractionation

(55–78 Gy, 1.2 Gy per fraction) by POG (Paediatric Oncology Group), CCG (Children's Cancer Group), UCSF (University College of San Francisco), and CHOP (Children's Hospital of Philadelphia). No clear survival advantage could be proven in this relatively large cohort of children. High doses (> 72 Gy) led to more radiation-related brain damage (e.g. intralesional necrosis). Results of further (randomized) trials (e.g. POG) have to be awaited before recommendation of any aggressive, hyperfractionated, high-dose radiotherapy for standard treatment (Heideman *et al.* 1997).

Adjuvant or neoadjuvant multiagent chemotherapy (e.g. CCNU, VCR) did not prove to be of significant value.

At present, the effects of simultaneous radiochemotherapy are under investigation, using chemotherapeutic agents (e.g. platinum) for their well-known radiosensitizing effect, in order to increase the local efficacy of radiotherapy (current POG trial).

Other low-grade gliomas

Low-grade gliomas comprise a heterogeneous group with regard to histological subtypes, anatomical location, and biological behaviour.

Roughly half of supratentorial, low-grade gliomas are located in the cerebral hemispheres, and the remainder occur in the deep midline structures of the diencephalon and basal ganglia. Pilocytic and diffuse astrocytomas are the most frequently encountered gliomas, although other variants, such as the ganglioglioma, pleomorphic xanthoastrocytoma, and oligodendroglioma, must also be considered in the differential diagnosis. Surgical excision remains the primary therapy for the majority of low-grade gliomas. Since at least 50% of children with low-grade gliomas of the cerebral hemispheres present with seizures, the goal of surgery includes the alleviation of an associated seizure disorder, when intractable. It is now possible to appropriately target the operative approach to a subcortical lesion or a superficial lesion that is located within 'eloquent' cortex, using a combination of functional studies and stereotactic localization. Provided a total excision can be achieved, no further therapy is warranted. For those lesions that are incompletely resected, conservative management with routine imaging follow-up is appropriate, since childhood tumours rarely progress histologically to more malignant lesions. Reoperation is necessary, if recurrence is documented, and radiotherapy is utilized for those lesions that are incompletely resected following recurrence (Berger 1996).

Until recently, thalamic astrocytomas were considered to be largely unresectable. However, with the implementation of computer-assisted stereotactic approaches, perioperative morbidity and mortality have dropped substantially, and near complete resection has become an attainable goal in many children with pilocytic, low-grade, and cystic astrocytomas. In such cases, adjuvant therapy can often be deferred. For patients in whom a subtotal resection is performed to avoid the risk of incurring neurological deficit, long-term, disease-free survival can occur with certain indolent, low-grade astrocytomas which correspond histologically to pilocytic astrocytoma of the cerebellum or optic pathway. Adjuvant therapy, be it radiation (e.g. stereotactic procedures) or chemotherapy, is utilized in those cases of low-grade lesions that are unresectable and have documented disease progression.

High-grade gliomas—anaplastic astrocytoma and glioblastoma

Most malignant gliomas, other than brain-stem gliomas, are supratentorial in location and are among the most difficult tumours to treat in children. With a combination of surgery and irradiation, the median survival for children with malignant gliomas is only 9 months. In a randomized CCSG trial (1985–90), a multidrug regimen ('eight in one') was tested against CCNU, vincristine, and prednisone which had been evaluated in the first trial (1976–81). No difference was detected. However, both groups had outcomes superior to standard irradiation and surgery. For anaplastic astrocytoma and glioblastoma, respectively, 5-year-survival was 42% and 27% for patients with greater than 90% resection, compared with only 14% and 4% with less resection. However, it remains uncertain whether this survival advantage is a direct result of surgery, or merely reflects the fact that certain tumours, by virtue of their less aggressive growth characteristics or more favourable location, are amenable to more extensive resection (Lyden *et al.* 1996).

PNET

Medulloblastoma

Medulloblastoma is a distinctive, embryonal brain tumour originating in the posterior fossa and disseminating early through the cerebrospinal fluid (CSF).

The diagnosis of medulloblastoma is usually suspected from preoperative MRI. Dissemination via the CSF (20–30%) must be investigated by MRI and CSF cytology before starting postoperative therapy. A surgically based staging system tries to classify tumour stage (T1–T4)—location, volume, and extension into neighbourhood structures—and stage of metastatic disease (M0–M4). Disease classified as T1–T3a M0 is regarded as early stage (favourable), and T3b–4 as locally advanced high stage (unfavourable).

Some prognostic factors are commonly described in series dealing with medulloblastoma. The most significant adverse factor is subarachnoid spread at diagnosis and presence of metastatic disease (M1–M4). Further important prognostic factors are the age of the child, with worse outcome in young children (< 2 years), and tumour resectability, which is correlated to local stage.

Surgery and postoperative radiotherapy are the standard treatments. Chemotherapy is indicated for high-risk patients, but its role has yet to be clearly established for low-risk patients.

Surgery aims at total tumour removal, which can now be achieved in the vast majority of cases (including 'near total' removal). However, in general, no major surgery-related, permanent, neurological deficits are acceptable.

After surgery a 'posterior fossa syndrome' (e.g. truncal ataxia, cerebellar mutism) may occur. This may be transient but also may take months to recover. Its presence should not delay postoperative treatment (Sutton *et al.* 1996).

Postoperative craniospinal irradiation (CSI), with an additional field to the posterior fossa, remains obligatory for the cure of medulloblastoma. The dose to the posterior fossa should be above 50 Gy. The current consensus is for a total dose of about 55 Gy, using 160–180 cGy per fraction.

There is some controversy about the adequate dose for prophylactic irradiation (spinal and supratentorial). In series with a final outcome of more than 50% 5-year survival, the most frequently reported doses have been about 35 Gy. In favourable cases, radiation-dose reduction alone has led to inferior results. Trials are underway to compare (in favourable cases) 24 Gy CSI plus chemotherapy with 36 Gy CSI alone. In overt, disseminated disease, the CSI dose should be increased to 40 Gy, with additional boost doses of up to 45–50 Gy (Jenkin 1996).

Careful designing of target volumes is mandatory (CSI and posterior fossa boost), based on all the information available—e.g. surgical and histopathological reports, MRI—and on institutional experience. CSI is one of the most complicated radiation treatment techniques in a young child. Bad results may be due to inadequate radiation treatment planning and performance, and therefore very careful attention must be paid to this treatment.

Chemotherapy (with platinum, vincristine, CCNU, alkylating agents) is accepted as standard for high-risk patients: locally advanced medulloblastoma, disseminated disease, and young children under 3 years of age. Five-year progression-free survival rates of up to 80% are reported in unfavourable local disease, but these figures need confirmation. Many trials are currently underway, trying to clarify chemotherapy schedules and timing of their delivery within a combined treatment approach (CCG, POG, SIOP, GPOH, CHOP). The current SIOP protocol is shown in Fig. 12.2.

In different series, survival rates have been reported after surgery and radiotherapy ranging from 50–70% at 5 years, and 30–60% at 10 years. Single institutions even report survival rates of about 80% at 5 years (Cohen and Duffner 1994; Kaye and Laws 1995).

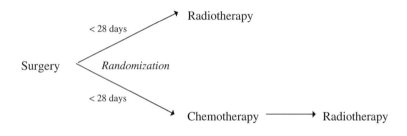

Chemotherapy   Radiotherapy

Vincristine 1.5 mg/m^2 bolus injection   Craniospinal 35 Gy.1.67 Gy/fraction.
Day 1, 7, 14, 21, 28, 35, 42, 49, 56, 63.

Carboplatin 500 mg/m^2 iv infusion over 1 hour   Post fossa boost 20 Gy.1.67 Gy/fraction.
in 5% Dexotrose. Days 1 and 2, 42 and 43.

Etoposide 100 mg/m^2 iv infusion over 1 hour in normal saline
Days 1, 2, 3;   21, 22, 23;   42, 43, 44;   63, 64, 65.

Cyclophosphamide 1500 mg/m^2 iv infused over 4 hours
Days 21, 63.

MESNA 750 mg/m^2 15 minutes before,+ 4 hours and 8 hours
after cyclophosphamide.

Fig. 12.2 Medulloblastoma SIOP III trial design protocol.

Other PNET

PNETs arising in the supratentorial region are associated with a different outcome, even when treatment similar to that given for medulloblastoma is used. These tumours occur often between birth and 5 years. They are found predominantly in the cerebral hemispheres, most commonly in the frontal and temporal lobes. On imaging, they may appear as well circumscribed masses, but there is often widespread microscopic extension. Glial, neuronal, or ependymal differentiation may be seen. Leptomeningeal spread is uncommon compared with medulloblastoma and is less frequent at presentation than with medulloblastoma. Patients present with non-specific signs of raised intracranial pressure, with seizures or motor impairment. Investigations should include imaging of the whole ventricular system and spine to exclude seeding. Surgical resection is often difficult because of their size and position. Craniospinal irradiation has been recommended, but results in progression-free survival rates of only 30%. Primary chemotherapy is being tested in current studies.

Ependymoma and choroid plexus neoplasms

Ependymomas arise from ependymal cells lining the ventricles and the central canal of the spinal cord. Nearly two-thirds occur in the infratentorial compartment. Anaplastic tumours tend to be more common in the posterior fossa than in the supratentorial region of young children. Tumour cells in the CSF are described in 5–15%; the rate of drop metastases is higher in anaplastic ependymoma.

Prognostic factors are the age of the patient, tumour location, tumour stage, histology, extent of resection, and radiation dose.

For optimal treatment planning, MRI of the brain and spinal cord at the time of diagnosis are mandatory.

Surgery, radiotherapy, and chemotherapy are used in treatment. Surgery is the most effective treatment, but is rarely curative. There are three indications for surgery: for tumour resection at diagnosis; for resection of residual disease after adjuvant therapy; for resection of a relapse, usually at the primary site. The primary goal is to remove the tumour totally and re-establish CSF flow.

If significant morbidity is to be avoided, total removal is often not possible in posterior fossa tumours, because of the specific growth pattern of ependymomas with invasion of the fourth ventricular floor and encasement of lower cranial nerves and regional arteries.

Although the role of postoperative radiotherapy is well established, there are many controversies regarding the appropriate extent of radiotherapy. Currently, postoperative CSI (35 Gy, 1.6 Gy per fraction) and boost to the primary tumour site (55 Gy, 1.8–2 Gy per fraction) are considered appropriate for anaplastic infratentorial ependymomas. CSI is also the standard basic treatment for disseminated tumours. In low-grade ependymoma, involved field radiotherapy alone (45–55 Gy) with broad margins (> 2 cm) seems to be sufficient after total resection (Halperin *et al.* 1994).

The role of chemotherapy is unclear. In current clinical trials, chemotherapy with vincristine, cisplatin, etoposide, and cyclophosphamide is being investigated. There seems to be an indication for children younger than 3 years, but neither the St Jude study nor 'Baby POG' has shown improved long-term outcome.

Overall, 5-year-survival rates, mostly after combination treatment, range from 28–60%, depending on prognostic factors (Cohen and Duffner 1994; Kaye and Laws 1995). The frequent local recurrence (within 18–24 months after diagnosis) is almost always incurable. Nevertheless, local palliative treatment procedures may improve symptoms for the limited life expectancy (Fig. 12.3).

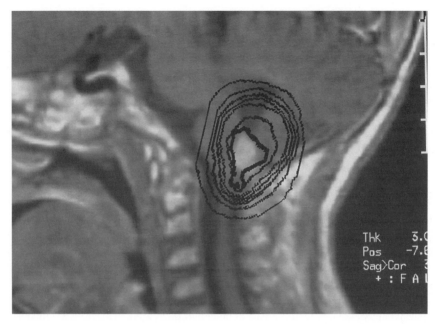

Fig. 12.3 Ependymoma recurrence: radiation dose distribution from stereotactic radiotheraphy using multiple arcs.

Choroid plexus neoplasms occur in all age-groups but represent 10–20% of brain tumours seen in children during the first year of life. The treatment of the benign choroid plexus papilloma is total surgical excision, which is usually curative. Surgery, however, can be difficult in these tumours due to their high vascularity. The likelihood of achieving gross total resection is less in the more aggressive and anaplastic choroid plexus carcinoma due to local invasion. The usefulness of radiotherapy, beyond that of slowing disease progression, is uncertain. In the young child, postoperative chemotherapy, with alkylator- and platinum-containing combinations, is the most promising approach.

Pineal tumours and germ-cell tumours

Tumours arising in the region of the pineal gland are rare, and can be classified into three groups: germ-cell tumours, pineal parenchymal tumours, and gliomas.

Primary CNS germ-cell tumours (40–65% of all pineal tumours) mainly arise in the pineal or suprasellar region. Their incidence is substantially higher in Japan than in Western countries. Their peak age-incidence is in the second or third decades of life. Germ-cell tumours are pathologically heterogeneous tumours, reflecting varied cell types of origin. At least half to two-thirds are pure germinomas. The remaining patients have non-germinomatous tumours, which may be classified, depending upon their predominant constituent cell type(s), into embryonal carcinoma, endodermal sinus (or yolk-sac) tumour, choriocarcinoma, malignant teratoma, or malignant, mixed germ-cell tumours. The histological appearance of these tumours is identical to similar tumours occurring outside the CNS. Rare patients are found with immature or mature teratomas, without any malignant germ-cell elements.

Once the presence of a pineal region mass has been demonstrated radiographically, CSF and serum should be examined for tumour markers such as alpha-fetoprotein (AFP) and the beta subunit of human chorionic gonadotrophin (β-HCG), which are produced by intracranial yolk-sac tumours and choriocarcinoma, respectively. This is important because in patients with significant marker elevation (β-HCG > 50 IU 1^{-1}, AFP > 25 ng ml^{-1}), surgery is not necessary to establish a tissue diagnosis before starting therapy. In all other patients, however, a histologically verified diagnosis is mandatory. Benign teratomas and dermoids are often surgically completely resectable, and thereby cured. In patients with malignant germ-cell tumours, leptomeningeal seeding may be present, and spinal MRI and CSF cytology are required for clinical staging.

For pure germinomas, radiotherapy alone leads to cure rates of up to 100% (e.g. GPOH trial). Dose (40–50 Gy local treatment and 22–35 Gy CSI) and volume, however, remain issues for debate. Some groups (e.g. SFOP) use platinum-based, multidrug regimens in combination with local radiotherapy and achieve equally good results.

Non-germinomatous germ-cell tumours are rarely cured with radiotherapy alone, and the addition of platinum-based chemotherapy is essential. Preoperative chemotherapy has been shown to be effective in facilitating complete resection of large or infiltrating tumours and in diminishing the risk of a primary operation. Local radiotherapy, however, is important for local control, even in patients with complete response to chemotherapy.

The pineal parenchymal tumours consist of pineoblastomas and pineocytomas. Pineoblastomas develop in the younger patient and belong to the primitive neuroectodermal tumours (PNET). The high malignancy suggests that the approach to treatment should be similar to medulloblastoma and include aggressive resection, CSI with a local boost, and chemotherapy. Pure pineocytomas are more slowly growing, relatively well-circumscribed masses, and have a benign course. Complete surgical removal represents the definitive treatment. Careful evaluation of the histology must exclude malignant components revealing a mixed tumour, which should be treated according to its most malignant part (Cohen and Duffner 1994).

Craniopharyngiomas

Craniopharyngiomas are histologically benign tumours originating in the sellar and suprasellar area from embryonic squamous cell rests of the pharyngeal-hypophyseal duct. Their macroscopic and neuroradiological appearance is that of a cystic, solid, or mixed-mass lesion, typically with calcifications.

Since they are slow growing tumours, they may reach large sizes before they become symptomatic, with endocrine dysfunction, visual problems, or signs of ICP with obstructive hydrocephalus in about 30%.

The best management of craniopharyngioma in children remains controversial. Treatment options for this tumour include microsurgery, fractionated conformal radiotherapy, stereotactic procedures, intracavitary radiotherapy, and intracavitary chemotherapy.

Surgery is performed with either an attempt at radical total removal, or more conservatively followed by radiotherapy. Total removal is possible in 60–90% of cases. Even in these recent series, however, recurrence rates between 7% and 34%, with an average of 23%, are reported, and even in experienced hands, major morbidity remains a concern. Morbidity not only relates to a deterioration of visual and pituitary function, but even more importantly to complex and severe cognitive and neurobehavioural disturbances. If the tumour is totally removed, no further imme-diate treatment is indicated (Epstein and Handler 1991).

Recurrence is treated by reoperation followed by radiotherapy, or radiotherapy alone. As approximately 70% of patients with partial resection will show tumour progression, these patients should be irradiated with conformal or stereotactic techniques (50–55 Gy). Occasionally, radi-ation will be deferred in a young child, but these patients require close follow-up. With a definitely lower mortality and morbidity, the long-term tumour control with this combined approach com-pares well with initial, aggressive, total resection alone, with about 20% recurrent tumour growth.

Intracavitary radiotherapy with ^{32}P or ^{90}Y in experienced centres has given excellent results in monocystic tumours. Intracystic application of bleomycin has not only been shown to facilitate sub-sequent resection due to fibrosis of the capsule, but can also lead to shrinkage and long-term control.

Intramedullary spinal cord tumours

Spinal cord tumours account for only 3–6% of primary CNS tumours in children. Of intra-medullary tumours, up to 60% are astrocytomas, and 20–30% ependymomas. Oligodendro-gliomas and gangliogliomas are less frequent. In general, these tumours are well differentiated, low-grade tumours, with only 10% having high-grade or anaplastic features. The tumours may be focal or extend to involve multiple segments. The most common symptom is local pain along the spinal axis, alteration of a previously normal gait, and other signs of spinal cord malfunction occurring later in the course of the disease. Hydrocephalus may complicate the clinical picture in as many as 15% of patients with spinal cord tumours.

Surgery for diagnosis and resection, if possible, is mandatory. Complete surgical resections are difficult in astrocytomas and appear to be possible more frequently in ependymomas, which tend to have a clearer cleavage plane.

Postoperative orthopaedic follow-up and monitoring for spinal deformity are important.

No controlled trial of radiation or chemotherapy has been carried out for intramedullary tumours, and evidence for their usefulness has to be inferred from the treatment of similar tumours in other CNS sites, such as cranial low-grade glioma, and ependymomas. If radiotherapy is performed, it is targeted to the tumour region, with a total dose of 40–50 Gy, and seems to improve functional recovery.

The overall survival rates of low-grade astrocytomas, with various degrees of resection and post-operative radiation therapy, are 66–70% at 5 years and 55% at 10 years. Local recurrence rates as high as 33–86% have been reported. In ependymomas, survival rates—depending on the amount of resection—vary from 50–100% at 5 years and 50–70% at 10 years (Epstein and Constantini 1995).

In the rare anaplastic, or high-grade tumours, postoperative total neuraxis irradiation and adju-vant chemotherapy are recommended. However, patients usually succumb to their disease due to local progression or dissemination along CSF pathways.

Management of brain tumours in very young children

Brain tumours in infants and very young children have unique properties with regard to clinical pre-sentation, anatomical location, histology, and prognosis that distinguish them from brain tumours occurring in the older child. By the time of diagnosis, most tumours in infants are quite large.

Delay in diagnosis occurs, in part, because the infant skull can expand to accommodate ICP, hence masking for some time the typical signs and symptoms associated with a mass lesion. Infants may present with failure to thrive (despite good appetite and food intake), endocrinopathies, developmental delay, vomiting, decreased visual acuity, and nystagmus accompanied by expanding head circumference.

Infants with brain tumours have the worst prognosis of any age-group. Although delay in diagnosis, tumour type and size, and the tendency for early dissemination may be important factors, the poor outcome probably reflects the limitations of treatment. Surgery is more difficult in the young child, due to tumour size, fragility of the immature brain, and problems related to neuroanaesthesia. In addition, radiation is known to be very toxic in this age-group. Therefore, the dose is routinely reduced by at least 10–20%. This reduction in dose is probably inadequate for tumour control. Nevertheless, even with reduced radiation dose, major long-term effects, including learning disabilities, mental retardation, endocrinopathies, leukoencephalopathy, and vasculopathy, are to be expected in a significant number of patients. These concerns have resulted in interest in delaying or eliminating radiation in this young population by postoperative chemotherapy. The largest study of prolonged postoperative chemotherapy and delayed radiation in infants with brain tumours has come from the POG. 198 children, less than 3 years of age with malignant brain tumours, were treated with a combination of cyclophosphamide, vincristine, cis-platinum, and VP16. Thirty-nine per cent of all patients with measurable disease postoperatively had complete or partial responses following two cycles of cyclophosphamide and vincristine. Response rates were highest for medulloblastoma (48%), malignant glioma (60%), and ependymoma (48%). Brain-stem gliomas and PNETs showed little or no response. The 1-year, progression-free survival was 42–47% in ependymomas, medulloblastomas, and high-grade gliomas, which compared favourably with historical controls using standard postoperative radiation. Most failures occurred within the first year, with few late failures.

Treating infants and very young children with medulloblastoma, ependymoma, and malignant glioma with primary post-operative chemotherapy and delayed radiation has become the standard approach for the majority of these patients (Duffner *et al.* 1993).

Late effects in children treated for brain tumours

As 5- and 10-year survival rates of children with CNS tumours have increased, so has concern over late effects of treatment. Many long-term survivors have intellectual, endocrine, and neurological deficits that lead to significant social handicaps as well as diminished quality of life. Damage to the CNS from several sources may play a role in these deficits. Direct destruction of normal brain tissue by tumour, as well as surgical trauma, may cause some degree of irreversible neurological damage. Likewise, chemotherapy, especially in combination with radiation, appears capable of inducing encephalopathy. However, it is radiation therapy that has been implicated as the main cause of adverse, long-term sequelae, particularly intellectual impairment. Some reports suggest that most children receiving whole-brain radiation have some form of cognitive deficits in various intelligence quotients, visual/perceptual skills, learning abilities, and adaptive behaviour. Prospective, controlled studies have found a younger age at diagnosis, radiotherapy, methotrexate chemotherapy, tumour location, and time interval to testing to be important and related to a high risk of subsequent cognitive deficits. Dose, fractionation, and volume of radiation influence the development of these deficits, with more severe sequelae occurring at higher doses and larger volumes (Halperin *et al.* 1994). Thus, current cooperative group studies are treating infants and very young children with brain tumours with prolonged postoperative chemotherapy in an attempt either to delay or to eliminate cranial radiation entirely.

Detailed studies have revealed a wide range of endocrine dysfunction following cranial irradiation which includes the hypothalamic-pituitary region. The most common impairment is growth failure due to growth hormone deficiency (Cohen and Duffner 1994). Although growth hormone replacement therapy will improve longitudinal growth, it has not been as effective as in children with idiopathic growth hormone deficiency. Another factor contributing to decreased growth is spinal irradiation. The younger the child at the time of spinal irradiation, the more severe the adverse effects on vertebral body growth.

Hypothyroidism may also occur, and if not corrected may lead to poor linear growth, learning difficulties, and lethargy. Evaluation of T4 and TSH function will allow early treatment of this problem. Gonadal dysfunction has only recently been reported in children with brain tumours. Radiation to the sacral spine, as well as a number of cytotoxic drugs, particularly alkylating agents, are associated with gonadal damage and can cause ovarian failure, oligospermia, or azoospermia in these patients. As more chemotherapy is used and the patients are followed longer, it is likely that a much higher incidence of these side-effects will be noted. Thus, several risk factors need to be addressed by future studies, and careful planning of drug-radiation combinations is essential to maximize survival while reducing long-term local and systemic sequelae.

It is therefore of paramount importance that these children remain under long-term surveillance so that problems are anticipated and therapeutic strategies are instituted as early as possible (see also Chapter 7).

References

Barkovoch, A.J. (1993), Paediatric neuroimaging. *Contemporary Neuroimaging*, Volume 1, 2nd Edition. Raven Press, New York.

Berger, M.S. (1996), The impact of technical adjuncts in the surgical management of cerebral hemispheric low-grade gliomas of childhood. *Journal of Neuro-Oncology*, 28, 129–55.

Campbell, J.W. and Pollack, I.F. (1996), Cerebellar astrocytoma in children. *Journal of Neuro-Oncology*, 28, 223–31.

Cohen, M.E. and Duffner, P.K. (eds.) (1994), Brain tumours in children. Principles of Diagnosis and Treatment. 2nd Edition, Raven Press, New York: principles of radiotherapy pp. 95–116 (L. Kun), principles of chemotherapy pp. 177–146 (M.L. Brecher), medulloblastomas pp. 177–201, ependymomas, pp. 219–39, pineal region tumours, pp. 329–46, long-term clinical effects pp. 455–81.

Duffner, P.K., Horowitz, M., Krischer, J., Friedman, H.S., Burger, P.C., Cohen, M.E., *et al.* (1993). Post-operative chemotherapy and delayed radiotherapy in children less than 3 years of age with malignant brain tumours. *New England Journal of Medicine*, 328, 1725–30.

Epstein, F.J. and Constantini, S. (1995), Spinal cord tumours of childhood. *Disorders of the pediatric spine* (ed. D. Pang), Raven Press Ltd, New York, pp. 371–88.

Epstein, F.J. and Handler, M.H. (eds.) (1991), Craniopharyngioma: The Answer, *Paediatric Neurosurgery*, 21, (Suppl. 1), 1–130.

Halperin, E.C., Constine, L.E., Tarbell, N.J., and Kun, L.E. (1994), Paediatric Radiation Oncology. 2nd edition, Raven Press, New York, pp. 40–139.

Heideman, R.L., Packer, J., Albright, L.A., Freeman, C.R., and Rorke, L.B. (1997), Tumours of the central nervous system. *Principles and Practice of Paediatric Oncology* (eds. P.A. Pizzo and D.G. Poplack), 3rd edition, pp. 633–698. J.B. Lippincott Company, Philadephia.

Jenkin, D. (1996), The radiation treatment of medulloblastoma. *Journal of Neuro-Oncology*, 29, pp. 45–54.

Kaye, A.H. and Laws Jr., E.R. (eds.) (1995), Brain Tumours. Churchill Livingstone: Glioma of the optic pathways pp. 665–671, intracranial ependymomas pp. 493–504, medulloblastoma and primitive neuroectodermal tumours, pp. 561–74.

Kleihues, P., Burger, P.C., and Scheithauer, B.W. (1993), Histological typing of tumours of the central nervous system. 2nd edition, Berlin-Heidelberg-New York-London-Paris-Tokyo-Hong Kong-Barcelona-Budapest, Springer.

Lyden, D.C., Mason, W.P., and Finlay, J.L. (1996), The expanding role of chemotherapy for supratentorial malignant gliomas. *Journal of Neuro-Oncology*, 28, 185–91.

Pollack, I.F. (1994), Brain tumours in children. *The New England Journal of Medicine*, 331, No. 22, pp. 1500–07.

Raffel, C. (1996), Molecular biology of paediatric gliomas. *Journal of Neuro-Oncology*, 28, 121–28.

Sutton, L.N., Phillips, P.C., and Molloy, P.T. (1996), Surgical management of medulloblastoma, *Journal of Neuro-Oncology*, 29, pp. 9–21.

Thomas, D.G.T. and Graham, D.I. (eds) (1995), Malignant brain tumours, Springer-Verlag.

13 Rhabdomyosarcoma

M.C.G. Stevens

Introduction and perspective

Rhabdomyosarcoma (RMS) is the commonest form of soft-tissue sarcoma encountered in child-hood, and accounts for approximately 4–5% of all childhood malignancy. It is rare in adults, and the peak incidence is seen early in childhood with a median age at diagnosis of about 5 years. Males (60%) are more frequently affected than females. The heterogeneity with which RMS presents at different anatomical sites has been a particular factor in determining strategies for treatment. The additional prognostic influence of histological subtype and the more recent emergence of important biological factors, add to the complexities of treatment planning.

Any attempt to read and understand the literature relating to RMS is complicated by the different terminologies used for staging and pathological classification. Recent collaboration between the North American Intergroup Rhabdomyosarcoma Study (IRS) Group and their European counterparts, the International Society of Paediatric Oncology (SIOP), German (CWS), and Italian soft-tissue sarcoma groups, has begun to resolve some of these difficulties by agreeing a standard approach to the criteria used for staging and pathological classification (Rodary *et al.* 1989; Newton *et al.* 1995).

Aetiology and biology

The histological classification (see below) of RMS is based on the resemblance of the tumour to normal foetal muscle. The mature elements (rhabdomyoblasts) share patterns of expression of muscle-specific regulatory genes consistent with skeletal muscle differentiation. RMS is, however, not restricted to sites of skeletal muscle development, and it is clear that these tumours are more broadly of mesenchymal tissue origin, characterized to a greater or lesser degree by evidence for myogenic differentiation.

The aetiology is unclear, but an association with both familial cancer risk in the Li Fraumeni syndrome (Li and Fraumeni 1969), and the more recent identification of genetic mechanisms to account for tumourogenicity (Loh *et al.* 1992; Shapiro *et al.* 1993), have created considerable interest in possible genetic factors in its causation. This may be further supported by the evidence for an association between RMS and congenital abnormalities (Ruymann *et al.* 1988) and other genetic conditions, including neurofibromatosis type 1. Additional aetiological theories may emerge from data suggesting links between RMS and various environmental factors, as diverse as parental smoking habits and use of 'recreational' drugs, fetal-alcohol syndrome, and occupational chemical exposures (Ruymann and Grufferman 1991).

The link between RMS and risk of breast cancer in female relatives may be of particular importance in highlighting previously unrecognized familial cancer risk in a small number of families for whom cancer control or screening strategies could be implemented. The link between these different malignancies may result from germ-line expression of mutant *p53* (Malkin *et al.* 1990).

Pathology

Classically, RMS is distinguished histologically in two main forms, the embryonal (which accounts for approximately 80% of all RMS) and alveolar subtypes (15–20% of RMS). A third group, pleomorphic RMS, is described but is virtually never encountered in a paediatric setting and no longer forms part of a paediatric classification. This classical definition has been further subdivided by the identification of three important subtypes within these two major groups. Botryoid RMS and a spindle-cell variant are both morphological variants of embryonal RMS, and solid alveolar RMS is a variant of classical alveolar RMS.

Embryonal rhabdomyosarcoma

This is characterized by a spindle or spindle and round cell tumour in a loose myxoid or dense collagenous stroma. Rhabdomyoblastic differentiation is expressed in the presence of strap-like cells, but cellularity, pleomorphism, and the number of mitoses vary considerably. Cross-striations are seen in more differentiated forms, and ultrastructural examination with electron microscopy demonstrates the presence of features such as sarcomeric Z bands, and thin and thick filaments. The botryoid subtype is typically found at vaginal or nasopharyngeal sites where tumour grows into organ cavities. It is histologically similar to embryonal RMS, with the additional feature of a condensed layer of tumour cells under the overlying mucosa, the so called cambium layer. The spindle-cell variant presents either as a collagen-poor leiomyomatous form or as a collagen-rich form with a storiform pattern. Distinction from other forms of soft-tissue sarcoma relies on the presence of well-differentiated rhabdomyoblasts in the spindle cell population.

Alveolar rhabdomyosarcoma

Classically, this shows an alveolar architecture, i.e. well-defined, alveolar-like spaces separated by thick collagenous bands, and lined with round tumour cells showing variable myogenic features. It is now generally accepted that the percentage of cells showing an alveolar pattern is unimportant and that even its focal presence is sufficient to justify the diagnosis. However, attention has also been paid to the cytological features of alveolar RMS which are distinct from embryonal RMS, and a diagnosis of alveolar RMS can be made in the absence of an overt alveolar pattern if the characteristic cytological features are present. This is the basis for the diagnosis of the so-called solid alveolar variant.

International classification of rhabdomyosarcoma

More recently, pathologists from the major international soft-tissue sarcoma groups have published a consensus for a new International Classification of Rhabdomyosarcoma (ICR) (Newton *et al.* 1995). This has been tested in multivariate analysis and shown to be strongly predictive of survival in addition to the established clinical risk factors. This classification system should now be used by all pathologists and cooperative groups in order to provide comparability between and within multi-institutional studies (Table 13.1). In this classification, the definition of alveolar RMS includes the solid alveolar subtype. There remain, however, areas of uncertainty, particularly with tumours which do not demonstrate clear cytological evidence for myogenic differentiation (Undifferentiated Sarcoma), or which cannot be adequately classified (Sarcoma NOS). There are also tumours, such as those with rhabdoid features, where it is not clear whether these form a distinct and separate group, or if they represent morphological variants of the major subtypes.

New diagnostic techniques

Immunohistochemistry (particularly for desmin and myoD1) is used to support or clarify morphological evidence for myogenesis, and now forms a routine aspect of the pathological diagnosis of RMS; but this is never a completely reliable technique (particularly in poorly differentiated embryonal tumours), and is open to subjective variation in its interpretation. Other technologies, particularly molecular genetic detection of the expression of myogenic transcription factors (for example, the *MYF* genes from the myoD protein family) and the presence of cytogenetic abnormalities representing abnormal fusion genes, are likely to become increasingly important in clarifying the diagnosis of RMS, in distinguishing it from other soft-tissue or small round cell tumours, and in confirming histological subtype. Most alveolar RMS demonstrate t(2,13) (q35;q14) or, less frequently, a variant t(1,13) (Turc-Carel *et al.* 1986), while many embryonal RMS show genetic loss on chromosome 11p15.5 (Scrable *et al.* 1989). Techniques to demonstrate such abnormalities are available, and although not yet robust enough for routine use, or reliable in paraffin-fixed tissue, their development may result in the need for a further review of existing classification schemes.

Table 13.1 Proposed International Pathology Classification for childhood rhabdomyosarcoma

Prognostic group	Histological subtypes
I (Superior prognosis)	Botryoid RMS
	Spindle-cell RMS
II (Intermediate prognosis)	Embryonal RMS
III (Poor prognosis)	Alveolar RMS
	Undifferentiated sarcoma
IV (Prognosis uncertain)	RMS with rhabdoid features

(Source: Newton *et al.* 1995)

Clinical presentation and diagnosis

RMS is encountered at almost all anatomical sites, although the head and neck and genitourinary locations are the most common (Fig. 13.1). Presentation is strongly influenced by site: for example, tumours within the orbit tend to present early with obvious displacement of the globe and are rarely associated with regional lymph-node or distant metastatic spread (Fig. 13. 2), while tumours in the nasopharynx may result in a relatively long history of nasal discharge and obstruction, and frequently involve local extension into the base of the skull or the posterior aspect of the orbits with the potential for associated cranial nerve palsies or visual loss. (Fig. 13.3). The definition of certain head and neck sites as 'parameningeal' (Table 13.2) relates to the risk of direct tumour extension into the meninges and beyond. Such tumours carry a risk of intracranial extension and, in some cases, CSF involvement. Tumours within the genitourinary tract may present with urinary obstruction (in bladder and prostate sites) (Fig. 13.4), as a scrotal mass (paratesticular), or as a vaginal polyp or discharge (vaginal and uterine tumours). Elsewhere, presentation is usually associated with development of a mass, and often the child is not unwell unless there is metastatic disease. In rare cases, widespread metastatic disease is encountered without clear evidence of a primary tumour, and the diagnosis is confirmed by bone marrow examination.

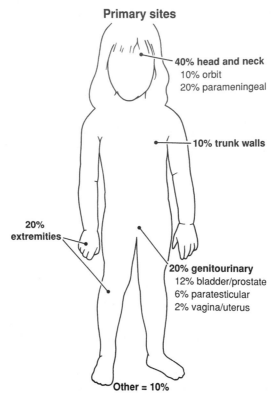

Primary sites

40% head and neck
10% orbit
20% parameningeal

10% trunk walls

20% extremities

20% genitourinary
12% bladder/prostate
6% paratesticular
2% vagina/uterus

Other = 10%

Fig. 13.1 Distribution of sites of disease.

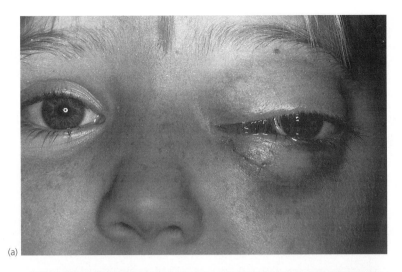

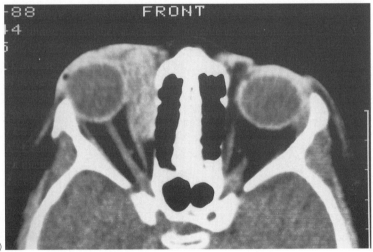

Fig. 13.2 Orbital tumour (a) clinical presentation with proptosis and deviation of globe. (b) CT scan shows large anteromedial soft-tissue mass without bone erosion.

Diagnostic and staging investigations must include adequate imaging of the primary site (CT or MRI) and accurate assessment of sites of potential metastatic spread (lungs, bones, and bone marrow). CSF should be sampled in the case of parameningeal tumours. The involvement of regional lymph nodes depends on the primary site, but the frequency with which positive lymph-node spread is reported also depends on the manner in which this is investigated. This remains a source of some controversy and, for example, the strategies promoted by the North American IRS Group have always encouraged more systematic use of surgicopathological lymph-node assessment than in the European SIOP studies, for which clinical and radiological evaluation has been the standard approach.

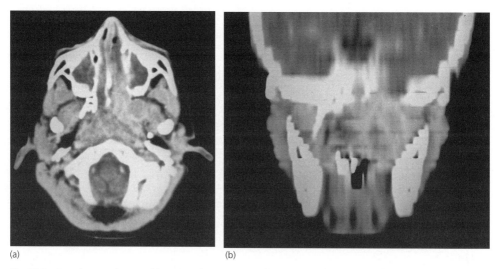

(a)   (b)

Fig. 13.3 Nasopharyngeal tumour (a) CT scan showing large soft-tissue mass filling the nasopharynx and nasal cavities with destruction of the pterygoid plate. (b) CT scan reconstruction showing tumour extension through the base of skull.

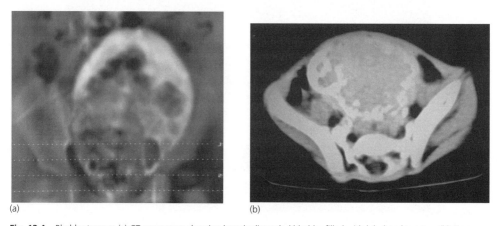

(a)   (b)

Fig. 13.4 Bladder tumour (a) CT scanogram showing hugely distended bladder filled with lobulated tumour. (b) Cross-sectional CT image showing lobulated tumour filling bladder and outlined by contrast excretion into surrounding urine.

Diagnosis must be confirmed histologically, and although needle biopsy may be the simplest approach and is favoured by some clinicians, it has the disadvantage of limiting tissue available for conventional histological examination, including immunohistochemistry, and may restrict access to fresh and frozen tissue for cytogenetic and molecular genetic investigation—techniques which may be of considerable importance in guiding diagnosis in difficult cases. Open biopsy is therefore frequently preferred and should, if possible, be undertaken at the oncology centre, where the optimal use of diagnostic material can be achieved and the initial surgical approach determined by the multidisciplinary team responsible for the child's subsequent treatment. As site is such an important determinant of prognosis and of treatment strategy, classification by site has been standardized by international agreement into seven major groups (Table 13.2) (Donaldson *et al.* 1986).

Table 13.2 Definition of sites of involvement in childhood rhabdomyosarcoma

Head and neck	Orbit
Head and neck	Non-parameningeal
Head and neck	Parameningeal[1]
Genitourinary	Bladder—prostate
Genitourinary	Non-bladder—prostate[2]
Limbs	
Other[3]	

[1] Parameningeal sites include nasopharynx, nasal cavity, paranasal sinuses, middle ear, mastoid, pterygoid fossa, and any non-parameningeal site with extension into a parameningeal position (e.g. orbital tumour extending intracranially into ethmoid sinus).
[2] Genitourinary, non-bladder prostate sites include paratesticular, vaginal, and uterine tumours.
[3] Other sites include trunk, chest, and abdominal walls, intraabdominal, intrapelvic, perineal, and paravertebral tumours.

Staging

The purpose of staging is to classify tumours into categories from which treatment can be planned and prognosis predicted. It is also important to be able to compare the outcome of different treatment strategies within groups of patients with similar disease. Two main approaches have been used in staging RMS—the postsurgical, clinical grouping system developed by the North American IRS Group (Lawrence *et al.* 1987) and a TNM system used by the SIOP MMT committee (Rodary *et al.* 1989) (Table 13.3 and 13.4). Attempts to compare and standardize the systems used have been discussed between the major collaborative treatment groups in international workshops (Rodary *et al.* 1989). The key issue in any staging system is to ensure a classification that allows patients to be allocated to a treatment strategy according to prognostic

Table 13.3 IRS clinical grouping system

Group	Description of disease
I	Localized disease, completely resected
	a) confined to organ or muscle of origin
	b) infiltration outside organ or muscle of origin
	Regional nodes not involved
II	Compromised or regional resection of three types:
	a) grossly resected tumours with microscopic residual, no evidence of regional lymph-node involvement
	b) regional disease, completely resected, in which nodes may be involved, and/or extension of tumour into an adjacent organ but with no microscopic residual
	c) regional disease with involved nodes, grossly resected, but with evidence of microscopic residual
III	Incomplete resection or biopsy only with gross (macroscopic) residual disease
IV	Distant metastases present at diagnosis

grouping. The features selected must not only take into account the extent of the disease at first presentation, but also the impact of any initial surgery and the amount of residual disease before starting chemotherapy, i.e. a consideration of both pre- and postsurgical staging factors. This is incorporated in the staging system promoted by the SIOP group (Tables 13.4a and 13.4b).

At presentation, most patients do not have evidence of regional lymph-node or distant metastases (Fig. 13.5). Prior to effective multiagent chemotherapy, there was a much greater emphasis on radical primary surgery, but the value of chemotherapy and the possibility of delaying surgery (where feasible) until later in the course of treatment has reduced the number of patients in whom primary tumour resection is attempted. The great majority of patients (approximately 75%) will have macroscopic residual disease at the primary site (postsurgical pT3bc in the SIOP TNM staging system; IRS Clinical Group III) at the start of chemotherapy, whether or not they also have node or distant metastases (Table 13.5 and Fig. 13.6).

Treatment strategies

The importance of multiagent chemotherapy has been clearly demonstrated for RMS as part of coordinated, multimodality treatment. Cure rates have improved from approximately 25% in the

Table 13.4a   SIOP pretreatment TNM staging

Stage	TNM characteristics		
I	T1a, T1b	N0, NX	M0
II	T2a, T2b	N0, NX	M0
III	Any T	N1	M0
IV	Any T	Any N	M1

T = Primary tumour
T0   No evidence of primary tumour
T1   Tumour confined to the organ or tissue or origin
        T1a   Tumour 5 cm or less in its greatest dimension
        T1b   Tumour more than 5 cm in its greatest dimension
T2   Tumours involving one or more contiguous organs or tissues or with adjacent malignant effusion, or multiple tumours in the same organ
        T2a   Tumour 5 cm or less in its greatest dimension
        T2b   Tumour more than 5 cm in its greatest dimension

N = Regional lymph nodes (see Table 13.5)
N0   No evidence of regional lymph-node involvement
N1   Evidence of regional lymph-node involvement

M = Distant metastases
M0   No evidence of distant metastases
M1   Evidence of distant metastases

Table 13.4b SIOP Postsurgical histopathological (pTNM) classification

pT = Primary tumour

pT0	No evidence of tumour found on histological examination of specimen
pT1	Tumour limited to organ or tissue of origin
	Excision complete and margins histologically free
pT2	Tumour with invasion beyond the organ or tissue of origin
	Excision complete and margins histologically free
pT3	Tumour with or without invasion beyond the organ or tissue of origin
	Excision incomplete
pT3a	Evidence of microscopic residual tumour
pT3b	Evidence of macroscopic residual tumour or biopsy only
pT3c	Adjacent malignant effusion regardless of the size

pN = Regional lymph nodes

pN0	No evidence of tumour found on histological examination of regional lymph nodes
pN1	Evidence of invasion of regional lymph nodes
pN1a	Evidence of invasion of regional lymph nodes
	Involved nodes considered to be completely resected
pN1b	Evidence of invasion of regional lymph nodes
	Involved nodes considered to be incompletely resected

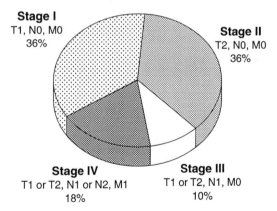

Stage I
T1, N0, M0
36%

Stage II
T2, N0, M0
36%

Stage IV
T1 or T2, N1 or N2, M1
18%

Stage III
T1 or T2, N1, M0
10%

Fig. 13.5 Pie chart showing distribution of clinical (TNM) stage at diagnosis.

early 1970s when combination chemotherapy was first implemented. It has been subsequently explored in a series of multicentre clinical trials in both North America and Europe (Pappo *et al.* 1995). Nevertheless, overall prognosis remains less than satisfactory, with 5-year survival rates of approximately 70%. Strategies have evolved which match the complexity of treatment against known prognostic factors—site, stage, and pathological subtype. These are utilized in stratifying treatment intensity and can select patients with good or poor predicted outcomes. Developments

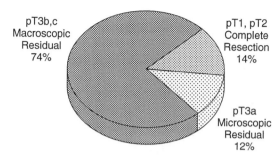

Fig. 13.6 Pie chart showing distribution of postsurgical stage (pTNM) before chemotherapy.

Table 13.5 Definition of regional lymph notes

Primary tumour site	Regional lymph nodes
Head and neck	Cervical and supraclavicular
Orbit	Preauricular
Abdominal and pelvic	Subdiaphragmatic, intraabdominal, and iliac according to site (e.g. for bladder prostate tumours, iliac nodes are the regional nodes and lumbo (para) aortic nodes are second-level nodes)
Paratesticular	External iliac and paraaortic
Perineum	Inguinal and iliac
Upper limbs	Epitrochlear and axillary
Lower limbs	Popliteal and inguinal

1. Regional lymph-node involvement = stage III disease in the SIOP classification.
2. In the case of unilateral tumours, all contralateral-involved lymph nodes are considered to be distant metastases (except in the head and neck).
3. Node involvement beyond the regional site represents stage IV disease.

in understanding the biology of RMS may offer additional prognostic variables which could be useful in further refining treatment stratification. There remain, however, anxieties about the possible overtreatment of patients with a good prospect for cure, as well as the persistently unacceptable cure rates for patients with less favourable disease. It is in this context that some important differences in treatment philosophy have emerged.

Prognostic factors

Stage, site, and pathology

These three variables remain the most consistent factors of prognostic significance across all major studies of RMS, but they are also interdependent.

Stage alone is a strong independent prognostic factor (Lawrence *et al.* 1987), and the IRS clinical grouping system shows a clear stratification of outcome through clinical groups I–IV (Table 13.7).

Site influences both tumour stage and histology. For example, orbital tumours are almost exclusively of the embryonal subtype, while limb tumours are overrepresented amongst those with alveolar histology. Tumours with favourable histological subtypes include those at bladder and vaginal sites, many of which show botryoid features, and paratesticular tumours which are often characterized by the spindle-cell variant of embryonal RMS. The interrelationship between site and clinical stage is shown in Fig. 13.7. Limb and (in some series) head and neck tumours are associated with a high incidence of regional lymph-node involvement (TNM Stage III), and limb tumours are also those most frequently associated with metastatic (stage IV) disease.

The prognostic importance of site is well recognized, and tumours arising from the orbit and genitourinary tract have the best outcome, followed by non-parameningeal head and neck tumours. Tumours arising in limbs and at 'other' sites have the worst prognosis, but outcome by site will also vary according to treatment strategy, particularly in relation to the use of local therapy.

The influence of histology on outcome has been less clear, although the adverse effect of alveolar histology was recognized in the first two IRS studies. However, IRS III did not identify this as an independent prognostic factor in patients with localized tumours (Crist *et al.* 1995). Inevitably, changes in intensity of treatment must also be considered as prognostic variables, and it is likely that intensification of treatment for patients with alveolar histology in IRS III eliminated its independent prognostic importance. The importance of alveolar histology has been observed in other studies (Stevens *et al.* 1995; Flamant, in press), influencing treatment stratification in the more recent MMT 95 study.

Biological variables

The importance of biological factors as aids to diagnosis has already been discussed, particularly in relation to the use of cytogenetics and molecular genetics to aid clarification of the histological

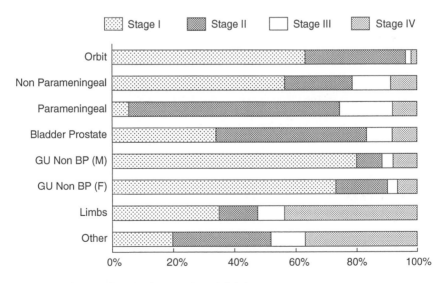

Fig. 13.7 Histogram showing relationship between site and clinical stage.
GU = genitourinary; BP = bladder prostate.

subtype (e.g. t(2;13) in alveolar RMS). This may, of course, have a direct impact on the precision of treatment stratification, and perhaps even become therapeutically important in the future development of gene therapy interventions. There are other biological 'markers' of disease behaviour which may enter consideration as additional factors in determining treatment strategies. In particular, there has been interest in the significance of DNA content utilizing techniques to measure tumour-cell ploidy and proliferative activity (S phase) (Pappo *et al.* 1995; Niggli *et al.* 1994). Tumours with hyperdiploid DNA content appear to have a better outcome, and those with tetraploid content do badly but are also overrepresented amongst patients with alveolar histology. The value of determining DNA content has yet to be established by multivariate analysis in the context of a large clinical trial.

Many of the patients who subsequently relapse have usually demonstrated a good response to initial chemotherapy, raising the possibility that acquired or intrinsic drug resistance mechanisms may be important in determining outcome. A single report (Chan *et al.* 1990) has identified cellular expression of p-glycoprotein (as a marker of multiple drug resistance—MDR) as a prognostic factor in RMS, and suggests that the possibility of therapeutic intervention to overcome MDR may be a way forward in circumventing treatment failure. This requires further evaluation.

The prognostic relevance of other molecular genetic changes, such as identification of *p53* mutations and expression of *myc* oncogenes within RMS, remains uncertain.

Treatment philosophies

Local tumour control is central to the possibility of cure for patients with non-metastatic disease. Controversies here relate to the method and timing of local treatment, and, more specifically, to the place of radiotherapy in guaranteeing local control for patients who appear to achieve complete remission with chemotherapy with or without surgery. This represents an important philosophical difference between the SIOP MMT studies and those of the IRS Group and, to some extent, those of the German and Italian cooperative groups. Local relapse rates are higher in the SIOP studies than those experienced elsewhere, although the SIOP experience has also made it clear that a significant number of patients who relapse may be cured with alternative treatment (Flamant, in press) (although the prospect for survival after relapse is seriously diminished if the patient has failed locally after previous radiotherapy). In the context of such differences in approach to local treatment, overall survival rather than disease-free or progression-free survival becomes the most important criterion for measuring outcome. The 'cost' of survival must, however, take into account the predicted late sequelae of treatment and the total burden of therapy experienced by an individual patient. This must include an assessment of all the treatment used, including that used for treatment of relapse. Although strategies which increase the intensity of initial chemotherapy may successfully limit local therapy in some patients, the use of agents such as iphosphamide and the anthracycline drugs are of particular concern, and the sequelae from the use of chemotherapy, particularly the risks of nephrotoxicity, cardiotoxicity, and second malignancy, cannot be ignored.

Surgery

At diagnosis

Biopsy is required for diagnosis, but primary tumour resection should be undertaken only if there is no evidence of lymph-node or metastatic disease, and if the tumour can be excised with good margins without danger, functional impairment, or mutilation. An attempt at surgical resection which leaves microscopic residual disease is possibly the worst outcome of all, as the patient is then unassessable for the efficacy of chemotherapy and may still require further local treatment.

Primary re-excision (i.e. a second surgical resection before chemotherapy) may be worthwhile in a minority of cases if there is confidence that clear margins of excision can be achieved without functional or cosmetic disadvantage (Hays *et al.* 1989). Histological assessment of tumour margins is not always consistent with the surgical findings because of the diffuse infiltration of some tumours into adjacent tissues.

The importance of surgical evaluation of lymph nodes at diagnosis is controversial. Clinically and radiologically, suspicious nodes should be sampled (fine needle aspiration may be a useful technique in such circumstances), but radical lymph node dissections are rarely justified and it is now generally accepted that routine surgical staging of regional (para-aortic) nodes in patients with localized, paratesticular tumours is unnecessary (Olive *et al.* 1984).

Secondary (delayed) surgery

Secondary surgery to achieve local control after initial chemotherapy remains an important aspect of treatment but depends on the site of disease — e.g. surgery has little or no role in the primary management of orbital, and only a selective place in local control of head and neck tumours in general. Surgery at this point in treatment should generally be conservative, whatever the site of disease, anticipating that the morbidity of radiotherapy may be more acceptable than radical operations which result in important functional (e.g. total cystectomy) and/or cosmetic (e.g. amputation) consequences. In some circumstances, however, the morbidity of radical surgery to achieve local control may be preferred, e.g. to avoid pelvic irradiation in very young children.

The value of secondary operations to *achieve* CR should be distinguished from procedures undertaken merely to *confirm* clinical or radiological complete response. Confirmatory procedures are generally unhelpful, although still utilized in some treatment strategies, and a significant minority of patients thought to be in PR after initial chemotherapy in the IRS III study were shown actually to be in CR at second-look surgery (Crist *et al.* 1995).

Chemotherapy

Philosophy of use

Chemotherapy is an essential component of treatment for all children with RMS. Experience since the 1970s has defined the efficacy of a variety of individual chemotherapeutic agents, the value of multiagent chemotherapy combinations, and the importance of adjuvant therapy in patients without macroscopic residual disease after initial surgery (Heyn *et al.* 1974; Wilbur 1974). It has long been recognized that chemotherapy given to more extensive (primarily unresectable) tumours could reduce the extent of subsequent surgery or radiation therapy, and this was the main conclusion from the first European study (SIOP RMS 75) (Flamant *et al.* 1985). However, the role of intensified chemotherapy in reducing or avoiding the need for local therapy remains controversial. This has been most consistently explored by the SIOP MMT studies (Stevens *et al.* 1995; Flamant in press). The strategies of the IRS Group (Maurer *et al.* 1988, 1993; Crist *et al.* 1995) and of the other European (German and Italian) cooperative groups (Treuner *et al.* 1991) still tend to retain a systematic approach to local therapy regardless of chemotherapy response, except in patients who achieve complete primary tumour resection with initial surgery. Overall, it seems likely that some patients who achieve complete tumour control with chemotherapy can be spared local treatment, but it is important to recognize that local recurrence is the predominant pattern of relapse in non-metastatic disease, and clinicians must not disregard the relevance of local therapy for many patients.

Active agents and combination therapies

Vincristine(V), actinomycin D(A), cyclophosphamide (C), and adriamycin (Adr) have been the most frequently utilized agents in the treatment of RMS, and have been used in various combinations (VA; VAC; VACAdr) in the sequential IRS studies. Adriamycin is an active agent when used alone, but its place in initial therapy remains uncertain, since the addition of adriamycin in the VAC combination did not appear to offer any advantage in terms of survival in the IRS II study (Maurer *et al.* 1993), and potential cardiotoxicity may justify a cautious approach to its use as part of primary treatment.

The introduction of newer drugs has not always been accompanied by clear evidence of their benefit as single agents within phase II studies, although such data is available for cisplatin, etoposide, and DTIC, all of which were introduced into IRS III. However, it was not possible to show that cisplatin, with or without etoposide, offered any survival advantage in this, although the combination of cisplatin with adriamycin in MMT 84 produced significant response rates in patients who failed to show an adequate response to (iphosphamide, vincristine, and actinomycin D) (IVA) (Flamant, in press).

The substitution of cyclophosphamide by iphosphamide in primary chemotherapy combinations with vincristine and actinomycin D (with or without adriamycin) has been the hallmark of all the recent European studies, particularly those initiated by SIOP. The evidence for the use of iphosphamide has been based on good phase-II data for its efficacy in RMS, both as a single agent and in combination with vincristine and with etoposide. The superiority of iphosphamide over cyclophosphamide is unproven, although data from the German group has suggested that iphosphamide is a more effective agent (Treuner *et al.* 1989). However, iphosphamide was introduced into treatment schedules at doses which were significantly greater (6–9 g m^{-2} per course) than those then used for cyclophosphamide (rarely > 1.5 g m^{-2} per course) in terms of dose-toxicity equivalence. The current IRS IV study is exploring iphosphamide in direct comparison with higher dose cyclophosphamide, and the recognition that it is now possible to support a dose increase using G or GM-CSF may overcome the limitations previously imposed by the myelosuppressive toxicity of cyclophosphamide. Both drugs require concurrent administration of mesna to avoid haemorrhagic cystitis, but iphosphamide carries a risk of renal toxicity not experienced with cyclophosphamide (Suarez *et al.* 1991).

Melphalan is another alkylating agent for which there is evidence of efficacy against RMS (Horowitz *et al.* 1988), but it is difficult to schedule in conventional chemotherapy combinations and most of its use has been in high dose as consolidation therapy for patients with metastatic disease, although it is also being evaluated in conventional dose in the IRS IV study.

A collaborative, European protocol for patients with metastatic disease introduced carboplatin and epirubicin (epiadriamycin) into first-line therapy as part of an intensive, six-drug schedule (with iphosphamide, vincristine, actinomycin D, and etoposide) designed to overcome drug resistance (Carli *et al.* 1993). The choice of carboplatin and epirubicin was based on preferential toxicity profiles (compared to cisplatin and adriamycin), and there is, so far, no single agent phase-II data for either, although their use in combination, with vincristine, produced excellent initial response rates (Frascella *et al.* 1996). This chemotherapy strategy was also incorporated into MMT 89 for the treatment of high-risk patients with lymph-node disease, and produced a significant improvement in outcome compared to historical data from similar patients treated in the previous study (MMT 84). The current MMT 95 protocol is exploring this six-drug combination in a direct, randomized comparison with conventional IVA (iphosphamide, vincristine, and actinomycin D) for patients with non-metastatic disease (Stevens *et al.* 1995).

New agents under examination for future studies include topotecan (in a pilot study in IRS V), taxotere, and taxol, both of which are awaiting completion of phase I and II evaluation in North America.

High-dose therapies

The place of high-dose chemotherapy strategies, necessitating autologous bone marrow or peripheral blood-stem-cell rescue, remains unclear. Some experience has been gained in individual institutions with a variety of chemotherapy schedules and, predominantly, in the treatment of patients with relapsed disease. More recently, the European collaborative groups agreed a shared strategy for the treatment of newly diagnosed patients with metastatic disease (Carli *et al.* 1993). This study initially intended to explore the value of high-dose chemotherapy only amongst patients with incomplete response to initial chemotherapy, but a modification to the study design in 1991 encouraged the use of high-dose melphalan as consolidation therapy for all patients who achieved CR after two cycles (six courses) of the six-drug chemotherapy schedule (described above). Preliminary analysis suggests that there is no survival advantage for those who received consolidation chemotherapy with melphalan compared with those, treated in the earlier phase of the study, who did not. Further studies with different drugs or drug combinations will be required if the question of intensive chemotherapy is to be resolved, but at present its use to consolidate remission, achieved with conventional treatment, does not appear to offer any advantage to patients with metastatic disease.

Radiotherapy

General principles

Early experience with radiation therapy demonstrated local control in up to 90% of patients with RMS using doses between 50 and 60 Gy. Subsequent experience in the IRS studies has confirmed that doses in excess of 50 Gy are not usually required when given by conventional (once a day) fractionation. However, there is also evidence that doses < 40 Gy may be insufficient to achieve local control, particularly in patients with macroscopic, residual disease. Current guidelines for therapy within the IRS Group studies vary the prescribed dose between 40 and 55 Gy, depending on the site, size, and histology of the tumour, and on the age of the child. Patients with localized and completely resected tumours (IRS Clinical Group I) do not receive radiotherapy unless they show unfavourable (alveolar) histology. The dose used in the SIOP studies is 45 Gy, regardless of site or age (although particular efforts are made to avoid irradiation in young children), with the possibility of a boost to 50 or 55 Gy to a reduced field if there is bulky, residual, macroscopic disease at the start of therapy. Radiotherapy is not used in the SIOP studies if the patient has achieved complete remission with chemotherapy, with or without surgery, except at parameningeal sites.

Treatment must always be given using megavoltage equipment. Electron treatment may be useful for superficial tumours, either as a direct electron field or as a boost to a linear accelerator planned field. There are well-recognized, but rare, indications for the use of brachytherapy in RMS (see below). Adequate margins must be used (usually 2–3 cm), and treatment is normally planned to the initial tumour volume in parameningeal disease, but in tumours at other sites, which show a good response to initial chemotherapy, treatment planned to the residual volume (with margins) is satisfactory.

Conventional treatment is usually given as a single daily fraction of 1.8 Gy. Interest in hyperfractionated schedules has been explored in both the IRS IV and MMT 89 studies. The rationale for this approach is to increase the prospect for local tumour control, without increasing late effects of treatment. Results are not yet available from the IRS study, but experience in MMT 89 (although this was not a randomized comparison because of logistical difficulties in adhering to a twice-daily schedule in many treatment centres) suggested that no benefit in disease control was achieved by the use of hyperfractionation. Toxicity was, however, enhanced, particularly in terms of acute mucosal damage in children with head and neck tumours (Habrand *et al.* 1996).

Parameningeal tumours

Early experience in the treatment of parameningeal tumours was discouraging. Local failure rates were high and there was a high incidence of local extension into the adjacent meninges, often with spinal subarachnoid spread, and high mortality. Investigation suggested that these patients were receiving inadequate dose and volume of radiation treatment, and the IRS studies were modified to include earlier introduction of radiotherapy, wider fields (extending to whole brain and spine in some cases), increased dose to the site of bulk disease, and the concurrent administration of intrathecal chemotherapy. This resulted in a much improved survival rate (Raney *et al.* 1987). Subsequently, these guidelines have been liberalized a little, particularly in relation to the volume of treatment, which now avoids whole-brain treatment whenever possible. Intrathecal chemotherapy remains part of the IRS treatment strategy but has never been used routinely in the SIOP studies, and there seems little justification to do so in patients (the majority) who do not demonstrate evidence of CSF or spinal dissemination. All groups agree, however, that patients with parameningeal disease require systematic radiotherapy, regardless of response to chemotherapy. This is especially important as assessment of complete response can be difficult at these sites, and surgery rarely offers a valid alternative approach to local control.

Brachytherapy

Interstitial radiotherapy using intracavitary moulds or implanted wires may be of particular relevance for small tumour residues at selected sites, notably in the vagina and perineum (Flamant *et al.* 1979). Occasionally this technique is utilized at other genitourinary sites, including tumours of the bladder base and prostate, and there is limited experience in its application to head and neck sites.

Outcome

Survival

The most recently published IRS Group study (IRS III) reported outcome for 1062 patients recruited between 1984 and 1991 (Crist *et al.* 1995). Overall, the 5-year, progression-free survival of 65% was significantly better than in the previous study (IRS II, PFS = 55%) (Maurer *et al.* 1993). This compares with 5-year, overall and event-free survivals of 66% and 47% in SIOP MMT 84 (recruiting patients from 1984–1989), and of 71% and 57% in SIOP MMT 89 (recruiting patients from 1989–1995) (Stevens *et al.* 1995; Flamant, in press). As discussed previously, these studies used significantly different approaches to local treatment, and the difference between overall and event-free survival in the SIOP studies reflects a higher relapse rate, with salvage possible for some patients.

By site

Table 13.6 gives details of the outcome of treatment by site in both the IRS III and MMT 89 studies. These confirm the prognostic effect of site, with an obvious difference between the favourable outcome associated with orbital and genitourinary sites, and the poor results achieved with tumours presenting in the limbs and at 'other' sites. The results for treatment of orbital tumours are better in the IRS experience, but nearly all such patients received systematic radiation therapy in comparison to MMT 89, where the strategy was designed to avoid local therapy in patients who achieved complete response with chemotherapy alone, in an attempt to spare the side-effects of radiotherapy. This was consistent with a similar strategy in MMT 84 in which approximately 45% of patients were apparently cured without local therapy (Rousseau *et al.* 1994). The potential benefit of avoiding local treatment must be balanced against the risk of local relapse, the toxicity of additional treatment required after relapse, and the chance of reduced survival: this is not an easy assessment.

By stage

The staging systems used were different in these two studies and it is difficult to draw a clear comparison between equivalent groups of patients (Table 13.7). Nevertheless, those with less

Table 13.6   Survival by site of primary tumour

Site	5-year survival (%) Data from IRS III	Data from MMT 89
Orbit	95	88
Genitourinary, non-bladder prostate	89	93
Genitourinary, bladder prostate	81	84
Non-parameningeal head and neck	78	71
Parameningeal head and neck	74	59
Limbs	74	65
Other	67	63

Table 13.7 Survival by stage

IRS clinical group	5-year survival (%) Data from IRS III	TNM stage	5-year survival (%) Data from MMT 89
I	84	I	78
II	74	II	65
III	66	III	57
IV	28	IV	26

advanced disease fared better than those with more advanced disease, and patients with distant metastases at diagnosis (Group IV/Stage IV) had a particularly disappointing outlook. Patients with lymph-node involvement (SIOP Stage III) are not selected as a separate group within the IRS studies. However, the results for these patients in MMT 89 show a substantial improvement over those achieved in MMT 84 (57% *vs* 42% 5-year, overall survival), and it is assumed that this reflects the benefits of more intensive chemotherapy.

Late effects of treatment

'Cure at what cost?' is the difficult, yet essential, judgement required when reviewing the outcome for survivors of all forms of cancer in childhood, particularly when survival relates to different philosophies and modalities of treatment. The importance of an accurate prognostic assessment at diagnosis is as much to ensure that patients with a good prognosis are not overtreated as to identify those with a poorer prognosis who require a more aggressive approach. Much concern has been focused on the late sequelae of local treatment for rhabdomyosarcoma, particularly after radiotherapy and after the types of aggressive surgery which result in significant functional or cosmetic problems (for example, orbital exenteration, retroperitoneal lymph-node dissections, and total cystectomy) (Heyn *et al.* 1986, 1992; Raney *et al.* 1993). Chemotherapy is also associated with significant sequelae in some patients, and the concept that more intensive chemotherapy may reduce the use of local treatment must be balanced against the additional toxicity this may bring. The more recent use of iphosphamide has raised concern about long-term renal damage (Suarez *et al.* 1991), and the continuing use of high doses of alkylating agents and, more recently, etoposide, may result in second malignancies (Heyn *et al.* 1993).

Long-term follow-up and prospective evaluation of all survivors is required in order to document the frequency and functional significance of all types of late effects of therapy.

References

Carli, M., Pinkerton, C.R., Frascella, E., Flamant, F., Oberlin, O., Koscienlniak, E., *et al.* (1993) Intensive chemotherapy for metastatic sarcoma in children. SIOP European Intergroup Study MMT89. *Proceedings of the American Society of Clinical Oncology*, 12, 410 (abstract).

Chan, H.S.L., Thorner, P.S., Haddad, G and Ling, V, (1990). Immunohistochemical detection of p-glycoprotein: prognostic correlation in soft tissue sarcoma. *Journal of Clinical Oncology*, 8, 689–704.

Crist, W., Gehan, E.A., Ragab, A.H., Dickman, P.S., Donaldson, S.S., Fryer, C., *et al.* (1995). The third Intergroup Rhabdomyosarcoma Study. *Journal of Clinical Oncology*, 13, 610–630.

Donaldson, S.S., Draper, G.S., Flamant, F., Gerard-Merchant, R., Mouriesse, H., Newton, W.A. *et al.* (1986). Topography of childhood tumours. Pediatric coding system. *Pediatric Hematology & Oncology*, 3, 249–258.

Flamant, F., Chassagne, D., Cosset, J.M., Gerbaulet, A., and Lemerle, J. (1979). Embryonal rhabdomyosarcoma of the vagina in children: conservative treatment with curietherapy and chemotherapy. *European Journal of Cancer*, 15, 527–532.

Flamant, F., Rodary, C., Voute, P.A., and Otten, J. (1985). Primary chemotherapy in the treatment of rhabdomyosarcoma in children: trial of the International Society of Pediatric Oncology (SIOP) preliminary results. *Radiotherapy & Oncology*, 3, 227–236.

Flamant, F., Rodary, C., Rey, A., Praquin, M-T., Sommelet, D., Quintana, E., *et al.* (1997). Treatment of non metastatic rhabdomyosarcomas in childhood and adolescence. Results of the second study of the International Society of Paediatric Oncology: MMT 84. *European Journal of Cancer*, in press.

Frascella, E., Pritchard Jones, K., Modak, S., Mancini, A.F., Carli, M., and Pinkerton, C.R. (1996). Response of previously untreated metastatic rhabdomyosarcoma to combination chemotherapy with carboplatin, epirubicin and vincristine. *European Journal of Cancer*, 32, 821–5

Habrand, J.L., Spooner, D., Barrett, A., Rey, A., Stevens, M., Oberlin, O. On behalf of SIOP MMT Committee. (1996). Radiotherapy in the initial management of localised malignant mesenchymal tumours. Update of the SIOP MMT 89 study. *Medical & Pediatric Oncology*, 27, 236 (abstract).

Hays, D.M., Lawrence, W., Wharam, M., Newton, W. Jr., Ruymann, F.B., Beltangady, M., *et al.* (1989). Primary re excision for patients with microscopic residual tumour following initial excision of sarcomas at trunk and extremity sites. *Journal of Pediatric Surgery*, 24, 5–10.

Heyn, R., Holland, R., Newton, W.A. Jr., Tefft, M., Breslow, N., and Hartmann, J.R. (1974). The role of combined chemotherapy in the treatment of rhabdomyosarcoma in children. *Cancer*, 34, 2128–2142.

Heyn, R., Ragab, A., Raney, R.B. Jr., Ruymann, F., Tefft, M., Lawrence, W. Jr., *et al.* (1986). Late effects of therapy in orbital rhabdomyosarcoma in children. A report from the Intergroup Rhabdomyosarcoma Study. *Cancer*, 57, 1738–1743.

Heyn, R., Raney, R.B., Hays, D.M., Tefft, M., Gehan, E., Webber, B., *et al.* (1992). Late effects of therapy in patients with paratesticular rhabdomyosarcoma. *Journal of Clinical Oncology*, 10, 614–623.

Heyn, R., Haeberlen, V., Newton, W.A., Ragab, A.H., Raney, R.B., Tefft, M., *et al.* (1993). Second malignant neoplasms in children treated for rhabdomyosarcoma. *Journal of Clinical Oncology*, 11, 262–270.

Horowitz, M., Etcubanas, E., Christensen, M.L., Houghton, J.A., George, S.L., Green, A.A., *et al.* (1988). Phase II testing of melphalan in children with newly diagnosed rhabdomyosarcoma: a model for anti cancer drug development. *Journal of Clinical Oncology*, 6, 308–314.

Lawrence, W., Gehan, E.A., Hays, D.M., Beltangady, M., and Maurer, H.M. (1987). Prognostic significance of staging factors of the UICC staging system in childhood rhabdomyosarcoma: A report from the Intergroup Rhabdomyosarcoma Study (IRS II). *Journal of Clinical Oncology*, 5, 46–54.

Li, F.B. and Fraumeni, J.F. Jr. (1969) Rhabdomyosarcoma in children; epidemiologic study and identification of a familial cancer syndrome. *Journal of the National Cancer Institute*, 43, 1365–1373.

Loh, W.E., Scrable, H.J., Livanos, E., Arboleda, M.J., Cavenee, W.K., Oshimura, M., *et al.* (1992). Human chromosome 11 contains two different growth suppressor genes for embryonal rhabdomyosarcoma. *Proceedings of the National Academy of Science USA*, 89, 1755–1759.

Malkin, D., Li, F.P., Strong, L.C., Fraumeni, J.F. Jr., Nelson, C.E., Kim, D.H., *et al.* (1990). Germ line p53 mutations in a familial syndrome of breast cancer, sarcoma and other neoplasms. *Science*, 250, 1233–1238.

Maurer, H.M., Beltangady, M., Gehan, E.A., Crist, W., Hammond, Hays, D.M., *et al.* (1988) The Intergroup Rhabdomyosarcoma Study-I: a final report. *Cancer*, 61, 209.

Maurer, H.M., Gehan, E.A., Beltangady, M., Crist, W., Dickman, P.S., Donaldson, S.S., *et al.* (1993). The Intergroup Rhabdomyosarcoma Study-II. *Cancer*, 71, 1904–1922.

Newton, W.A., Gehan, E.A., Webber, M.D., Marsden, H.B., van Unnik, A.J.M., *et al.* (1995). Classification of rhabdomyosarcoma and related sarcomas. *Cancer*, 76, 1073–85.

Niggli, F.K., Powell, J.E., Parkes, S.E., Ward, K., Raafat, F., Mann, J.R., *et al.* (1994). DNA ploidy and proliferative activity (S-phase) in childhood soft-tissue sarcomas: their value as prognostic indicators. *British Journal of Cancer*, 69, 1106–10.

Olive, D., Flamant, F., Zucker, J.M., Voute, P.A., Brunat-Mentigny, M., Otten, J., *et al.* (1984). Para aortic lymphadenectomy is not necessary in the treatment of localised paratesticular rhabdomyosarcoma. *Cancer*, 54, 1283–1287.

Pappo, A.S., Shapiro, D.N., Crist, W.M., and Maurer, H.M. (1995). Biology and therapy of rhabdomyosarcoma. *Journal of Clinical Oncology*, 13, 2123–2139.

Raney, R.B., Tefft, M., Newton, W.A., Ragab, A.H., Lawrence, W. Jr., Gehan, E.A., *et al.* (1987). Improved prognosis with intensive treatment of children with cranial sarcoma arising in non orbital parameningeal sites: a report of the Intergroup Rhabdomyosarcoma Study. *Cancer*, 59, 147–155.

Raney, R.B., Heyn, R., Hays, D., Tefft, M., Newton, W. Jr., Wharam, M., *et al.* (1993). Sequelae of treatment in 109 patients followed for five to fifteen years after diagnosis of sarcoma of the bladder and prostate: a report from the Intergroup Rhabdomyosarcoma Committee. *Cancer*, 71, 2387–2394.

Rodary, C., Flamant, F., and Donaldson, S.S. (1989). An attempt to use a common staging system in rhabdomyosarcoma: A report of an international workshop initiated by the International Society of Pediatric Oncology (SIOP). *Medical and Pediatric Oncology*, 17, 210–215.

Rousseau, P., Flamant, F., Quintana, E., Voute, P.A., and Gentel, J.C. (1994). Primary chemotherapy in rhabdomyosarcoma and other malignant mesenchymal tumours of the orbit: results of the International Society of Pediatric Oncology MMT 84 Study. *Journal of Clinical Oncology*, 12, 516.

Ruymann, F., Maddux, H., Ragab, A., Soule, E.H., Palmer, N., Beltangady, M., *et al.* (1988). Congenital anomalies associated with rhabdomyosarcoma; a report from the Intergroup Rhabdomyosarcoma Study. *Medical and Pediatric Oncology*, 16, 33–39.

Ruymann, F.B. and Grufferman, S. (1991). Introduction and epidemiology of soft tissue sarcomas. In Rhabdomyosarcoma and related tumours in children and adolescents (eds. HM Maurer, FB Ruymann, C Pochedly), pp. 3–18. CRC Press, Boca Raton, Florida.

Scrable, H.J., Witte, D.P., Shimada, H., Seemayer, T., Sheng, W.W., Soukup, S., *et al.* (1989). Molecular differential pathology of rhabdomyosarcoma. Genes Chromosomes *Cancer*, 1, 23–25.

Shapiro, D.N., Sublett, J.E., Li, B., Downing, J.R., and Naeve, C.W. (1993) Fusion of PAX 3 to a member of the forkhead family of transcription factors in human alveolar rhabdomyosarcoma. *Cancer Research*, 53, 5108–5112.

Stevens, M.C.G., Oberlin, O., Rey, A., and Praquin, M.T. for the SIOP MMT Committee (1995). Non metastatic rhabdomyosarcoma (RMS): Update from the SIOP MMT 89 study and implications for SIOP MMT 95. *Medical and Pediatric Oncology*, 25, 256 (abstract)

Suarez, A., McDowell, H., Niaudet, P., Comoy, E., and Flamant, F. (1991). Long term follow up of Iphosphamide renal toxicity in children treated for malignant mesenchymal tumours: an International Society of Pediatric Oncology report. *Journal of Clinical Oncology*, 9, 2177–2182.

Treuner, J., Koscielniak, E., and Keim, M. (1989). Comparison of rates of response to Iphosphamide and Cyclophosphamide in primary unresectable rhabdomyosarcoma. *Cancer Chemother Pharmacol*, 24 (suppl.), 48–50.

Treuner, J., Flamant, F., and Carli, M. (1991). Results of treatment of rhabdomyosarcoma in the European studies. In Rhabdomyosarcoma and related tumours in children and adolescents (eds. HM Maurer, FB Ruymann, C Pochedly), pp. 227–241. CRC Press, Boca Raton, Florida.

Turc-Carel, C., Lizard-Nacol, S., Justrabo, E., Favrot, M., Philip, T., and Tabone, E. (1986). Consistent chromosomal translocations in alveolar rhabdomyosarcoma. *Cancer Genetics and Cytogenetics*, 19, 361–362.

Wilbur, J.R. (1974). Combination chemotherapy of embryonal rhabdomyosarcoma. *Cancer Chemotherapy Reports*, 58, 281–284.

14 Osteosarcoma

A.W. Craft

Osteosarcoma is one of the two common bone tumours occurring in childhood. Although it has been reported in a child of 3 years and can occur at almost any time during adult life, the peak age is between 10 and 20 years. Many of the tumours which occur in later life complicate Paget's disease, which does not occur in children. The annual incidence has been reported as 1.6–2.8 per million children under 15 years. It occurs more commonly in males (male to female ratio 1.6: 1).

Aetiology

There is evidence that age, sex, and the anatomical site of osteosarcoma correlate well with periods of rapid growth in man (Fig. 14.1) and in animals. Large dogs, for example, Saint Bernards, have an incidence of up to 200 times that of smaller breeds (Tjalma 1966). As many tumours arise in the front legs as the hind legs in dogs, whereas in humans more tumours are found in the lower extremities. Subclinical trauma may therefore be of significance. Radiation, from both internal and external sources, can be an aetiological agent in some cases, as seen in the increased incidence of the tumour within the radiation field of children treated for retinoblastoma, and the very high risk for children given [224] Ra for the treatment of tuberculosis in the late 1940s (Speiss 1969). Osteosarcoma is the commonest second malignancy reported by the Late Effects Study Group (Meadows *et al.* 1985) and by the Childhood Cancer Research Group (Hawkins *et al.* 1996). Although many of these are undoubtedly radiation induced, there is a greatly increased incidence of osteosarcoma outside the radiation field in patients with bilateral retinoblastoma, who are estimated to have a 400- fold increased risk of this tumour (Hawkins *et al.* 1996). This is almost certainly associated with the retinoblastoma gene *RB-1* (Abramson *et al.* 1976).

Heterozygosity for the retinoblastoma gene locus on chromosome 12q14 has been observed in some osteosarcoma tumour cells and cell lines. Deletions, rearrangements of the *RB* gene, or altered expression of the gene product have also been found. The mechanism for tumourogenesis may involve the unmasking of recessive mutations at a locus exerting pleiotropic tissue effects, so that defects in both retinoblastoma alleles occurring in an appropriate bone cell may lead to osteosarcoma. Other osteosarcomas and cell lines express normal RB protein and normal *RB* alleles, suggesting that an alternative pathway independent of *RB* inactivation may exist. *P53* may also be involved, since deletion of the *p53* locus, loss of heterozygosity, and mutations of MDM2, a cellular phosphoprotein from the murine double minute 2 gene which binds to p53

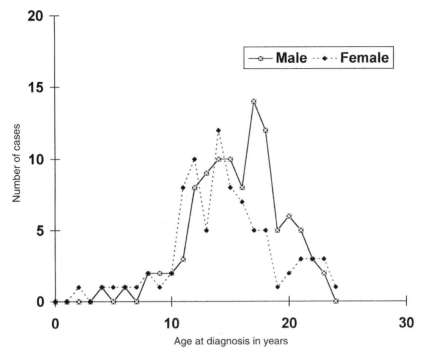

Fig. 14.1 Age and sex distribution of osteosarcoma at diagnosis, 1968–85, n = 185 (data from North of England Children's Malignant Disease Registry and Manchester Children's Tumour Registry).

protein, are also seen. The region of the human *MDM2* gene on chromosome 12q-13-14 is amplified in approximately 20% of osteosarcomas, and it is believed that high levels of MDM2 may inactivate the tumour-suppressor activity of p53 (Link and Eilber 1997).

Presentation

The commonest mode of presentation is with bone pain, usually with swelling of the affected part and some locomotor disability, which is more prominent if there is a pathological fracture. There is rarely any systemic upset, in contrast with Ewing's sarcoma. The majority of tumours arise around the knee joint in the metaphysis of the femur or tibia. Together these account for 60% of all sites, although the tumour can arise in virtually any bone (Fig. 14.2). Tumours arising outside the bone (extraosseous tumours) are extremely rare. The major sites of metastatic spread at presentation are the lungs and, less often, other bones. It is not certain whether such bone lesions represent metastases or a multifocal primary process.

Diagnostic evaluation

A definitive diagnosis can only be made by an adequate tissue biopsy, but certain investigations may be usefully performed before this.

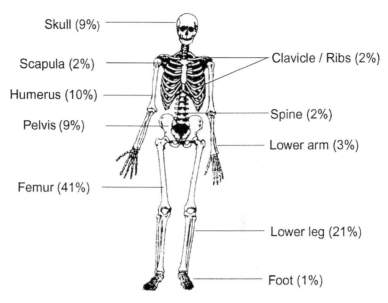

Skull (9%)

Scapula (2%)

Humerus (10%)

Pelvis (9%)

Femur (41%)

Clavicle / Ribs (2%)

Spine (2%)

Lower arm (3%)

Lower leg (21%)

Foot (1%)

Fig. 14.2 Skeleton showing major sites of osteosarcoma.

Radiology

A plain radiograph of the affected bone often shows the characteristic, but not diagnostic, appearance of osteosarcoma. The typical radiological features are destruction of bone with a consequent loss of normal trabeculae and the appearance of radiolucent areas. New bone formation, both within the bone itself and in the soft-tissue extension, are typical features, but some tumours may be almost completely lytic whilst others are predominantly sclerotic. The frequently seen 'sunburst' appearance occurs where the tumour penetrates the cortex and elevates the periosteum (Fig. 14.3). Tomography of the affected bone may give additional information on the extent of the tumour, both within the medullary cavity and in the soft tissues, and demonstrate whether or not 'skip' lesions are present in the more proximal part of the bone. Computed tomography of the bone and the non-affected limb should be carried out before any surgical intervention. This investigation can prove invaluable when the definitive surgical management of the child is being planned. The typical appearances are shown in Fig. 14.4. Magnetic resonance imaging may be a more valuable examination (Fig. 14.5; see also Figs 14.6 and 14.7). Radiological investigations are important in the detection of metastatic disease, and the presence of secondary spread influences both the prognosis and the management. A chest X-ray may demonstrate obvious metastases, but either conventional whole-lung tomography or computed tomography detects much smaller lesions more effectively; the latter is preferable. Metastases to bone also occasionally occur, and these can be demonstrated by radiographic survey of all bones or, more appropriately, by isotope scintigraphy using a bone-seeking isotope, e.g.^{99}Tc (Fig. 14.8).

Laboratory studies

The blood count and erythrocyte sedimentation rate are often normal in this disease, and these are therefore not helpful in diagnosis. Serum alkaline phosphatase may be elevated in some cases and

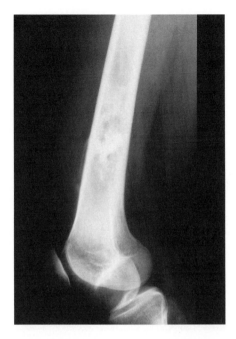

Fig. 14.3 Radiograph showing typical appearance of osteosarcoma at lower end of femur.

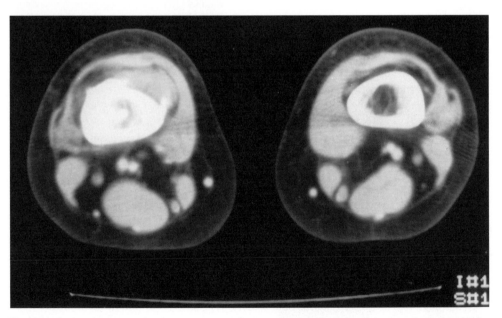

Fig. 14.4 Computer tomogram showing osteosarcoma of same patient as in Fig. 14.3 with tumour extending outside the bone.

in such individuals can be helpful as a 'tumour marker', which may indicate the presence of persistent or recurrent disease. Other investigations are necessary once the diagnosis has been made, and before chemotherapy is started (see below).

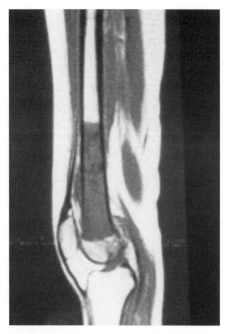

Fig. 14.5   Magnetic resonance image of same patient as in Fig. 14.3 showing extent of bone-marrow involvement by tumour.

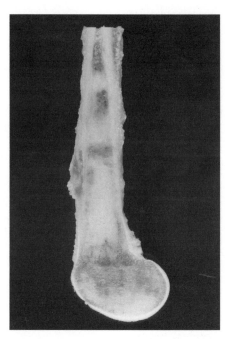

Fig. 14.6   Photograph of resected specimen of patient in Fig. 14.3 showing extent of tumour involvement following removal of soft tissues.

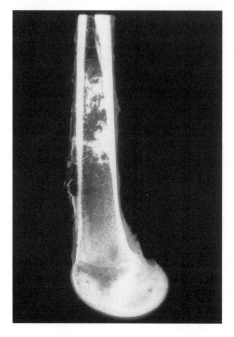

Fig. 14.7   Radiograph of resected specimen of patient in Fig. 14.3 following removal of soft tissues.

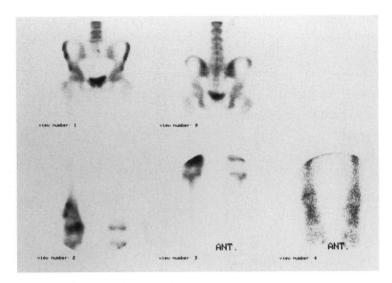

Fig. 14.8 Bone scan using ⁹⁹Tc showing high uptake in tumour.

Surgical biopsy

The biopsy area, including stitch and drain tracks, may prove to be contaminated with tumour. The biopsy must therefore be planned so that during the definitive operation the entire biopsy scar can be excised en bloc with the tumour. The incision should be as short as possible and made in a straight line parallel to the axis of the affected bone. The biopsy specimen should contain tissue from the extraosseus component, as well as extending through the cortex and into the bone. A needle biopsy is now often used, but most pathologists still prefer the more generous amount of tissue obtained from open biopsy. This is not only for histological examination but also for cytogenetic and other biological investigations.

Histological evaluation

Osteosarcoma is a heterogeneous term and includes various subtypes. The World Health Organization defines osteosarcoma as the presence of malignant cells producing osteoid. The major varieties are osteoblastic, chondroblastic, and telangiectatic. With current chemotherapy regimes there is no evidence that prognosis depends on the type of pathology, and all should be treated identically. Periosteal osteosarcoma is uncommon, but should also be treated in the same way. The other major type is parosteal; this appears to be a much lower grade of tumour, which rarely metastasizes and can often be cured by surgery alone.

Treatment

Once the diagnosis of osteosarcoma has been made, a plan of management can be formulated for the particular patient. The exact treatment depends on the age of the patient, the site of the tumour, and the presence or absence of metastases. However, the management plan should include a pretreatment evaluation. The following investigations should be carried out in all patients:

- clinical history
- examination
- measurement of tumour with an estimate of volume
- full blood count
- urea and electrolytes
- liver function tests
- alkaline phosphatase
- calcium
- magnesium
- creatinine or ^{51}Cr-EDTA clearance
- electro and echocardiogram
- pure tone audiometry
- anteroposterior and lateral X-ray of tumour
- computed tomogram or magnetic resonance image of tumour
- computed tomogram of lungs
- ^{99}Tc-Labelled isotope bone scan.

Prior to the advent of chemotherapy, only about 20% of patients with osteosarcoma could be cured, usually by amputation. Controlled trials of chemotherapy *versus* no chemotherapy have shown a clear advantage for those patients who receive drug therapy, and demonstrated that disease-free survival in the group without chemotherapy is similar to that in the prechemotherapy era (Link *et al.* 1986).

As with most childhood tumours, it is advisable that the patient be referred to a specialist centre and, where appropriate, entered into a clinical study aimed at defining the best treatment for osteosarcoma. There is no doubt that surgical removal of the primary tumour is required if the patient is to be cured, but the optimum type of surgery varies among patients. Chemotherapy is now given for all patients, and there is a steady move towards preoperative drug treatment. The rationale behind the use of preoperative chemotherapy is three-fold. The early institution of chemotherapy means that any micrometastases which are present at the time of diagnosis receive treatment before the inevitable delay which would occur if the surgery were carried out immediately. Secondly, it may make the definitive surgery easier, particularly if endoprosthetic replacement is to be considered. On the other hand, tumours which do not respond to the chemotherapy may grow during treatment and theoretically make surgery more difficult. However, in practice this rarely happens; nevertheless, very careful observation is required during initial chemotherapy to determine whether the tumour is growing. Rapid tumour necrosis occurring during chemotherapy can result in considerable oedema, and this must be distinguished from true tumour growth. Regular measurement of the tumour size at a set distance from fixed bony landmarks is essential. Finally, as discussed below, the histological response of the tumour to chemotherapy may be of prognostic value.

Radiotherapy has no part to play in the management of primary osteosarcoma, but may be of value as a palliative measure in metastatic disease (see below). Whole-lung radiation does not appear to prevent occurrence of lung metastases (Burgers *et al.* 1988).

Chemotherapy

In 1970, Marcove *et al.* (1970), reporting on the Sloan-Kettering experience of the prechemotherapy era, reported a 5-year, disease-free survival of 17% in a consecutive series of 145 cases. Jaffe *et al.* (1978) were among the first to report the benefit of high-dose methotrexate with folinic acid rescue in this disease, although the early, very optimistic results have not been sustained. Since then, the efficacy of adriamycin (Bellani *et al.* 1979), cisplatin (Ochs *et al.* 1978), and iphosphamide (Brade *et al.* 1985) as single agents has been demonstrated. Various combinations of these active drugs have subsequently been used, sometimes with the addition of bleomycin, cyclophosphamide, and actinomycin (BCD) (Rosen *et al.* 1982). A randomized, controlled trial of immediate against delayed chemotherapy showed a clear advantage for chemotherapy (Link *et al.* 1986).

As is seen below, there are many important prognostic variables in osteosarcoma, but Rosen *et al.* (1982) believe that the most important factor is the pathological response of the primary tumour to chemotherapy. In their T10 study, they developed a chemotherapeutic regimen which was tailored to the pathological response. In this protocol, all patients receive a common preoperative chemotherapy based on methotrexate. They then have definitive surgery and, depending on the amount of tumour necrosis present, either continue with the same therapy, if there has been more than 50% necrosis, or change to a platinum-based regimen if there has been a poor response. Details of the T10 protocol are given by Rosen *et al.* (1982), and an outline scheme is shown in Fig. 14.9. A recent update of the early T10 results shows a 76% 5-year, disease-free survival (Meyers *et al.* 1992), and similar results have been reported in Europe using methotrexate-based regimes. A German/Austrian group is also using a very similar protocol, with encouraging results (Winkler *et al.* 1988). A large European cooperative osteosarcoma study group (EOI) has developed a shorter two-drug chemotherapy (Fig. 14.10) using cisplatin and adriamycin, and the results of a large, randomized, controlled trial of this against a regime similar to T10 has shown them to be equivalent, although overall survival is less than that reported by Rosen (Souhami *et al.* 1996). Table 14.1 shows the very similar results obtained by different chemotherapy regimes.

Each of the four most active chemotherapeutic agents used in this disease has potentially very serious side-effects. High-dose methotrexate therapy must be monitored very carefully, with routine measurement of drug levels and appropriate adjustment of the dose of folinic acid. This treatment should be given only in centres in which a very rapid analysis of blood levels of methotrexate is available. Adriamycin is cardiotoxic, and most treatment regimens restrict the cumulative dose of the drug to 400–450 mg/m^2. Cisplatin and iphosphamide are nephrotoxic, and routine monitoring of renal function should be carried out before each dose of cisplatin.

^{51}Cr-labelled EDTA clearance is the most accurate method of assessment, but a creatinine clearance on a 24-hour urine collection is an alternative. Cisplatin is also toxic to the acoustic nerve, and high-tone hearing loss may occur. Disturbances in magnesium and calcium homeostasis may occur, and tetany is not uncommon during the later stages of therapy. Iphosphamide

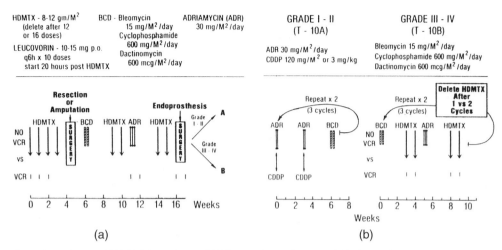

Fig. 14.9   T10 protocol (a) initial chemotherapy, (b) follow-on therapy (HDMTX = high-dose methotrexate, VCR = vincristine, CDDP = cisplatin, ADR = adriamycin (doxorubicin), BCD = bleomycin, cyclophosphamide, actinomycin D).

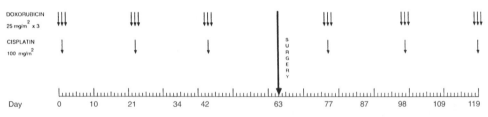

Fig. 14.10   EOI two-drug chemotherapy for osteosarcoma.

Table 14.1   Adjuvant chemotherapy for osteosarcoma; relapse-free survival for multiagent chemotherapy

Group/centre	Number of evaluable patients	Relapse-free survival (%)
Memorial Sloan-Kettering (Meyers *et al.* 1992)	279	65
German Cooperative Osteosarcoma Studies		
COSS 80 (Winkler *et al.* 1984)	91	72
COSS 82 (Winkler *et al.* 1988)	125	58
Multi-institutional Osteosarcoma Study (Link *et al.* 1986)	18	71
University of California, Los Angeles (Eilber *et al.* 1987)	24	55
Bologna (Bacci *et al.* 1990)	57	66
European Osteosarcoma Intergroup 2 drug arm (Bramwell *et al.* 1992; Souhami *et al.* 1997)	298	57

can cause a tubular nephropathy with loss of electrolytes and subsequent acidosis. There is no consistent evidence that intra-arterial chemotherapy is superior to the conventional intravenous route, and it is more difficult to administer and more expensive.

Surgery

Radical surgical removal of the primary tumour is mandatory if there is to be any hope of cure. Fortunately, most tumours arise in long bones, where removal is possible, but even for those arising in the pelvis or jaw, cure can be achieved with aggresive surgery. This does not have to be mutilating, and careful planning and cooperation among the various surgical disciplines can lead to a cosmetically very satisfactory result (Fig. 14.11). The type of surgery required depends on the age of the child and the site of the tumour. Resection or amputation are the two options available. In young children with a tumour located around the knee joint, the remaining expected growth should be estimated. If this is more than 5 cm, the potential functional results of resection, which in effect means no further growth of the limb, usually preclude resection and prosthetic replacement as a surgical option, although expanding prostheses are now being tried. However, if the total height is already reasonable, stapling of the epiphyses of the normal limb to prevent disproportionate growth can also be considered.

Amputation

The theoretical possibility of skip lesions in the more proximal bone has led in the past to the suggestion that very high amputation, or disarticulation, should be the treatment of choice.

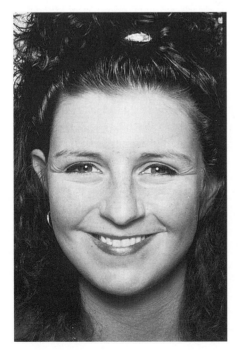

Fig. 14.11 A 17-year-old girl 8 years after hemimaxillectomy for osteosarcoma.

However, there has been a move in recent years to carry out cross-bone amputation, leaving a reasonable, usually 8 cm, segment of normal bone between the amputation line and the tumour. Computed tomography or magnetic resonance imaging will guide the level at which it is safe to carry out the amputation.

Resection

In a child of a suitable age, in whom subsequent growth will not be a problem, resection can be considered; for those children who are still growing, some centres are developing 'growing' prostheses (Lewis 1986). The size of the tumour and the involvement of soft tissues, especially nerves and blood vessels, can greatly influence the feasibility of this type of surgery. The advent of preoperative chemotherapy has also influenced the situation (Rosen *et al.* 1982). It may well be that a tumour which, at initial evaluation appears unresectable, shrinks dramatically under the influence of the drugs, becoming amenable to conservative surgery rather than amputation. The decision about resectability must therefore be deferred until the time of surgery, and no strict guidelines can be laid down. It is largely a matter of individual judgement and experience, which is yet another reason why children with bone cancer should be treated in specialist centres.

Infection, either locally or elsewhere, is a contraindication to this type of surgery. Pathological fracture is in itself not a contraindication, providing that the whole of the tumour mass is excised along with the haematoma and other contaminated tissue. All soft tissues, including muscles which are invaded by tumour, should be excised, although resection of parts of muscles is acceptable. If subsequent histological examination reveals that resection has not been complete, amputation should be carried out as soon as possible, and certainly within 4 weeks. If the insertion of the capsule of the joint is involved by tumour, then resection of the entire joint should be included.

There are three main types of procedure which have been used to replace the resected bone. A metal prosthesis, which usually includes bone and one or more joints, is the most widely used method. The availability of an appropriate prosthesis may determine whether or not this type of surgery can be performed. Meticulous preoperative planning is mandatory if the operation is to be successful. Modular prostheses (Kotz and Ritsch 1987) are now available which can be assembled at the time of operation. Figure 14.12 shows a prosthesis *in situ*, along with the external appearance (Fig. 14.13). Autologous bone transplants can be used in appropriate circumstances; for example, the fibula can be used to replace part of a humerus. However, there is less experience with these techniques, and it is recommended that immediate resection and replacement with autologous bone be avoided; it is better to insert a 'spacer' to bridge the gap, and carry out a further operation later. The occasional poor functional results and long rehabilitation time involved with prosthetic surgery for tumours in the femur have led to renewed interest in resection of the tumour with preservation of the vessels and then a tibial rotationplasty (Kotz and Salzer 1982). Figure 14.14 shows the result of such a procedure which, although cosmetically far from ideal, gives an extremely good functional result with a prosthetic lower limb attached to the plantar flexed foot. This operation is suitable principally for young children in whom considerable growth has still to occur. At the time of surgery the ankle is placed lower than the contralateral knee, so that by the time growth is completed the reversed ankle and the knee are at the same level.

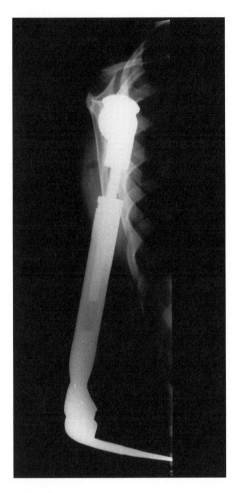

Fig. 14.12 X-ray of prosthesis *in situ*: expanding prosthesis in place of humerus.

Rehabilitation

The management of osteosarcoma is based upon the expectation that children will be longterm survivors. It is very important that adequate rehabilitation services are available as part of the team of specialists who care for the child. Early mobilization and fitting of artificial limbs are an essential part of the management. Growing children may require many changes of prosthesis to accommodate their changing stature. The physiotherapist and prosthetist should be involved at the earliest possible opportunity, and certainly before surgery. The psychological rehabilitation of the child must also be considered, although children do cope surprisingly well with amputation.

Management of metastases

Before the chemotherapy era, pulmonary metastases occurred in approximately 80% of patients within 18 months of presentation, and were the usual cause of death. Chemotherapy has changed

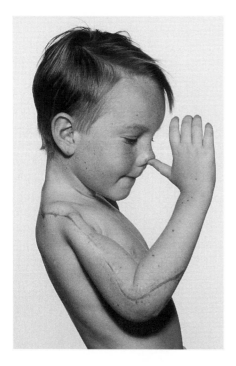

Fig. 14.13 8-year-old boy with X-ray shown in Fig. 14.12, showing preservation of a functional limb.

this clinical picture, and many more patients now suffer no metastases. Of those who do, the lesions occurring in the lung can appear much later, and it is not uncommon for them to appear up to 4 or more years after diagnosis of the primary tumour. More bone metastases are now being seen than previously. The presence of pulmonary metastases at the time of diagnosis, or their subsequent development, was previously regarded as an untreatable situation, but more aggressive surgery and chemotherapy have rendered many such patients curable. Patients who have pulmonary metastases present at diagnosis should have thoracotomy and metastatectomy added to the conventional protocol (Rosen *et al.* 1978). At operation, more metastases may be found than were visible by imaging. A midline sternotomy enables both lungs to be examined and all palpable disease removed. For those who develop these lesions later, intensive investigation, including bone scan and computed tomography of lungs, should be carried out. Treatment should then be designed with regard to the patient's previous therapy. If the patient has not previously received one of the drugs of known activity, this drug can be used, or methotrexate can be used at an even higher dose than before. However, thoracotomy should be considered even if the lesions have apparently disappeared on chest X-ray. In patients who develop metastases in bone, the disease takes a progressive course and is not generally curable, unless the lesion is solitary and can be resected. However, good palliation can be achieved with radiotherapy.

Prognosis

The overall prognosis for patients with osteosarcoma has improved in recent years, but the extent to which this has been achieved varies. Single-institution studies generally report the best results,

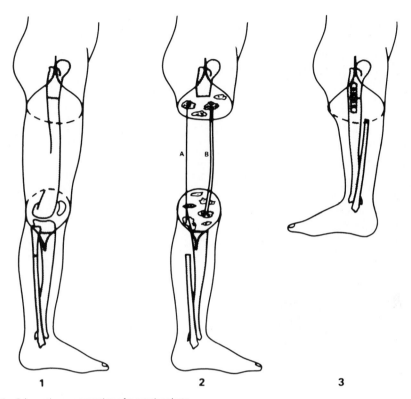

Fig. 14.14 Schematic representation of a rotationplasty.

although there is a remarkable consistency in multicentre studies, with 55–65% of patients being long-term survivors. Some of these studies are shown in Table 14.1. One of the reasons for the discrepancy in the studies using apparently similar treatment is that there are several prognostic factors which must be taken into account when trying to assess the comparability of different studies (Craft 1985). Some of these are discussed below.

Pathological subtype

Osteoblastic and telangiectatic osteosarcoma probably have a similar prognosis, although the latter has been reported by some to have a worse outlook. There is general agreement that parosteal tumors have a better prognosis and can be cured by surgery alone.

Metastasis

The presence of metastases at diagnosis is the single most important prognostic factor, but they do not signify an inevitably fatal outcome. Up to 30% of patients with metastases can still be cured.

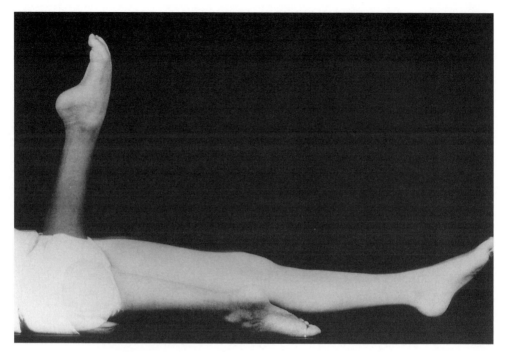

Fig. 14.15   Double-exposure photograph of results of rotationplasty.

Duration of disease

A longer duration of disease had a favourable effect on prognosis in some earlier series. However, it is likely that the advent of chemotherapy, along with earlier referral, has eliminated this as a prognostic factor.

Age and sex

There is no general agreement on the prognostic significance of age or sex, although, in a study in which other variables were controlled, there was a consistently improved chance of survival for patients aged 15–21 years, compared with those who were younger. A more favourable prognosis has been reported for female patients (Rosen *et al.* 1984).

Site and size of tumour

Osteosarcoma can occur in almost any bone. However, those in the axial skeleton are generally less amenable to surgery and therefore have a worse prognosis. Those in the jaw seem to have a more favourable outlook. Of those in the limbs, the femur not only is the commonest site but also has the worst prognosis. The larger the tumour, the worse is the prognosis.

Alkaline phosphatase

Jurgens *et al.* (1981) reported that an elevated serum alkaline phosphatase level, which falls to normal with treatment, indicates a good response to chemotherapy, and that this correlates with a favourable outcome.

Response to chemotherapy

The histological response to chemotherapy may be the most important prognostic factor, the findings of Rosen *et al.* (1982) having been confirmed in other studies (Souhami *et al.* 1996).

P-glycoprotein

Tumours expressing p-glycoprotein have been reported to have a worse prognosis (12% survival) than p-glycoprotein-negative tumours (80%) (Baldini *et al.* 1995).

Follow-up

Metastases are most likely to occur in the lungs, and if they are detected at an early stage, the patient may still be curable. During treatment and for the next 6 months, a chest X-ray should be carried out once per month. The frequency can be reduced to once every 2 months for the next year, every 3 months during the third year, every 4 months during the fourth year, and every 6 months in the fifth year. After that, an annual chest X-ray can be carried out. In patients who initially have an elevated serum alkaline phosphatase level which falls to normal with treatment, it may be worthwhile measuring this routinely at follow-up, as it may give early evidence of metastases.

Chondrosarcoma

The general view is that chondrosarcoma is very rare in the first two decades of life. When it does occur, it is likely to be in a pre-existing osteochondroma, and only rarely in an enchondroma. It is very important to differentiate it from a chondroblastic osteosarcoma, and if a chondrosarcoma is suspected on the basis of a biopsy in a child, serious consideration should be given to a rebiopsy to exclude the possibility of an osteosarcoma. The commonest sites of involvement are pelvis and femur. Chondrosarcoma rarely metastasizes at an early stage, and in many cases can be cured by radical surgical removal.

References

Abramson, D.H., Ellsworth, R.M., and Zimmerman, L.E. (1976), Nonocular cancer in retinoblastoma survivors. *Trans Am Acad Ophthalmol Otolarynogol*, 81, OP454.

Bacci, G., Picci, P., Ruggieri, P., Mercuri, M., Avella, M., *et al.* (1990). Primary chemotherapy and delayed surgery (neoadjuvant chemotherapy) for osteosarcoma of the extremities. The Instituto Rizzoli experience in 127 patients treated preoperatively with intravenous methotrexate (high versus moderate doses and intraarterial cisplatin). *Cancer*, 65: 2539–2553.

Baldini, N., Scotlandi, K., Barbanti-Brodano, G., Manara, M.C., Maurici, D., Bacci, G., *et al.* (1995). Expression of P-glycoprotein in high-grade osteosarcomas in relation to clinical outcome. *The New England Journal of Medicine*, 21, 1380–83.

Bellani, F.F., Gasparini, M., Gennari, L., Fontanillas, L., and Bonnadonna, G. (1979). Adjuvant treatment with adriamycin in primary operable osteosarcoma. *Cancer Treatment Reports*, 63, 1621–1627.

Brade, W.P., Herdrich, K., and Vapini, M. (1985). Iphosphamide—pharmacology, safety and therapeutic potential. *Cancer Treatment Reviews*, 12, 1–47.

Bramwell, V.H.C., Burgers, M., Sneath, R., Souhami, R., van Oosterom, A.T., Voute, P.A., *et al.* (1992). A comparison of two short intensive adjuvant chemotherapy regimens in operable osteosarcoma of limbs in children and young adults. Doxorubicin/cisplatinum vs high dose methotrexate + doxorubicin/cisplatinum. The first study of the European Osteosarcoma Intergroup. *Journal of Clinical Oncology*, 10(10): 1579–1591.

Burgers, J.M.V., Van Glabbeke, M., Busson, A., Cohen, P., Mazabraud, A.R., Abbatucci, J.S., *et al.* (1988). Osteosarcoma of the limbs. Report of the EORTC-SIOP 03 trial 20781 investigating the value of adjuvant treatment with chemotherapy and/or prophylactic lung irradiation. *Cancer*, 61, 1024–1031.

Craft, A.W. (1985). Controversies in the management of bone tumours. *Cancer Surveys*, 3, 733–750.

Eilber, F., Giuliano, A., Edkardt, J., Patterson, K., Moseley, S., and Goodnight, J. (1987). Adjuvant chemotherapy for osteosarcoma: a randomised prospective trial. *Journal of Clinical Oncology*, 5, 21–26.

Hawkins, M.M., Kinnear-Wilson, L.M., Burton, H.S., Potok, M.H.N., Winter, D.L., Marsden, H.B., *et al.* (1996). Radiotherapy, alkylating agents and risk of bone cancer after childhood cancer. *Journal of National Cancer Institute*, 88, 270–278.

Jaffe, N., Frei, E., Watts, H., and Traggis, D. (1978). High dose methotrexate in osteogenic sarcoma: a five year experience. *Cancer Treatment Reports*, 62, 259–264.

Jurgens, H., Kosloff, C., Nirenberg, A., Mehta, B., Huvos, A.G., and Rosen, G. (1981). Prognostic factors in the response of primary osteogenic sarcoma to preoperative chemotherapy (high dose methotrexate with citrovorum factor). *National Cancer Institute of Monography*, 56, 221–226.

Kotz, R. and Ritsch, P. (1987). Modular replacement of femur and tibia in 'Bone Tumour Management' ed. Coombs R, Friedlander G–London–Butterworths.

Kotz, R. and Salzer, M. (1982), Rotationplasty for childhood osteosarcoma of the distal part of the femur. *Journal of Bone and Joint Surgery [Am]*, 64, 959–969.

Lewis, M. (1986). The use of expendable and adjustable prostheses in the treatment of childhood malignant bone tumours of the extremity. *Cancer*, 57, 499.

Link, M.P. and Eilber, F. (1997) Osteosarcoma in 'Principles and Practice of Paediatric Oncology', ed. Pizzo, P.A. and Poplack, D.G. Lippincott Raven Publishers, Philadephia. p 889–892.

Link, M.P., Goorin, A.M., Miser, J., Green, A.A., Pratt, C.B., Belasco, J.B., *et al.* (1986). The effect of adjuvant chemotherapy on relapse free survival in patients with osteosarcoma of the extremity. *New England Journal of Medicine*, 314, 1600–1606.

Marcove, R.C., Mikem, V., Hajek. J.V., Levin, A.G., and Hutter, R.V.P. (1970). Osteogenic sarcoma under the age of twenty one. A review of one hundred and forty five operative cases. *Journal of Bone and Joint Surgery [Am]*, 52, 411–423.

Meadows, A.T., Baum, E., Fossati-Bellini, F., Green, D., Jenkin, R.D., Marsden, B., *et al.* (1985). Second malignant neoplasms in children: an update from the Late Effects Study Group. *Journal of Clinical Oncology*, 3, 532–538.

Meyers, PA., Heller, G., Healey, J., Huvos, A., Lane, J., Marcone, R., *et al.* (1992) Chemotherapy for non-metastatic osteosarcoma: the Memorial Sloane Kettering experience. *Journal of Clinical Oncology*, 10, 5–15.

Ochs, J.J., Freman, A.I., Douglass, H.O. Jr, Higby, D.S., Mindell, E.P., and Sinks, L.F. (1978). cis-Dichlorodiamineplatinum (II) in advanced osteogenic sarcoma. *Cancer Treatment Reports*, 62, 239–245.

Rosen, G., Caparros, B., Groshen, S., Nirenberg, A., Cacavio, A., Marcove, R.C., *et al.* (1984). Primary osteogenic sarcoma of the femur: a model for the use of preoperative chemotherapy in high risk malignant tumours. *Cancer Investigations*, 2, 181–192.

Rosen, G., Caparros, B., Huvos, A.G., Kosloff, C., Nirenberg, A., Cacavio, A., *et al.* (1982). Preoperative chemotherapy for osteogenic sarcoma. *Cancer*, 49, 1221–12308.

Rosen, G., Huvos, A., Mosende, C., Beattie, E.J., Exelby, P.R. Jr, Capparos, B., *et al.* (1978). Chemotherapy and thoracotomy for metastatic osteogenic sarcoma. A model for adjuvant chemotherapy and the rationale for the time of thoracic surgery. *Cancer*, 41, 841–849.

Souhami, R.L., Craft, A.W., Van der Eijken, J., Nooy, M., Spooner, D., *et al.* (1997). Randomized trial of two regimens of chemotherapy in operable osteosarcoma. *Lancet*, 350, 911–917.

Souhami, R.L., Craft, A.W., Nooy, M., and van der Eijken, J. (1996) A randomised trial of two regimens of chemotherapy in operable osteosarocoma. A study of the European Osteosarcoma Intergroup. *Proceedings of the American Society of Clinical Oncology*, 15, p. 520.

Speiss, H. (1969), [224]Ra-induced tumours in children and adults. In: Mays, C.W., Jee, W.S.S., Lloyd, R.D., Stover, B.J., Dougherty, J.H., Taylor, G.N. (eds) Delayed effects of bone seeking radionuclides. University of Utah Press, Salt Lake City, pp. 227–246.

Tjalma, R.A. (1966). Canine bone sarcoma: estimation of relative risks as a function of body size. *Journal of National Cancer Institute*, 36, 1137–1150.

Winkler, K., Beron, G., Kotz, R., Salzer-Kuntschik, M., Beck, J., Beck, W., *et al.* (1984). Neoadjuvant chemotherapy for osteogenic sarcoma. Results of a co-operative German/Austrian study. *Journal of Clinical Oncology*, 2, 617–624.

Winkler, K., Beron, G., Delling, U., Heise, U., Kabisch, H., Purfurst, C., *et al.* (1988). Neoadjuvant chemotherapy of osteosarcoma: results of a randomized cooperative trial (COSS-82) with salvage chemotherapy based on histological tumor response. *Journal of Clinical Oncology*, 6/2, 329–337.

15   Ewing's sarcoma

H. Jürgens, A. Barrett, B. Dockhorn-Dworniczak, and W. Winkelmann

Ewing's sarcoma is a malignant bone tumour characterized histologically by a uniform pattern of small cells with round nuclei but without distinct cytoplasmic borders or prominent nucleoli (Campanacci 1990; Huvos 1991). Following initial description and case reports by Lücke (1866) and Hildebrand (1890–91), various reports published by Ewing between 1921 and 1939 on 'diffuse endothelioma' or 'endothelial myeloma' defined this tumour as a distinct entity (Ewing 1921, 1939).

Epidemiology

Ewing's sarcoma accounts for 10–15% of all primary malignant bone tumours (Huvos 1991). The annual incidence is estimated at 0.6 per million population (Price and Jeffree 1977). Ewing's sarcoma rarely occurs in persons under the age of 5 years or over the age of 30 years; peak incidence is between the ages of 10 and 15 years. The overall male:female ratio is 1.5:1; the male predominance is not demonstrable in children, but increases with age (Fig. 15.1) (Glass and Fraumeni 1970). Epidemiologically, it is remarkable that there is a low incidence in Black and Chinese populations (Glass and Fraumeni 1970; Li et al. 1980; Huvos 1991).

Clinical appearance and diagnosis

As with other primary malignant bone tumours, the most common symptoms are increasing, persistent pain and swelling of the affected area, with impairment of function. The patient usually presents with a palpable, painful, and tender swelling, rapidly increasing but quite variable in size and consistency. Involvement of peripheral nerves may produce neurological symptoms (Rosen 1976). Slight to moderate fever is reported in about one-third of patients, and occurs more often in those with metastatic disease at diagnosis, accounting for the prognostic significance of these non-specific systemic symptoms (Huvos 1991; Dahlin 1996). The most common sites of the primary lesion are pelvis, femur, tibia, fibula, ribs, scapula, vertebra, and humerus (Fig. 15.2). In comparison to the skeletal distribution of osteogenic sarcoma, the flat bones of the trunk are more often affected. In long bones, the tumour originates from the diaphysis, either centrally or towards the ends, but is definitely distinct from the typical metaphyseal presentation of osteosarcoma (Campanacci 1990; Huvos 1991; Dahlin 1996).

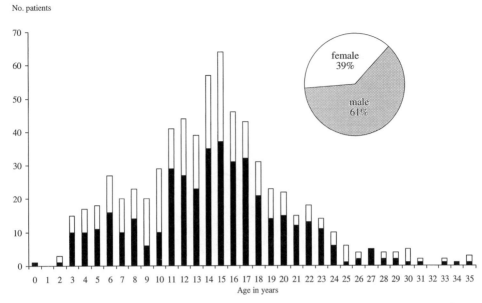

Fig. 15.1 Age and sex distribution in Ewing's sarcoma based on 692 patients from the consecutive (E1)CESS studies.

The initial diagnostic steps usually involve conventional X-ray evaluation, where the typical appearance of Ewing's sarcoma often includes a patchy, 'moth-eaten' pattern of bone destruction with poorly defined margins and a parallel 'onion-skin' periostial lamellation with a varying degree of soft-tissue extension of tumour (Fig. 15.3). A pathological fracture is noted in about 5% of cases. Rib lesions are often associated with pleural effusion (Fig. 15.4). However typical the radiographic image may be, especially in a patient in the first two decades of life, the X-ray findings cannot be considered pathognomonic. Histological confirmation is required in all cases.

The diagnostic work-up includes an exact description of the primary lesion and a search for metastases: X-ray of the primary lesion in two planes, preferably with additional computed tomograms and/or magnetic resonance imaging and/or angiography; whole-body radionuclide bone scan to determine the extent of the primary tumour and to detect other sites of bony involvement; PA (postero-anterior) and lateral chest X-ray to demonstrate pulmonary metastases, preferably complemented with full-chest tomography and/or computed tomogram of the chest. Bone marrow aspiration and/or biopsy, preferably obtained from several sites, is required to detect bone-marrow involvement. Conventional, light-microscopic evaluation should be complemented by modern molecular techniques, e.g. RT-PCR (reverse transcription-polymerase chain reaction) to detect minimal dissemination (Dockhorn-Dworniczak *et al.* 1995). Approximately 20% of patients present with visible metastases at diagnosis. Of these, about 50% have lung metastases and about 40% multiple bone involvement and diffuse bone-marrow involvement. Lymphatic spread is seen in fewer than 10% of cases. CNS involvement in the form of either meningeal spread or CNS metastases is extremely uncommon at initial presentation, but may occur in advanced disease (Kulick and Mones 1970; Mehta and Hendrickson 1974).

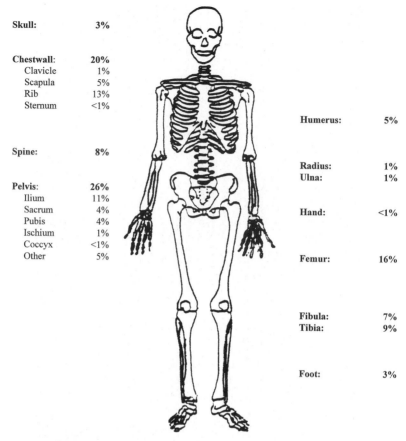

Skull: 3%

Chestwall: 20%
Clavicle 1%
Scapula 5%
Rib 13%
Sternum <1%

Spine: 8%

Pelvis: 26%
Ilium 11%
Sacrum 4%
Pubis 4%
Ischium 1%
Coccyx <1%
Other 5%

Humerus: 5%

Radius: 1%
Ulna: 1%

Hand: <1%

Femur: 16%

Fibula: 7%
Tibia: 9%

Foot: 3%

Fig. 15.2 Skeletal distribution in Ewing's sarcoma. Percentages based on 1281 patients entered into the consecutive (EI)CESS trials. Central, 55%; proximal, 22%; distal, 23%.

Laboratory studies usually show a moderately elevated erythrocyte sedimentation rate and may reveal some degree of anaemia and leucocytosis. An elevated serum level of lactate dehydrogenase (LDH) is thought to be of prognostic significance (Glaubiger *et al.* 1980; Dahlin 1996), probably due to its correlation with tumour burden. Elevation of serum neuron-specific enolase is seen in some patients, possibly related to more neurally differentiated, small round-cell sarcomas. Its relationship to prognosis has yet to be determined.

Pathology

The intraosseous component of the tumour is usually of firm consistency, while the extraosseous component is often soft, with areas of haemorrhage and cystic degeneration (Rosen 1976; Huvos 1991). The histological appearance of Ewing's sarcoma is characterized by a structureless array of small hyperchromatic cells (Fig. 15.5) (Remagen and Salzer-Kuntschik 1981; Campanacci

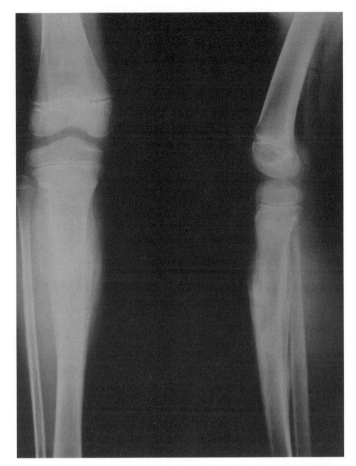

Fig. 15.3 Typical tibial Ewing's sarcoma with medullary bone destruction and periostial lamellation in a 9-year-old boy.

1990; Huvos 1991). Special stains demonstrate glycogen by periodic acid-Schiff and diastase reactions in about 90% of all cases (Schajowicz 1959; Salzer-Kuntschik and Wunderlich 1971). The presence of glycogen cannot be considered pathognomonic for Ewing's sarcoma since this has also been demonstrated in other small-cell sarcomas (Triche and Rosse 1978). The categorization into different microscopic patterns, such as diffuse, lobular, filigree, and pseudofiligree (Kissane *et al.* 1983), has not universally been shown to be of prognostic significance (Schmidt *et al.* 1987). A large-cell variant of Ewing's sarcoma, distinct from the common small-cell appearance, has also been described, and according to some reports this is associated with a poorer prognosis (Llombart-Bosch *et al.* 1978; Nascimento 1980).

Routine pathological examination has now been supplemented by additional diagnostic procedures; in particular immunocytochemistry has become invaluable in distinguishing Ewing's sarcoma from other small round-cell tumours (Schmidt and Harms 1990). The typical pattern of immune reactivity of Ewing's sarcomas and other small round-cell tumours is listed in Table 15.1 (also see 'Differential Diagnosis' p. 240) (Miser *et al.* 1989; Schmidt and Harms 1990; Jürgens

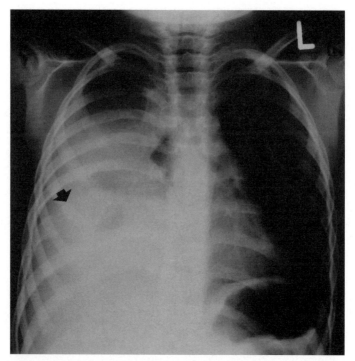

Fig. 15.4 Ewing's sarcoma of the rib (arrow) with extensive soft-tissue mass and pleural effusion in a 7-year-old girl.

1994). In particular, Ewing's sarcoma cells are found to express a surface p-glycoprotein, 30/32 MIC2, encoded by the *MIC2* gene within the pseudo-autosomal region of X and Y chromosomes (Ambros *et al.* 1991; Fellinger *et al.* 1991; Weidner and Tjoe 1994). Against this protein the monoclonal antibody HBA-71 has been developed and found positive in 98% of Ewing tumours. The product of the *MIC2* gene is involved in cellular adhesion processes (Gelin *et al.* 1989). The *MIC2* gene is not associated with specific chromosomal translocations found in Ewing's sarcoma, and must be considered an independent characteristic of this group of tumours which is shared with ependymal and endocrine cells as well as some cells of the lymphatic system (Ladanyi *et al.* 1993).

Immunohistochemistry is also used for the description of biological properties. Resistance to cytostatic drugs may be associated with multidrug resistance due to the expression of a channel-forming transport protein (p-glycoprotein), which acts as an energy-dependent efflux pump of the outer cell membrane, eliminating compounds such as anthracyclines, vinca alkaloids, and other hydrophobic antineoplastic agents (Endicott and Ling 1989). An earlier report has shown evidence that small round-cell tumours, carrying p-glycoprotein, are associated with poorer outcome (Roessner *et al.* 1993).

With the introduction of immunocytochemistry into the differential diagnosis of small round-cell tumours of bone, some Ewing-like, small round-cell tumours of bone were found to react positively with markers of neural differentiation, such as neuron-specific enolase (NSE), S100, chromogranin A and B, secretogranin, or the protein gene product 9.5 (PGP 9.5) (Gelin *et al.* 1989;

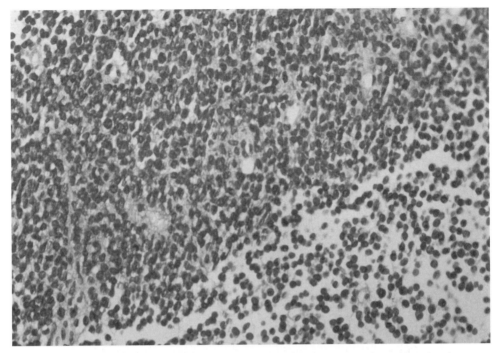

Fig. 15.5 Typical histological appearance of Ewing's sarcoma with round or oval nuclei and poor delineation of cytoplasm of cells.

Jürgens 1994). Round-cell tumours of the chest wall, occurring predominantly in adolescents as first described by Askin and colleagues, also fall into this category of primitive neuroectodermal tumours (Askin *et al.* 1979). The shared chromosomal characteristics (see below) and the observation that some Ewing's sarcoma cell lines in culture develop neural characteristics (van Valen *et al.* 1992) support the hypothesis that these two variants are closely related and represent different stages of differentiation of the same malignancy (Schmidt *et al.* 1989). The possible neural origin of these tumours has led to the use of 'Ewing tumour' or 'Ewing group of tumours' rather than 'Ewing's sarcoma' for this class of small round-cell tumours of bone. Some investigators have suggested using the term 'Ewing's sarcoma' for the variant with no immunohistochemical evidence of neural differentiation, the term 'atypical Ewing's sarcoma' for variants with one positive neural marker, and the term 'peripheral neuroectodermal tumour' for the variant with two or more positive neural markers. The term 'atypical Ewing's sarcoma' has, however, sometimes also been used for the large-cell variant of Ewing tumours (Nascimento 1980).

Cyto- and molecular genetics

The concept of Ewing tumour as a diagnostic and histogenetically distinct tumour entity has been supported by the discovery of a highly specific chromosome alteration t(11;22) (Turc-Carel *et al.* 1988). The t(11;22) (q24;q12) has been fully characterized at the molecular genetic level, and

Table 15.1 Immunological diagnosis of small round-cell tumours of bone

Agent	Ewing's sarcoma	Malignant PNET	Malignant lymphoma	Rhabdomyosarcoma	Small-cell osteosarcoma	Neuroblastoma
Vimentin	+	+	+/–	+	+	+
LCA	–	–	+	–	–	–
Desmin	–	–	–	+	–	–
Muscle actin	–	–	–	+	–	–
Osteonectin	–	–	–	–	+	–
HBA 71	+	+	–	–	–	–
Chromogranin A+B	–	–	–	–	–	+
Secretogranin	–	+/–	–	–	–	+
NSE	+/–	+	–	–	–	+
S-100	–	+	–	–	–	+

(Source: Jürgens 1994)
PNET, primitive neuroectodermal tumour.

subsequently the genes disrupted by the translocations have been cloned (Zucman *et al.* 1992). The translocation results in the formation of a chimeric gene between *EWS* (Ewing's sarcoma gene), a novel putative RNA-binding gene located on 22q12, and *FLI1*, a member of the ETS (erythroblastosis virus transforming sequence) family of transcription factors located at 11q24 (Delattre *et al.* 1992). Fusion of these two genes has been detected in roughly 90% of histologically defined Ewing tumours (Delattre *et al.* 1994; Dockhorn-Dworniczak *et al.* 1994*b*). Three variant translocations have been described, all members of the same family of ETS oncogenes: the t(11;22) (q12;q12) involving a gene on chromosome 21 *ERG*, the t(7;22) (p22;q12) with the *ETV1* (Ewing tumour variant 1) gene, at 7p22, and the t(17;22) (q12;q12) with *EIAF*, at 17q12 (Sorensen *et al.* 1994 Jeon *et al.* 1995, Kaneko *et al.* 1996). Whereas *EWS-ERG* chimeric transcripts account for 5% of Ewing tumours, *EWS-ETV1* and *EWS-EIAF* have been detected in single cases.

The molecular genetic characterization of these novel gene products as a result of chromosomal translocations has facilitated novel diagnostic approaches. Until recently, the detection of a recurrent translocation, such as the t(11;22) (q24;q12), was often hampered by the lack of suitable tumour cell karyotypes. This problem is largely solved by introducing two innovative techniques: FISH (fluorescence *in situ* hybridization) and PCR (polymerase chain reaction). FISH is a non-isotopic, slide-based technique that employs hybridizing DNA probes, specific to the chromosomal regions of interest, to cell preparations, and visualizes their location using fluorescent reporter molecules. Gene-specific cosmid probes flanking the translocation breakpoints at chromosome 22 and 11, respectively, have been used in interphase FISH for rapid and reliable diagnosis (Desmaze *et al.* 1994; McManus *et al.* 1995). Although FISH is an upcoming alternative to RT-PCR-based methods in the routine laboratory setting, detection and characterization of the translocations at the RNA level provide additional information of presumed clinical relevance.

At the DNA level, chromosomal breakpoints are scattered over 2 and 40 kilobase pairs in *EWS* and *FLI1* genes, resulting in the inclusion of variable portions of the constituents in the fusion protein, with a minimal region present in all *EWS-FLI1* and *EWS-ERG* products. This region consists of the domains encoded by *EWS* exon 1 to 7 and *FLI1* exon 9 or the respective portions of *ERG*, *ETV1*, or *EIAF*. At the RNA level, these regions move very closely together and are therefore detectable by RT-PCR-based methods. Only material containing the tumour-specific gene will result in a positive PCR signal, which can be visualized as a band in gel electrophoresis, and identified by Southern blotting with gene-specific probes. Tumour cell concentrations of 10^{-5}–10^{-4} in unprocessed tissue suffice for analysis. Using this approach, the diagnostic value of *EWS* rearrangement in Ewing tumours was confirmed on a large number of small round-cell tumours (Downing *et al.* 1993; Sorensen *et al.* 1993; Delattre *et al.* 1994; Dockhorn-Dworniczak *et al.* 1994*b*). So far, there is no convincing evidence for the occurrence of Ewing-tumour-specific rearrangements in other tumours, suggesting that the presence of the specific fusion transcripts defines a subgroup of small round-cell tumours, namely the Ewing tumour family.

So far, more than 15 different fusion transcripts have been described. It has been shown that the chimeric genes result in the production of very similar proteins, suggesting that the exact nature of the chromosomal breakpoint may probably be irrelevant to potential oncogenic behavior (Zucman *et al.* 1993). Other studies supported the concept that the heterogeneity of fusion transcripts may contribute to different clinical outcome (Delattre *et al.* 1994). Recently, a larger, European, multicenter study revealed a statistically significant advantage in relapse-free survival for patients with localized disease and a chimeric transcript fusing *EWS* exon 7 to *FLI1* exon 6

(Zoubek *et al.* 1996). Although this will require prospective validation with a larger number of patients and follow-up periods, these findings underline that detection of *EWS-FLI1* and *EWS-ERG* might not only improve diagnosis as an adjunct to surgical pathology, but may also help to identify prognostic parameters in Ewing tumour disease.

Furthermore, the high sensitivity of RT-PCR analysis allows the detection of circulating translocation-carrying tumour cells. Several studies have demonstrated the feasibility of using RT-PCR methodology for detecting small numbers of Ewing tumour cells in bone marrow and peripheral blood samples (Dockhorn-Dworniczak *et al.* 1994a, Dockhorn-Dworniczak *et al.* 1995, Peter *et al.* 1995, West *et al.* 1997). In addition, these assays have been utilized to demonstrate the presence of tumour cells in peripheral blood stem-cell grafts collected for progenitor cell rescue in high-dose chemotherapy treatment. At present, the true biological meaning and clinical relevance of disseminated tumour cells in blood or bone marrow samples of Ewing tumour patients is unknown. Large-scale studies are warranted to evaluate if RT-PCR detection of tumour cells in bone marrow and peripheral blood samples is suitable for identification of submicroscopical metastasis, and for monitoring residual disease in patients who are undergoing therapy.

Extraskeletal Ewing's sarcoma

Extraskeletal Ewing's sarcoma is uncommon, but can usually be distinguished from primitive or undifferentiated rhabdomyosarcoma, neuroblastoma, and lymphoma by histocytochemistry, electron microscopy, and molecular studies (Angervall and Enzinger 1975; Wigger *et al.* 1977; Meister and Gökel 1978; Soule *et al.* 1978; Berthold *et al.* 1982; Kinsella *et al.* 1983b). The major differential diagnosis includes Ewing's sarcoma of bone with extensive soft-tissue extension, and an inapparent intraosseous component (Angervall and Enzinger 1975). The predominant site of initial presentation is the trunk. As distinct from Ewing's sarcoma of bone, there is no predominance in boys. The same rules as for Ewing's sarcoma of bone apply for the investigation and systemic treatment of extraskeletal Ewing's sarcoma. However, as there appears to be a higher risk of lymphatic spread, the local therapy, especially radiation, must be planned according to the same principles as applied to embryonal rhabdomyosarcoma (Raney *et al.* 1997).

Differential diagnosis (see Table 15.1)

The most important clinical differential diagnosis in Ewing's sarcoma is osteomyelitis (Huvos 1991). The radiological appearance may be very similar; in addition, however, Ewing's sarcoma of bone may be secondarily infected. On histological examination, Ewing's sarcoma must be differentiated from other small round-cell sarcomas; these include: (a) embryonal rhabdomyosarcoma, (b) neuroblastoma, (c) malignant, primitive (peripheral), neuroectodermal tumour (Askin's tumour), (d) small-cell osteogenic sarcoma, and (e) malignant lymphoma.

Myxoid changes and cross-striations, along with the typical ultrastructural appearance of thin or thick microfilaments arranged in Z-bands, lead to the diagnosis of rhabdomyosarcoma (Schmidt and Harms 1990). On immunocytochemistry, myogenous markers such as desmin, myoglobin, and myosin are usually positive, and help to support the diagnosis (see p. 235). In children younger than 5 years of age, the classical differential diagnosis is neuroblastoma (Berthold *et al.* 1982). This must be assumed when the 24-hour urinary catecholamine excretion is increased and histological examination reveals the presence of intercellular neurofibrillary matrix, while neurosecretory granules are seen on electron microscopy (Schmidt *et al.* 1989). In addition, immunocytochemistry shows a positive reaction with antibodies directed against neural markers such as neuron-specific enolase and S100 (Schmidt *et al.* 1987; Schmidt and Harms 1990).

The presence of extracellular matrix, particularly tumour osteoid, may suggest the diagnosis of small-cell osteosarcoma (Sim *et al.* 1979). Malignant cartilage may lead to the diagnosis of mesenchymal chondrosarcoma (Huvos *et al.* 1983). Another consideration in the differential diagnosis of Ewing's sarcoma is primary lymphoma of bone, although the absence of disseminated lymph nodes, and visceral, meningeal, or bone marrow involvement is atypical for the childhood lymphomas (Schmidt *et al.* 1987, Huvos 1991). Again, immunocytochemistry is essential to make the distinction; positive reactivity with lymphoid markers is characteristic for malignant lymphoma.

Treatment

The treatment of patients with primary Ewing's sarcoma includes the eradication of the primary lesion by high-dose radiation therapy and/or radical surgical removal, together with combination chemotherapy to control microscopic metastatic deposits (Chan *et al.* 1979; Gasparini *et al.* 1981; Jürgens *et al.* 1988; Perez *et al.* 1977; Razek *et al.* 1980; Rosen *et al.* 1981*a*). The scheduling and integration of these three treatment modalities must be carefully designed to provide a curative approach for the individual patient (Razek *et al.* 1980; Zucker *et al.* 1983; Jürgens *et al.* 1985). This is the subject of ongoing clinical trials. Prior to the era of adjuvant chemotherapy, the treatment results were universally poor, with 5-year survival rates in the range of 5–10% owing to rapid systemic spread of the disease, clinically evidenced by pulmonary and/or multiple bone metastases (Falk and Alpert 1967; Jürgens *et al.* 1988).

Radiotherapy

Conventionally, radiotherapy plays a major role in obtaining local control of Ewing's sarcoma, due to its radiosensitivity with SF_2 (Surviving Fraction at 2 Gy) values of 0.24–0.58 (Perez *et al.* 1977; Razek *et al.* 1980; Donaldson 1981; Jentzsch *et al.* 1981; Gonzales-Gonzales and Breur 1983; Kinsella *et al.* 1983*a*; Weichselbaum *et al.* 1989). The radiosensitivity of Ewing's sarcoma was already recognized by James Ewing himself (Ewing 1921), and since then has been confirmed by the experience of many investigators and cooperative studies (Razek *et al.* 1980; Perez *et al.* 1981; Thomas *et al.* 1984). However, since the widespread adoption of systemic chemotherapy, with increasing evidence of its success in prolonging disease-free survival, the problem of local failure following radiation has become more evident (Razek *et al.* 1980; Rosen *et al.* 1981*b*; Donaldson and Hendrickson 1983; Jürgens *et al.* 1985, 1988). The definite risk of local failure following radiation accounts for the ongoing controversy regarding the indications for radiotherapy (Pritchard 1981). Surgery has been shown to produce a survival advantage compared with radiotherapy in several series (Wilkins *et al.* 1986; Barbiera *et al.* 1990), but in some cases this may have just reflected the inherently better prognosis of those small peripheral lesions where surgery was more feasible. Prospective randomized studies regarding the optimal modality to achieve local control are lacking. In most recent studies, the favoured approach to obtain safe, local control is a combined modality approach of both surgery and radiotherapy. However, approximately 20% of Ewing's sarcoma will be inoperable because of position, size, or soft-tissue extension, and radiotherapy is the only option for local control. In view of this individualized approach to local control, the recent European CESS 86 study no longer showed a difference in survival rates according to local treatment. However, definitive radiotherapy only was limited to 25% of patients, whereas 22% of patients underwent surgery and 53% of patients received combined modality local treatment. Local relapse rates were highest in the group treated by radiotherapy alone. This advantage, however, was balanced by an increased rate of distant metastases (26%) in the group treated by surgery or after resection and radiotherapy (29%), compared with radiotherapy alone (16%). The overall survival was 69%, with relapse rates after radiotherapy of 30%, after radical surgery of 26%, and after combination therapy of 34%. The local relapse rates were 0% after surgery, 3% after surgery and radiotherapy, and 7% after radiotherapy alone. The combined relapse rates were 0% after surgery, 2% after surgery and radiotherapy, and 7% after radiotherapy alone (Dunst *et al.* 1995). In case of any doubt about the margins of excision, radiotherapy must be given following surgery (Jereb *et al.* 1986). As with osteosarcoma, persistence of active disease following chemotherapy is a poor prognostic factor. It is, however, difficult to conclude to what extent this increased risk can be minimized by the addition of radiotherapy. Whether distant metastases following surgery can be prevented by preoperative radiotherapy to further sterilize the tumour-bearing compartment is the subject of ongoing trials. However, pilot experience with preoperative radiotherapy in addition to upfront chemotherapy has shown that viable tumour was demonstrated in as many as 43% of surgical specimens that had received both chemotherapy and radiotherapy, indicating the definite hazard of local failure following radiotherapy (Jürgens *et al.* 1996).

An important improvement in outcome of local radiotherapy was seen between the CESS 81 and 86 studies which was attributed to improved quality control of radiotherapy delivery (Dunst *et al.* 1995). Similar findings have been published by the Paediatric Oncology Group in the United States, where local control rates were 63% if there were protocol deviations, compared with 88% if treatment was given according to protocol (Markus 1996).

Planning of radiotherapy

The recommended approach to the primary tumour requires meticulous evaluation of stage and extent of disease. In patients with biopsy-confirmed Ewing's sarcoma who receive chemotherapy prior to radiotherapy, treatment planning must be based upon the extent of initial tumour (Razek *et al.* 1980; Jürgens *et al.* 1988). Characteristically, intramedullary extension of the tumour visualized by radionuclear studies, computed tomography, and/or magnetic resonance imaging exceeds that visible by conventional X-ray techniques.

Dose and volume

Traditionally, whole-bone irradiation was advised because the tumour was thought to arise in the bone marrow, putting the whole bone marrow cavity at risk. The advent of good imaging with MRI to demonstrate clearly the extent of marrow involvement, and effective chemotherapy, call this approach into question, and in a POG randomized study completed in 1989 it has been shown that results of radiation to initial tumour volume with a 2 cm margin are as good as those obtained after whole-bone irradiation. Doses for local irradiation should exceed 50 Gy (Perez *et al.* 1977) for gross tumour and 45 Gy (Dunst *et al.* 1991) for microscopic disease. Meticulous attention must be paid to ensuring adequate margins around the initial volume of tumour (usually 2–5 cm). A strip of normal tissue should be left where possible on either side of the treatment field to prevent the late development of lymphoedema, and joints and epiphyses should be avoided whenever possible, in particular in growing children.

Surgery

Increasing awareness of the risk of local recurrence following radiotherapy has prompted the use of surgery or combined modality local treatment. Ewing's sarcoma of bone is rarely limited to the bony compartment. The presence of a soft-tissue component is common, classifying most tumours as highly malignant, extracompartmental tumours according to the Enneking classification (Enneking 1987). To allow comparison of surgical interventions, all surgical procedures should be classified according to the Enneking criteria (Enneking 1987) as intralesional, marginal, wide, or radical resection (Table 15.2).

According to the (EI)CESS experience, surgical margins and response to initial upfront therapy correlate with outcome, both with regard to the rate of local control and the rate of distant metastases (Fig. 15.6) (Salzer-Kuntschik *et al.* 1983; Enneking 1987).

Hence, whenever possible, good response to initial therapy and tumour-free margins must be achieved.

Situations in which surgical resections are preferable to radiation therapy include the following: (a) lesion in expendable bone, (b) pathological fracture, (c) distal extremity, (d) bulky primary tumour, and (e) poor response to initial chemotherapy. In addition, Ewing's sarcoma of the pelvis requires particular attention since this lesion has a poor prognosis (Pritchard 1981; Kinsella *et al.* 1984; Nesbit *et al.* 1990). Only in rare cases is the pelvic lesion small and so located as to be readily resectable; for example, a small lesion of the rim of the ilium or of the

Table 15.2   Enneking classification of surgical intervention

Intralesional resection	The tumour is opened during surgery, the surgical field is contaminated, there is microscopic or macroscopic residual disease.
Marginal resection	The tumour is removed en bloc. However, the line of resection runs through the pseudocapsule of the tumour. Microscopic residual disease is likely.
Wide resection	The tumour and its pseudocapsule are removed en bloc, surrounded by healthy tissue within the tumour-bearing compartment.
Radical resection	The whole tumour-bearing compartment is removed en bloc, e.g. above-knee amputation in tibial tumours.

(Source: Enneking 1987)

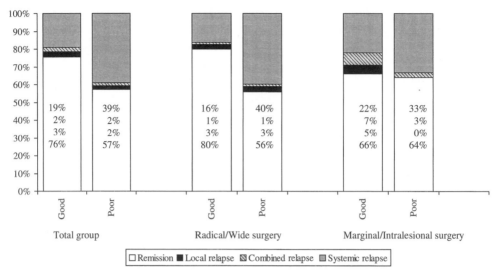

Fig. 15.6 Site of failure in surgically (± radiotherapy) treated Ewing's sarcoma patients according to surgical margins and response.

symphysis pubis may be completely resected without inducing any significant morbidity. Most pelvic lesions are large and not primarily resectable (Scully *et al.* 1995). There is, however, good evidence that the prognosis of extensive pelvic lesions can be improved if the residual disease is resected following tumour shrinkage induced by initial chemotherapy (Winkelmann and Jürgens 1989). It is the subject of current ongoing trials to define exact guidelines for the role of radiotherapy prior to, or following, resection in combination with initial debulking chemotherapy (Teff *et al.* 1977). Nevertheless, a team approach for the evaluation of these patients prior to local therapy is essential. The treatment plan must be individualized depending upon the location and size of the tumour and anatomical structures in the vicinity of the tumour which might be affected by the type of treatment selected (Sauer *et al.* 1987; Jürgens *et al.* 1988; Nesbit *et al.* 1990).

Chemotherapy

Single-drug data show the responsiveness of Ewing's sarcoma to various chemotherapeutic agents. Alkylating agents such as cyclophosphamide (Samuels and Howe 1967; Seeber *et al.* 1974), nitrogen mustard, chlorambucil, and iphosphamide are particularly effective (De Kraker and Voûte 1984; Bier *et al.* 1987; Jürgens *et al.* 1989*a,b*). The other agents studies include vincristine, etoposide, actinomycin D, 5-fluorouracil, and in particular doxorubicin (adriamycin) (Oldham and Pomeroy 1972).

The improved disease-free survival rates now reported have been brought about by the use of aggressive combination multicycle chemotherapy regimens (Razek *et al.* 1980; Gasparini *et al.* 1981; Rosen *et al.* 1981*a*; Jürgens *et al.* 1988). Although the optimal chemotherapeutic schedule in the treatment of this tumour remains to be established, the convincing data recorded in the

IESS have shown the superiority of a four-drug regimen with vincristine, actinomycin D, cyclophosphamide, and doxorubicin over a three-drug regimen with vincristine, actinomycin D, and cyclophosphamide in terms of disease-free survival (74% *versus* 54%) and effectiveness of local control (96% *versus* 86%) (Perez *et al.* 1977; Razek *et al.* 1980; Nesbit *et al.* 1990). Results reported by Rosen from the Memorial Sloan-Kettering Cancer Center (MSKCC) confirmed the effectiveness of the four-drug regimen and provided evidence that the use of these four effective agents in combination, rather than sequentially, may further improve the results (Rosen *et al.* 1981*a,b*). It must be taken into account that a considerable number of patients in earlier series received cumulative doxorubicin doses of over 700 mg/m^2 before its use was restricted to 500 mg/m^2 because of the risk of doxorubicin-related cardiomyopathy. The MSKCC and IESS experience led to the wide use of similar four-drug regimens in most ongoing therapeutic trials (Razek *et al.* 1980; Gasparini *et al.* 1981; Rosen *et al.* 1981*b*; Jürgens *et al.* 1988). Results of recently reported trials are listed in Table 15.3. Disease-free survival rates for over 3 years, obtained with chemotherapy and local control with radiation and/or surgery, range between 50% and 70%. Hence, chemotherapy has impressively improved the disease-free survival rate over that obtained with local therapy alone.

Table 15.3 Results of Ewing's sarcoma trials

Trial/Institution (Reference)	Number of patients	Treatment strategy	Follow-up (years)	NED (%)	Results of subgroups (%)
IESS I 1990 (Tefft *et al.* 1977)	342	Radiation, chemotherapy	> 6	48	VACA (59) VAC (55) VAC + pulmonary radiation (42) Pelvic sites (34) Non-pelvic sites (57)
IESS II 1990 (Burgert *et al.* 1990)	214	Radiation surgery, chemotherapy	1–9	64	VACA high dose (73) VACA moderate dose (56)
MSKCC Rosen *et al.* 1978)	67	T2, T6, T9 protocols; radiation, surgery	1–10	79	Axial tumours (65) Distal tumours (95) Proximal tumours (79) Radiation (76) Amputation (77) Surgery + radiation (85)
Istituto Nazionale, Italy (Gasparini *et al.* 1981)	34	Radiation, chemotherapy	2–6	59	Extremities (67) Axial skeleton (40) Adequate radiotherapy (76) Inadequate radiotherapy (33)
Villejuif, France (Zucker *et al.* 1983)	30	Radiation, chemotherapy	5–8	50	Long bones (69) Axial skeleton (35)

Table 15.3 *Continued*

Trial/Institution (Reference)	Number of patients	Treatment strategy	Follow-up (years)	NED (%)	Results of subgroups (%)
12 centres, France (Deméocq *et al.* 1984)	70	Radiation, chemotherapy	2–5	54	Long bones (78) Flat bones (37) Ribs (50)
Bologna, Italy (Gnudi *et al.* 1983; Bacci *et al.* 1989)	144	Radiation, surgery, chemotherapy	5–16	41	Sequential chemotherapy (32) Combination chemotherapy (54) Surgery + radiation (60) Radiation (28) Pelvic sites (24) Non-pelvic sites (46)
SJCRH, USA (Hayes *et al.* 1989)	50	Radiation, surgery, chemotherapy	3	80	< 8 cm (82) > 8 cm (64)
CESS 81, Germany (Jürgens *et al.* 1988)	93	Radiation, surgery, chemotherapy	2–6	55	Axial (53) Proximal (45) Distal (75) Surgery (64) Radiation + surgery (69) Radiation (50) < 100 ml tumour volume (80) > 100 ml tumour volume (32) histological response good (79) poor (31)
CESS 86, Germany (Jürgens 1991)	177	Radiation, surgery, chemotherapy	4–9	66	Axial (66) Proximal (76) Distal (55) Surgery (55) Surgery + radiation (63) Radiation (66) < 100 ml tumour volume (72) ≥ 100 ml tumour volume (62) histological response good (70) poor (55)

The impact of treatment intensity on further improvement of disease-free survival was shown by an analysis of IESS-II, in which high-dose, intermittent chemotherapy was compared to moderate-dose, continuous chemotherapy, resulting in a significant benefit from the more intensive regimen (68% *versus* 48% disease-free survival at 5 years) (Burgert *et al.* 1990). A first cooperative Ewing's sarcoma study of the German Society of Paediatric Oncology (CESS 81) had shown the prognostic significance of tumour burden at diagnosis and histological response to initial chemotherapy, and also stressed the impact of surgery on local control (Göbel *et al.* 1987; Sauer *et al.* 1987; Jürgens *et al.* 1988). In a follow-up study (CESS 86), patients with large primary tumours (> 100 ml) received a more intensive chemotherapy regimen in which conventional doses of cyclophosphamide (1200 mg/m^2 per course) were replaced by high doses of iphosphamide (6000 mg/m^2 per course) in combination with other agents.

The results show a significant benefit for high-risk patients from the more intensive regimen, again stressing the impact of treatment intensity on survival.

The combination of iphosphamide and etoposide has shown high response rates in patients who had failed previous chemotherapy and might add to the efficacy of first-line chemotherapy (Miser *et al.* 1987). The role of the addition of etoposide as fifth agent to conventional four-drug chemotherapy is currently under evaluation; the risk of late effects, such as increased risk of second malignant neoplasms, must be weighed against any potential benefit (Fig. 15.7) (Kobayashi and Ratain 1992).

In view of increasing knowledge about the mechanisms of treatment resistance (Goldie and Coldman 1979), for example, p-glycoprotein-mediated resistance against anthracyclines and vinca alkaloids (Gerlach *et al.* 1987), attention must be focused in future on further improving the

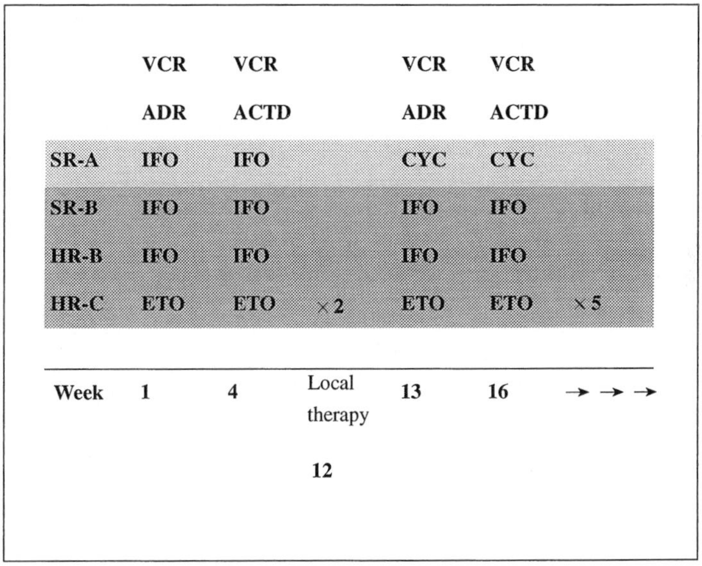

	VCR	VCR		VCR	VCR	
	ADR	ACTD		ADR	ACTD	
SR-A	IFO	IFO		CYC	CYC	
SR-B	IFO	IFO		IFO	IFO	
HR-B	IFO	IFO		IFO	IFO	
HR-C	ETO	ETO	× 2	ETO	ETO	× 5

Week	1	4	Local therapy	13	16	→ → →
			12			

Fig. 15.7 (EI)CESS 92 chemotherapy. Randomized allocation to four treatment arms: standard risk (tumour volume < 100 ml): four-drug chemotherapy regimen with vincristine (VCR), adriamycin (ADR; doxorubicin), actinomycin D (ACTD), and iphosphamide (IFO), followed by VCR, ADR, ACTD, and either cyclophosphamide (CYC) (treatment A) or IFO (treatment B); high risk (tumour volume > 100 ml and/or metastatic disease at diagnosis): either four-drug chemotherapy regimen with vincristine (VCR), adriamycin (ADR; doxorubicin), actinomycin D (ACTD), and iphosphamide (IFO) (treatment B), or VCR, ACTD, IFO, and etoposide (ETO) (treatment C).
VCR: 1.5 mg/m^2 push days 1, 21; ADR: 20 mg/m^2/day over 4 hours, days 1–3; ACTD: 0.5 mg/m^2/day push days 21–23; IFO: 2000 mg/m^2/day over 1 hour, days 1–3, 21–23; CYC: 1200 mg/m^2 over 1 hour, days 1, 21; ETO: 150 mg/m^2/day over 1 hour, days 1–3, 21–23.

prognosis of subgroups of patients who have not benefited from current treatment strategies, such as with intensive combination induction chemotherapy to eradicate systemic disease early, to obtain shrinkage of the primary tumour, and possibly to avoid and prevent chemotherapy resistance (Deméocq *et al.* 1984; Oberlin *et al.* 1985).

Metastatic disease

Of patients presenting with a diagnosis of Ewing's sarcoma, approximately 15–35% have detectable metastatic disease at diagnosis (Hayes *et al.* 1987; Wessalowski *et al.* 1988). The survival of these patients, even with multimodal therapy, has been disappointing, but it seems better for patients with pulmonary metastases than for those with multiple bone lesions (Wessalowski *et al.* 1988; Paulussen *et al.* 1993). Treatment includes combination chemotherapy, if pulmonary disease is present, as outlined for patients with primary Ewing's sarcoma, and radiation of both lungs at a dose of 14–20 Gy, given in 1.5-Gy fractions on 5 days a week. For multiple bone lesions, all involved areas must be irradiated. However, it may not be possible to irradiate the entire bone at all sites affected, since this would set a limit to the tolerance of chemotherapy (Pilepich *et al.* 1981; Wessalowski *et al.* 1988). Survival in patients with multiple bone lesions at diagnosis has been dismal despite initial response to intensive systemic and local treatment. The survival rates reported are below 10% at 2 years for patients with multiple bone disease, and are hence comparable to the prognosis for patients with disseminated neuroblastoma (Glaubiger *et al.* 1980; Wessalowski *et al.* 1988). Encouraging results have recently been reported with autologous or allogeneic bone marrow or peripheral stem-cell transplantation in first remission, particularly when a conditioning regimen combining total-body irradiation with mega-dose chemotherapy was used (Burdach *et al.* 1993). Consolidation with a megatherapy conditioning regimen, followed by bone marrow transplantation, is aimed solely at controlling residual, resistant, systemic disease. It is essential to obtain control of bulky disease in addition to such a procedure, since attempts to control bulky disease with such megatherapy regimens have been discouraging (Pinkerton *et al.* 1986).

   In patients who develop metastatic disease either on or off therapy, survival is poor and second remissions are usually short-lived (Craft 1987; Jürgens *et al.* 1988). Exceptions may be related to less intensive primary treatment (Hayes *et al.* 1989). Attempts are being made to increase salvage with the use of megatherapy approaches with stem-cell rescue (Pinkerton *et al.* 1986; Craft 1987; Burdach *et al.* 1993). In some patients, with relapses responding to reinduction chemotherapy, this might be of value. Results in patients with resistant disease have so far been disappointing (Craft 1987).

Prognostic factors

As noted above, the reported disease-free survival rate of 50–70% necessitates a recognition of patients characteristics related to prognosis, since knowledge of these factors may have important implications for treatment stratification. Factors related to prognosis are listed in Table 15.4.

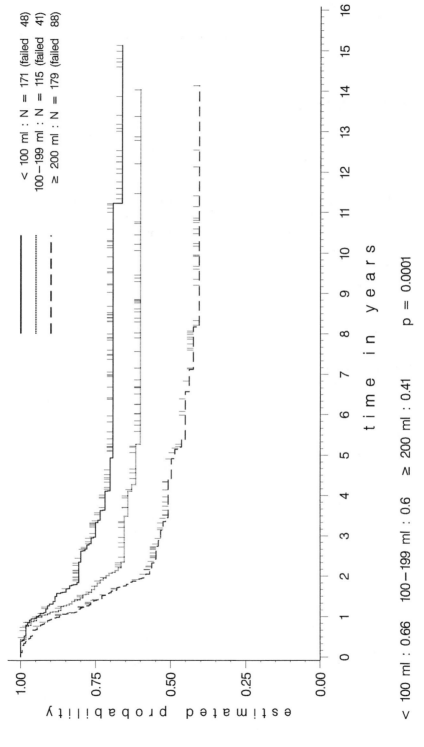

Fig. 15.8 Disease-free survival according to tumour burden (from CESS/EICESS data).

Table 15.4   Prognostic factors in Ewing's sarcoma (poor < good prognosis)

Sex	Male < female (Pomeroy and Johnson 1975; Gehan *et al.* 1981)
Age	Over 15 years < under 15 years
Tumour Site	Central < proximal < distal (Pomeroy and Johnson 1975; Glaubiger *et al.* 1980; Gehan *et al.* 1981)
Tumour size	Tumour extension above 8 cm < less than 8 cm (Mendenhall *et al.* 1983; Hayes *et al.* 1989)
	Tumour volume above 100 ml < below 100 ml (Jürgens *et al.* 1985, 1988)
	Soft-tissue extension present < absent (Mendenhall *et al.* 1983)
Metastases	Visible at diagnosis < undetectable (Glaubiger *et al.* 1980)
Histology	Large-cell variant < conventional histology (Nascimento 1980)
	Poor < good histological response to therapy (Jürgens *et al.* 1988)
Laboratory	Elevated serum LDH < normal serum LDH (Glaubiger *et al.* 1980)
Chemotherapy	Vincristine, actinomycin D, cyclophosphamide < vincristine, actinomycin D, cyclophosphamide, doxorubicin (Nascimento 1980) < vincristine, actinomycin D, iphosphamide, doxorubicin (Jürgens *et al.* 1988, 1989*b*)

Future prospects

Since Ewing's sarcoma is fundamentally a systemic disease, the combination of local control with radiation and/or surgery and systemic, multiagent, multicycle chemotherapy has improved the disease-free survival rate from approximately 10%, with local therapy alone, to a range of 50–70%. Careful analyses of patterns of failure and tailoring of the treatment approach to prognostic subgroups of patients appear to be the tasks for the future to overcome tumour resistance to both chemotherapy and radiation, and to minimize late side-effects of treatment, such as secondary neoplasms (Kuttesch *et al.* 1996) and infertility (Kliesch *et al.* 1996). Initial chemotherapy following biopsy-confirmed diagnosis prior to local therapy, leads to impressive tumour shrinkage in more than 90% of patients so treated. The optimal combination of agents and the length of the initial treatment are still under evaluation. There is evidence that high-dose iphosphamide with mesna uroprotection is more effective than conventional-dose cyclophosphamide as first-line treatment, at least for poor-prognosis subgroups (Jürgens *et al.* 1988). However, the risk of long-term renal toxicity of high cumulative doses of iphosphamide must be weighed against its benefit (Ashraf *et al.* 1994; Rossi *et al.* 1994). In view of the proven benefit of more intensive combination chemotherapy, the use of growth factors to ameliorate bone marrow toxicity may be of value (Andreeff and Welte 1989). *In vitro*, Ewing's sarcoma cell lines have responded to the combination of tumour necrosis factor alpha and gamma interferon (van Valen *et al.* 1994). This may start an era of effective treatment of Ewing's sarcoma using biological response modifiers. Finally, since intensive megatherapy regimens with stem-cell rescue are of benefit for some patients with disseminated disease, this might also be of value in poor-prognosis subgroups of patients with localized disease (Pinkerton *et al.* 1986; Craft 1987; Burdach *et al.* 1993).

In conclusion, the prognosis is determined primarily by tumour dissemination and tumour burden, as well as by response to treatment. While tumour burden can only be limited by early diagnosis, response is subject to iatrogenic intervention; other important factors for improvement are design of effective combinations, increased drug intensity with improved supportive care (e.g. cytokine or stem-cell support), and surgical removal of tumour to prevent recurrence, particularly in view of the high rate of viable tumour detected in previously irradiated surgical specimens (Jürgens *et al.* 1996). In addition, the determination of prognostic factors must result in the definition of different risk groups to stratify treatment intensity and to limit the risk of late effects from treatment.

Acknowledgements

The authors wish to thank Gabriele Braun-Munzinger for her invaluable help in preparing and editing the manuscript.

References

Ambros, I.M., Ambros, P.F., Strehl, S., Kovar, H., Gadner, H., and Salzer-Kuntschik, M (1991). MIC2 is a specific marker for Ewing's sarcoma and peripheral primitive neuroectodermal tumors. Evidence for a common histogenesis of Ewing's sarcoma and peripheral primitive neuroectodermal tumors from MIC2 expression and specific chromosome aberration. *Cancer*, 67, 1886–1893.

Andreeff, M. and Welte, K. (1989). Hematopoietic colony-stimulating factors. *Seminars in Oncology*, 16, 211–229.

Angervall, L. and Enzinger, F.M. (1975). Extraskeletal neoplasm resembling Ewing's sarcoma. *Cancer*, 36, 240–251.

Ashraf, M.S., Brady, J., Breatnach, F., Deasy, PF., and O'Meara, A. (1994). Ifosfamide nephrotoxicity in paediatric cancer patients. *European Journal of Pediatrics*, 153, 90–94.

Askin, F.B., Rosai, J., Sibley, R.K., Dehner, L.P., and McAlister, W.H. (1979). Malignant small cell tumor of the thoracopulmonary region in childhood. *Cancer*, 43, 2438–2451.

Bacci, G., Toni, A., Avella, M., Manfrini, M., Sudanese, A., and Ciaroni, M. (1989). Long-term results in 144 localized Ewing's sarcoma patients treated with combined therapy. *Cancer*, 63, 1477–1486.

Barbiera, E., Emiliani, E., Zini, G., Mancini, A., Toni, A., Frezza., G. *et al.* (1990). Combined therapy of localized Ewing's sarcoma of bone: Analysis of results in 100 patients. *International Journal of Radiation Oncology, Biology and Physics*, 19, 1165–1170.

Berthold, F., Kracht, J., Lampert, F., Millar, T.J., Müller, T.H., Reither, M., *et al.* (1982). Ultrastructural, biochemical, and cell-culture studies of a presumed extraskeletal Ewing's sarcoma with special reference to differential diagnosis from neuroblastoma. *J Cancer Res Clin Oncol*, 103, 293–304.

Bier, V., Jürgens, H., Etspüler, G., Exner, U., Kühl, J., Ritter, J., *et al.* (1987). 120-h continuous infusion of ifosfamide alone and in combination with cis-platinum in children and adolescents with recurrent Ewing's sarcoma. *Contr Oncol*, 26, 131–138.

Burdach, S., Jürgens, H., Peters, C., Nürnberger, W., Mauz-Körholz, C., Körholz C., *et al.* (1993). Myeloablative radiochemotherapy and hematopoietic stem-cell rescue in poor prognosis Ewing's sarcoma. *Journal of Clinical Oncology*, 11, 1482–1488.

Burgert, E.O., Nesbit, M.E., Garnsey, L.A., Gehan, E.A., Herrman, J., Vietti, R.J., *et al.* (1990). Multimodal therapy for the management of nonpelvic localized Ewing's sarcoma of bone: Intergroup Study IESS-II. *Journal of Clinical Oncology*, 8, 1514–1524.

Campanacci, M. (1990). Ewing's sarcoma. In: Campanacci M. (ed) Bone and soft tissue tumors. Springer, Vienna New York, pp. 309–538.

Chan, R.C., Sutow, W.W., Lindberg, R.D., Samuels, M.L., Murray, J.A., and Johnston, D.A. (1979). Management and results of localized Ewing's sarcoma. *Cancer*, 43, 1001–1006.

Craft, A.W. (1987). Chemotherapy of Ewing's sarcoma. Baillière *Clin Oncol* 1, 205–221.

Dahlin, D.C. (1996). Bone tumors, general aspects and data on 11 087 cases. Lippincott-Raven, Philadelphia New York.

De Kraker, J. and Voûte, P.A. (1984). Ifosfamide and vincristine in paediatric tumors. A phase II study. *European Paediatric Haematol Oncol*, 1, 47–50.

Delattre, O., Zucman, J., and Plougastel, B. (1992). Gene fusion with an ETS DNA-binding domain caused by chromosome translocation in human tumours. *Nature*, 359, 162–165.

Delattre, O., Zucman, J., and Melot, T. (1994). The Ewing family of tumors-a subgroup of small-round-cell tumors defined by specific chimeric transcripts *New England Journal of Medicine*, 331, 294–299, 1994.

Deméocq, F., Carton, P., Patte, C., Oberlin, O., Sarrazin, D., and Lemerle, J. (1984). Traitement du sarcome d'Ewing par chimiothérapie initiale intensive. *Presse Med*, 13, 717–721.

Desmaze, C., Zucman, J., Delattre, O., Melot, T., Thomas, G., and Aurias, A. (1994). Interphase molecular cytogenetics of Ewing's sarcoma and peripheral neuroepithelioma t(11;22) with flanking and overlapping cosmid probes. *Cancer Genet. Cytogenet.*, 74, 13–18.

Dockhorn-Dworniczak, B., Schäfer, K.L., Dantcheva, R., Blasius, S., Böcker, W., Winkelmann, W., *et al.* (1994*a*) Comments on 'Prognostic features of Ewing's sarcoma on plain radiograph and computed tomography scan after initial treatment'. *Cancer*, 74, 988–989.

Dockhorn-Dworniczak, B., Schäfer, K.L., and Dantcheva, R. (1994*b*) Diagnostic value of the molecular genetic detecton of the t(11;22) translocation in Ewing's tumors. *Virchows Arch A.*, 425, 107–112.

Dockhorn-Dworniczak, B., Pfleiderer, C., Schäfer, K.L., Zoubek, A., Burdach, S., Hoffmann, C., *et al.* (1995). Molecular staging of Ewing tumor patients using RT-PCR analysis of blood and bone marrow samples. ASCO Annual Meeting, Los Angeles, May 20–23, 1995; *Proceedings of ASCO*, 14, 620.

Donaldson, S.S. (1981). A story of continuing success—radiotherapy for Ewing's sarcoma. *Int J Radiat Oncol Biol Phys*, 7, 279–281.

Donaldson, S.S. and Hendrickson, M.R. (1983). Patterns of failure in childhood solid tumors: Wilms' tumor, neuroblastoma and rhabdomyosarcoma. *Cancer Treat Symp*, 2, 267–283.

Downing, J.R., Head, D.R., Parham, D.M., *et al.* (1993). Detection of the (11;22)(q24;q12) translocation of Ewing's sarcoma and peripheral neuroectodermal tumor by reverse transcription polymerase chain reaction. *Am. J. Pathol.*, 143, 1294–1300.

Dunst, J., Sauer, R., Burgers, J.M.V., Hawlicek, R., Kürten, R., Winkelmann, W., *et al.* (1991). Radiation therapy as local treatment in Ewing's sarcoma. Results of the Cooperative Ewing's Sarcoma Studies CESS 81 and CESS 86. *Cancer*, 67, 2818–2825.

Dunst, J., Jürgens, H., Sauer, R., Pape, H., Paulussen, M., Winkelmann, W., *et al.* (1995). Radiation therapy in Ewing's sarcoma: An update of the CESS 86 trial. *Int J Radiat Oncol Biol Phys*, 32, 919–930.

Endicott, J.A. and Ling, V. (1989). The biochemistry of p-glycoprotein-mediated multidrug resistance. *Ann Rev Biochem*, 58, 137–171

Enneking, W. (1987). A system of staging musculoskeletal neoplasms. Baillière's *Clinical Oncology*, 1, 97–110.

Ewing, J. (1921). Diffuse endothelioma of bone. *Proc NY Pathol Soc*, 21, 17–24.

Ewing, J. (1939). A review of the classification of bone tumors. *Surg Gynecol Obstet*, 68, 971–976.

Falk, S. and Alpert, M. (1967). Five-year survival of patients with Ewing's sarcoma. *Surg Gynecol Obstet*, 124, 319–324.

Fellinger, E.J., Garin-Chesa, P., Su, S.L., DeAngelis, P., Lane, J.M., and Retting, W.J. (1991). Biochemical and genetic characterization of the HBA71 Ewing's sarcoma cell surface antigen. *Cancer Res.*, 51, 336–340.

Gasparini, M., Lombardi, F., Gianni, C., and Fossati-Bellani, F. (1981). Localized Ewing's sarcoma: results of integrated therapy and analysis of failure. *Eur J Cancer Clin Oncol*, 17, 1205–1209.

Gehan, E.A., Nesbit, M., Burgert, O.E., Vietti, T.J., Tefft, M., Kissane, J., *et al.* (1981). Prognostic factors in children with Ewing's sarcoma. *Natl Cancer Inst Monogr*, 56, 273–278.

Gelin, C., Aubrit, F., and Phaliphon, A. (1989). The E2 antigen, a 32 kd glycoprotein involved in T-cell adhesion processes, is the MIC2 gene product. *EMBO J.*, 8, 3253–3259.

Gerlach, J.H., Bell, D.R., Karakousis, C., Slocum, H.K., Kartner, N., Rustum, Y.M., *et al.* (1987). P-glycoprotein in human sarcoma: evidence for multidrug resistance. *J Clin Oncol*, 5, 1452–1460.

Glass, A.G. and Fraumeni Jr, J.F. (1970). Epidemiology of bone cancer in children. *Journal of the National Cancer Institute*, 44, 187–199.

Glaubiger, D.L., Makuch, R., Schwarz, J., Levine, A.S., and Johnson, R.E. (1980). Determination of prognostic factors and their influence on therapeutic results in patients with Ewing's sarcoma. *Cancer*, 45, 2213–2219.

Gnudi, S., Picci, P., Gherlinzoni, F., Bacci, G., and Putti, C. (1983). Adjuvant chemotherapy for localized Ewing's sarcoma. Ten year experience at the Istituto Ortopedico Rizzoli in 121 cases. In: Spitzy KG, Karrer K (eds) *Proceedings of the 13*[th] International Congress of Chemotherapy, Vienna, Austria, part 251, pp. 19–22.

Göbel, V., Jürgens, H., Etspüler, G., Kemperdick, H., Jungblut, R.M., Stienen, U., *et al.* (1987). Prognostic significance of tumor volume in localized Ewing's sarcoma of bone in children and adolescents. *J Cancer Res Clin Oncol*, 113, 187–191.

Goldie, J.H. and Coldman, A.J. (1979). A mathematical model for relating the drug sensitivity of tumors to their spontaneous mutation rate. *Cancer Treat Rep*, 63, 1727–1733.

Gonzales-Gonzales, D. and Breur, K. (1983). Clinical data from irradiated growing long bones in children. *Int J Radiat Oncol Biol Phys*, 9, 841–846.

Hayes, F.A., Thompson, E.I., Parvey, L., Rao, B., Kun, L., Parham, D., *et al.* (1987). Metastatic Ewing's sarcoma: remission induction and survival. *J Clin Oncol*, 5, 1199–1204.

Hayes, F.A., Thompson, E.I., Meyer, W.H., Kun, L., Parham, D., Rao, B., *et al.* (1989). Therapy for localized Ewing's sarcoma of bone. *J Clin Oncol*, 7, 208–213.

Hildebrand (1890–1891). Über das tubuläre Angiosarkom oder Endotheliom des Knochens. *Dtsch Z Chir*, 31, 262–281.

Huvos, A.G. (1991). Ewing's sarcoma: In: Huvos, A.G. (ed) Bone tumors. Diagnosis, treatment and prognosis. Saunders, Philadelphia, pp. 523–552

Huvos, A.G., Rosen, G., Dobska, M., and Marcove, R.C. (1983). Mesenchymal chondrosarcoma. *Cancer*, 51, 1230–1237.

Jentzsch, K., Binder, H., Cramer, H., Glaubiger, D.L., Kessler, R.M., Bull, C., *et al.* (1981). Leg function after radiotherapy for Ewing's sarcoma. *Cancer*, 47, 1267–1278.

Jeon, I.S., Davis, J.N., Braun, B.S., *et al.* (1995). A variant Ewing's sarcoma translocation (7;22) fuses the EWS gene to the ETS gene ETV1. *Oncogene*, 10, 1229–1234.

Jereb, B., Ong, R.L., Mohan, M., Caparros, B., and Exelby, P. (1986). Redefined role of radiation in combined treatment of Ewings sarcoma. *Paed Hem and Oncol*, 3, 111–118.

Jürgens, H. (1991). CESS 86: updated Nov. 1, 1991, interim analysis (previously unpublished data).

Jürgens, H. (1994). Ewing's sarcoma and peripheral primitive neuroectodermal tumor. *Curr Opin Oncol*, 6, 391–396.

Jürgens, H., Göbel, V., Michaelis, J., Ramach, W., Ritter, J., Sauer, R., *et al.* (1985). Die cooperative Ewing-Sarkom-Studie CESS 81 der GPO—Analyse nach 4 Jahren. *Klin Pädiatr*, 197, 225–232.

Jürgens, H., Exner, U., Gadner, H., Harms, D., Michaelis, J., Sauer, R., *et al.* (1988). Multidisciplinary treatment of primary Ewing's sarcoma of bone: A 6-year experience of a European cooperative trial. *Cancer*, 61, 23–32.

Jürgens, H., Exner, U., Kühl, J., Ritter, J., Treuner, J., Weinel, P., *et al.* (1989*a*) High-dose ifosfamide with mesna uroprotection in Ewing's sarcoma. *Cancer Chemother Pharmacol*, 24, S40–S44.

Jürgens, H., Treuner, J., Winkler, K., and Göbel, U. (1989*b*) Ifosfamide in pediatric malignancies. *Sem Oncol*, 16, 46–50.

Jürgens, H., Hoffmann, Ch., Ahrens, S., Salzer-Kuntschik, M., Dworniczak, B., Winkelmann, W., *et al.* (1996). Radiocurability of Ewing's sarcoma: histological response following preoperative chemo-and radiotherapy. ASCO Meeting, May 1996, Philadelphia; *Proceedings of ASCO*, 15, 464.

Kaneko, Y., Yoshida, K., Handa, M., *et al.* (1996). Fusion of an ETS-family gene, EIAF, to EWS by t(17;22)(q12;q12) chromosome translocation in an undifferentiated sarcoma of infancy. *Genes Chromosomes-Cancer*, 15, 115–121.

Kinsella, T.J., Loeffler, J.S., Fraass, B.A., and Tepper, J. (1983*a*) Extremity preservation by combined modality therapy in sarcomas of the hand and foot: an analysis of local control, disease-free survival and functional results. *Int J Radiat Oncol Biol Phys*, 9, 1115–1119.

Kinsella, T.J., Triche, T.J., Dickman, P.S., Costa, J., Tepper, J.E., and Glaubiger, D. (1983*b*) Extraskeletal Ewing's sarcoma: results of combined-modality treatment. *Am J Clin Oncol*, 1, 489–495.

Kinsella, T.J., Lichter, A.S., Miser, J., Gerber, L., and Glatstein, E. (1984). Local treatment of Ewing's sarcoma: radiation therapy versus surgery. *Cancer Treat Rep*, 68, 695–701.

Kissane, J.M., Askin, F.B., Foulkes, M., Stratton, L.B., and Shirley, S.F. (1983). Ewing's sarcoma of bone: clinicopathologic aspects of 303 cases from the Intergroup Ewing's Sarcoma Study. *Hum Pathol*, 14, 773–779.

Kliesch, S., Behre, H.M., Jürgens, H., and Nieschlag, E. (1996). Cryopreservation of semen from adolescent patients with malignancies. *Med Pediatr Oncol*, 26, 20–27.

Kobayashi, K. and Ratain, M.J. (1992). New perspectives on the toxicity of etoposide. *Seminars in Oncology*, 19, 78–83.

Kulick, A. and Mones, J. (1970). The neurological complications of Ewing's sarcoma: incidence of neurologic involvement and value of radiotherapy. *Mt Sinai J Med (NY)*, 37, 40–59.

Kuttesch, J.F., Wexler, L.F., Marcus, R.B., Fairclough, D., Weaver-McClure, L., White, M., *et al.* (1996). Second malignancies after Ewing's sarcoma: Radiation dose dependency of secondary sarcomas. *J Clin Oncol*, 14, 2818–2825.

Ladanyi, M., Lewis, R., Garin-Chesa, P., *et al.* (1993). EWS rearrangement in Ewing's sarcoma and peripheral neuroectodermal tumor. Molecular detection and correlation with cytogenetic analysis and MIC2 expression. *Diagn. Mol Pathol*, 2, 141–146.

Li, F.P., Tu, J.T., Liu, F.S. *et al.* (1980). Rarity of Ewing's sarcoma in China. *Lancet*, 1, 1255.

Llombart-Bosch, A., Blache, R., and Peydro-Olaya, A. (1978). Ultrastructural study of 28 cases of Ewing's sarcoma: typical and atypical forms. *Cancer*, 41, 1362–1373.

Lücke, A. (1866). Beiträge zur Geschwulstlehre. III. Lympho-Sarcom der Achseldrüsen: embolische Geschwülste der Lungen: allgemeine Leukämie. *Virs chows Arch*, [A] 35, 524–539.

Markus Jr, R.B, (1996). Current controversies in pediatric radiation oncology, *Orthopedic Clinics of North America*, 27 (3), 551–557.

McManus, A.P., Gusterson, B.A., Pinkerton, C.R., and Shipley, J.M. (1995). Diagnosis of Ewing's sarcoma and related tumours by detection of chromosome 22q12 translocations using fluorescence in situ hybridization on tumour touch imprints. *J. Pathol*. 176, 137–142.

Mehta, Y. and Hendrickson, R. (1974). CNS involvement in Ewing's sarcoma. *Cancer*, 33, 859–862.

Meister, P. and Gökel, J.M. (1978). Extraskeletal Ewing's sarcoma. *Virchows Arch*, [A] 378, 173–179.

Mendenhall, C.M., Marcus, R.B., Enneking, W.F., Springfield, D.J., Thar, T.L., and Million, R.R. (1983). The prognostic significance of soft tissue extension in Ewing's sarcoma. *Cancer*, 51, 913–917.

Miser, J.S., Kinsella, T.J., Triche, T.J., Tsokos, M., Jarosinski, P., Forquer, R., *et al.* (1987). Ifosfamide with mesna uroprotection and etoposide: an effective regimen in the treatment of recurrent sarcomas and other tumors of children and young adults. *J Clin Oncol*, 5, 1191–1198.

Miser, J.S., Triche, T.J., Pritchard, D.J., and Kinsella, T. (1989). Ewing's sarcoma and the non-rhabdomyosarcoma soft tissue sarcomas of childhood. In: Pizzo, P.A., Poplack, D.G. (eds) Principles and practice of pediatric oncology. Lippincott, Philadelphia, pp. 659–688.

Nascimento, A.G. (1980). A clinicopathologic study of 20 cases of large-cell (atypical) Ewing's sarcoma of bone. *Am J Surg Pathol*, 4, 29–36.

Nesbit, M.E., Gehan, E.A., Burgert, E.O., Vietti, T.J., Cangir, A., Tefft, M., *et al.* (1990). Multimodal therapy for the management of Ewing's sarcoma of bone: a long-term follow-up of the first Intergroup Study. *J Clin Oncol*, 8, 1664–1674.

Oberlin, O., Patte, C., Deméocq, F., Lacomb,e M.J., Brunat-Mentigny, M., Demaille, M.C., *et al.* (1985). The response to initial chemotherapy as a prognostic factor in localized Ewing's sarcoma. *Eur J Cancer Clin Oncol*, 21, 463–467.

Oldham, R.K. and Pomeroy, T.C. (1972). Treatment of Ewing's sarcoma with adriamycin (NSC-123,127). *Cancer Chemother Rep*, 56, 635–639.

Paulussen, M., Braun-Munzinger, G., Burdach, St, Denecke, S., Dunst, J., Fellinger, E., *et al.* (1993). Treatment results in Ewing's sarcoma with pulmonary metastases at diagnosis: a retrospective analysis of 41 patients. *Klin Pädiatr*, 205, 210–216.

Perez, C.A., Razek, A., Tefft, M., Nesbit, M., Burgert, A.O., Kissane, J., *et al.* (1977). Analysis of local tumor control in Ewing's sarcoma. Preliminary results of a cooperative intergroup study. *Cancer*, 40, 2864–2873.

Perez, C.A., Tefft, M., Nesbit, M., Burger, E.O., Vietti, T.J., Kissane, J., *et al.* (1981). The role of radiation therapy in the management of non-metastatic Ewing's sarcoma of bone. Report of the Intergroup Ewing's sarcoma Study. *J Radiat Oncol Biol Phys*, 7, 141–149.

Peter, M., Magdelenat, H., Michon, J., *et al.* (1995). Sensitive detection of occult Ewing's cells by the reverse transcriptase-polymerase chain reaction. *Br J Cancer*, 72, 96–100.

Pilepich, M.V., Vietti, T.J., Nesbit, M.E., Tefft, M., Kissane, J., and Burgert, E.O. (1981). Radiotherapy and combination chemotherapy in advanced Ewing's sarcoma-Intergroup Study. *Cancer*, 47, 1930–1936.

Pinkerton, R., Philip, T., Bouffet, E., Lashford, L., and Kemshead, J. (1986). Autologous bone marrow transplantation in paediatric solid tumors. *Clin Hematol*, 15, 187–203.

Pomeroy, T.C. and Johnson, R.E. (1975). Prognostic factors for survival in Ewing's sarcoma. *Am J Roentgenol Radium Ther Nucl Med*, 123, 598–606.

Price, C.H.G. and Jeffree, G.M. (1977). Incidence of bone sarcoma in SW England, 1946–74, in relation to age, sex, tumor site and histology. *Br J Cancer*, 36, 511–522.

Pritchard, D.J. (1981). Surgical experience in the management of Ewing's sarcoma of bone. *Natl Cancer Inst Monogr*, 56, 169–171.

Raney, B.R., Asmar, L., Newton, W.A. Jr, Bagwell, C., Breneman, J.C., Crist, W., *et al.* (1997). Ewing's sarcoma of soft tissues in childhood: A report from the Intergroup Rhabdomyosarcoma Study, 1972 to 1991. *J Clin Oncol*, 15, 574–582.

Razek, A., Perez, C.A., Tefft, M., Nesbit, M., Vietti, T., Burgert, A.O., *et al.* (1980). Intergroup Ewing's sarcoma study. Local control related to radiation dose, volume and site of primary lesion in Ewing's sarcoma. *Cancer*, 46, 516–521.

Remagen, W. and Salzer-Kuntschik, M. (1981). Zur histopathologischen Problematik und Diagnose des Ewing-Sarkoms. *Klin Pädiatr*, 193, 171–174.

Roessner, A., Ueda, Y., Blasius, S., Dockhorn-Dworniczak, B., Peter,s A., Wuismann, P., *et al.* (1993). Prognostic implication of immuno-detection of p-glycoprotein in Ewing's sarcoma. *J Cancer Res Clin Oncol*, 119, 185–189.

Rosen, G. (1976). Management of malignant bone tumors in children and adolescents. *Pediatr Clin North Am*, 23, 183–213.

Rosen, G., Caparros, B., Mosende, C., McCormick, B., Huvos, A.G., and Marcove, R.C. (1978). Curability of Ewing's sarcoma and considerations for future therapeutic trials. *Cancer*, 41, 888–899.

Rosen, G., Caparros, B., Nirenberg, A., Marcove, R.C., Huvos, A.G., Kosloff, C., *et al.* (1981*a*) Ewing's sarcoma: ten years experience with adjuvant chemotherapy. *Cancer*, 47, 2204–2213.

Rosen, G., Jürgens, H., Caparros, B., Nirenberg, A., Huvos, A.G., and Marcove, R.C. (1981*b*) Combination chemotherapy (T-6) in the multidisciplinary treatment of Ewing's sarcoma. *Natl Cancer Inst Monogr*, 56, 289–299.

Rossi, R., Gödde, A., Kleinebrand, A., Riepenhausen, M., Boos, J., Ritter, J., *et al.* (1994). Unilateral nephrectomy and cisplatin as risk factors of ifosfamide-induced nephrotoxicity: analysis of 120 patients. *J Clin Oncol*, 12, 159–165.

Salzer-Kuntschik, M., Delling, G., Beron, G., and Sigmund, R. (1983). Morphological grades of regression in osteosarcoma after polychemotherapy study COSS 80. *Cancer Res Clin Oncol*, 106, 21–24.

Salzer-Kuntschik, M., and Wunderlich, M. (1971). Das Ewing-Sarkom in der Literatur: kritische Studien zur hitomorphologischen Definition und zur Prognose. *Arch Orthop Unfallchir*, 71, 297–306.

Samuels, M.L. and Howe, C.D. (1967). Cyclophosphamide in the management of Ewing's sarcoma. *Cancer*, 20, 961–966.

Sauer, R., Jürgens, H., Burgers, J.M.V., Dunst, J., Hawlicek, R., and Michaelis, J. (1987). Prognostic factors in the treatment of Ewing's sarcoma. *Radiother Oncol*, 10, 101–110.

Schajowicz, F. (1959). Ewing's sarcoma and reticulum cell sarcoma of bone. With special reference to the histochemical demonstration of glycogen as an aid to differential diagnosis. *J Bone Joint Surg*, [Am] 41, 349–356.

Schmidt, D., Harms, D., and Jürgens, H. (1987). Maligne periphere neuroektodermale Tumoren. Histologische und immunhistochemische Befunde an 41 Fällen. *Zentralbl Allg Pathol*, 135, 257–267.

Schmidt, D. and Harms, D. (1990). The applicability of immunohistochemistry in the diagnosis and differential diagnosis of malignant soft tissue tumors. A reevaluation based on the material of the Kiel Pediatric Tumor Registry. *Klin Pädiatr*, 202, 224–229.

Scully, S.P., Temple, H.T., O'Keefe, R.J., Scarborough, M.T., Mankin, H.J., and Gebhardt, M.C. (1995). Role of surgical resection in pelvic Ewing's sarcoma. *J Clin Oncol*, 13, 2336–2341.

Seeber, S., Gallmeier, W.M., Bruntsch, U., Osieka, R., and Schmidt, C.G. (1974). Fortschritte in der Therapie des Ewing-Sarkoms. *Dtsch Med Wochenschr*, 99, 883–887.

Sim, F.H., Unni, K.K., Beabout, J.W., and Dahli,n D.C. (1979). Osteosarcoma with small cells simulating Ewing's sarcoma. *J Bone Joint Surg*, [Am] 61A/2, 207–215.

Schmidt, D., Harms, D., and Pilon, V.A. (1987). Small-cell pediatric tumors: histology, immunohistochemistry and electron microscopy. *Clin Lab Med*, 7, 63–89.

Sorensen, P.H., Liu, X.F., and Delattre, O. (1993). Reverse transcriptase PCR amplification of EWS/FLI-1 fusion transcripts as a diagnostic test for peripheral primitive neuroectodermal tumors of childhood. *Diagn. Mol. Pathol*, 2, 147–157.

Sorensen, P.H., Lessnick, S.L., Lopez-Terrada, D., Liu, X.F., Triche, T.J., and Denny, C.T. (1994). A second Ewing's sarcoma translocation, t(21;22), fuses the EWS gene to another ETS-family transcription factor, ERG. *Nat. Genet*, 6, 146–151.

Soule, E.H., Newton, W. Jr, Moon, T.E., and Tefft, M. (1978). Extraskeletal Ewing's sarcoma: a preliminary review of 26 cases encountered in the Intergroup Rhabdomyosarcoma Study. *Cancer*, 42, 259–264.

Tefft, M., Chabora, B., and Rosen, G. (1977). Radiation in bone sarcomas. *Cancer*, 39, 806–816.

Thomas, P.R., Perez, C.A., Neff, J.R., Nesbit, M.E., and Evans, R.G. (1984). The management of Ewing's sarcoma: role of radiotherapy in local tumor control. *Cancer Treat Rep*, 68, 703–710.

Triche, T.J. and Rosse, W.E. (1978). Glycogen-containing neuroblastoma with clinical and histopathologic features of Ewing's sarcoma. *Cancer*, 41, 1425–1432.

Turc-Carel, C., Aurias, A., Mugneret, F., *et al.* (1988). Chromosomes in Ewing's sarcoma. I. An evaluation of 85 cases of remarkable consistency of t(11;22)(q24;q12). *Cancer Genet Cytogenet.*, 32, 229–238.

van Valen, F., Winkelmann, W., and Jürgens, H. (1992). Expression of functional Y_1 receptors for neuropeptide in human Ewing's sarcoma cell lines. *J Cancer Res Clin Oncol*, 118, 529–536.

van Valen, F., Hanenberg, H., and Jürgens, H. (1994). Expression of functional very late antigen-alpha 1, -alpha 2, -alpha 3, and -alpha 6 integrins on Ewing's sarcoma and primitive peripheral neuroectodermal tumour cells and modulation by interferon-gamma and tumour necrosis factor alpha. *Eur J Cancer*, 30A, 2119–2125.

Weichselbaum, R.R., Rotmensch, J., Ahmed-Swan, S., and Beckett M.A. (1989). Radiobiological characterization of 53 human tumor cell lines. *Int J Radiat Biol*, 56, 553–560.

Weidner, N. and Tjoe, J. (1994). Immunohistochemical profile of monoclonal antibody O13: antibody that recognizes glycoprotein p30/32MIC2 and is useful in diagnosing Ewing's sarcoma and peripheral neuroepithelioma. *Am. J. Surg. Pathol.*, 18, 486–494.

Wessalowski, R., Jürgens, H., Bodenstein, H., Brandeis, W., Gutjahr, P., Havers, W., *et al.* (1988). Behandlungsergebnisse beim primär metastasierten Ewing-Sarkom: eine retrospektive Analyse von 48 Patienten. *Klin Pädiatr*, 200, 253–260.

West, D.C., Grier, H.E., Swallow, M.M., Demetri, G.D., Granowetter, L., and Sklar, J. (1997). Detection of circulating tumor cells in patients with Ewing's sarcoma and peripheral primitive neuroectodermal tumor. *J Clin Oncol*, 15, 583–588.

Wigger, H.J., Salazar, G.H., and Blanc, W.A. (1977). Extraskeletal Ewing's sarcoma. An ultrastructural study. *Arch Pathol Lab Med*, 101, 446–449.

Wilkins, R.M., Pritchard, D.J., Burgert, E.O. Jr., and Unni, K.K. (1986). Ewings sarcoma of bone; experience of 140 patients, *Cancer*, 58, 2551–2555.

Winkelmann, W. and Jürgens, H. (1989). Lokalkontrolle beim Ewing-Sarkom. Vergleichende Ergebnisse nach intraläsionaler, marginaler bzw. Tumorresektion im Gesunden. *Z Orthop Grenzgeb*, 127, 424–426.

Zoubek, A., Dockhorn-Dworniczak, B., Delattre, O., *et al.* (1996). Does expression of different EWS chimeric transcripts define clinically distinct risk groups of Ewing tumor patients? *J. Clin. Oncol.*, 14, 1245–1251.

Zucker, J.M., Henry-Amar, M., Sarrazin, D., Blanche, R., Platte, C., and Schweisguth, O. (1983). Intensive systemic chemotherapy in localized Ewing's sarcoma in childhood. A historical trial. *Cancer*, 52, 415–423.

Zucman, J., Delattre, O., Desmaze, C., *et al.* (1992). Cloning and characterization of the Ewing's sarcoma and peripheral neuroepithelioma t(11;22) translocation breakpoints. *Genes Chromosom Cancer.*, 5, 271–277.

Zucman, J., Melot T., Desmaze, C., *et al.* (1993). Combinatorial generation of variable fusion proteins in the Ewing family of tumours. *EMBO.J*, 12, 4481–4487.

16 Nephroblastoma

B. de Camargo and S. Weitzman

Nephroblastoma (Wilms' tumour) is the commonest renal tumour in children comprising 90% of renal cancer in this age-group. The survival of Wilms' tumour patients has improved to 90% overall, allowing the focus of research to be on the reduction of morbidity in patients with good prognosis and the improvement in survival in those whose outlook remains poor.

Epidemiology and genetics

The annual incidence of Wilms' tumour has been found to average 7 per million children under age 16. A lower incidence has been noted in Asian countries such as Japan, India, and Singapore, as well as in Asian children living in more developed countries. In contrast, a higher incidence is found in Scandinavia, Nigeria, and Brazil, and in Black children generally (Parkin *et al.* 1988). Typically, Wilms' tumour (WT) is found in early childhood, with a median of 3.5 years of age at diagnosis. More than 80% of patients present under 5 years of age, but documented cases of Wilms' tumour have been described occasionally in adults. The frequency appears to be equal in males and females. Wilms' tumour is strongly associated with several congenital anomalies, notably aniridia, hemihypertrophy, and genitourinary anomalies (cryptorchidism, hypospadias, horseshoe kidney), and with some specific syndromes such as the Beckwith-Wiedemann, Denys-Drash, and WAGR (Wilms' tumour, aniridia, genitourinary abnormalities, mental retardation) syndromes (Miller *et al.* 1964; Beckwith 1969; Jadresic *et al.* 1990). The association of these anomalies has helped to identify a group of children at risk for development of Wilms' tumour, and recommendations for screening programmes are under study (Clericuzio and Johnson 1995).

In 1972, Knudson and Strong applied the two-step mutational model that had so successfully described the development of retinoblastoma to Wilms' tumour (Knudson and Strong 1972). The model suggests that WT is due to loss of both alleles of a WT-suppressor gene, and that children with a genetic susceptibility have a constitutional (germ-line) genetic change leading to the loss of one allele, either inherited from a parent or resulting from a spontaneous mutation, and require only one new genetic event for tumourogenesis. In sporadic cases, on the other hand, two, rare, independent somatic mutations are required. According to this model, children with inherited germ-line mutations would be predicted to develop tumours at an earlier age, and indeed children with associated anomalies such as aniridia and the WAGR syndrome and those with multifocal tumours develop WT at a significantly lower median age than do sporadic cases (Grundy *et al.*

1994). Those with hemihypertrophy, however, do not. Karyotypic analysis of children with the WAGR syndrome demonstrated a deletion within the short arm of one copy of chromosome 11, at band p13. This constitutional deletion was thought to represent the first hit in these children and provided the first clue to the location of a gene involved in the development of Wilms' tumour. It is now known that the WAGR deletion encompasses a number of contiguous genes, including the aniridia gene *PAX6* and the Wilms' tumour suppressor gene *WT1* (Coppes *et al.* 1994). Loss of one allele of the *PAX6* gene is responsible for aniridia, whereas mutation of one *WT1* allele may produce genitourinary defects, in addition to constituting the first event for the development of Wilms' tumour. The *WT1* gene has been cloned, and its protein product has been shown to be a transcriptional down-regulator. *WT1* expression is thought to be important for normal renal and genital development, explaining the frequent association of WT with GU anomalies (Madden *et al.* 1991).

Aniridia is found in 1% of WT and, conversely, approximately 33% of children with aniridia will develop WT2 (Miller *et al.* 1964). It has been recommended that all children with aniridia be screened with regular abdominal ultrasound, but more recently it has been suggested that children born with aniridia should undergo molecular characterization of germ-line DNA, and that screening be limited to those patients whose *PAX6* deletion includes also the neighbouring *WT1* gene (Grundy *et al.* 1994). The *WT1* gene has been confirmed as a tumour suppressor, but *WT1* abnormalities are only found in 10–20% of sporadic WT, suggesting that more than one locus is involved in the development of Wilms' tumour (Madden *et al.* 1991). The existence of a putative second Wilms' tumour locus was first suggested by the fact that a subset of Wilms' tumours undergoes loss of heterozygosity restricted to markers located at chromosome 11p15. This second putative gene has been designated *WT2*. As with the association between the 11p13 Wilms' tumour locus and the WAGR syndrome, the 11p15 locus has been linked to the Beckwith-Wiedemann syndrome (BWS) (Coppes *et al.* 1994), a syndrome characterized by prenatal and postnatal overgrowth, congenital anomalies such as omphalocoele, macroglossia, abdominal organomegaly, and ear pits or creases. BWS is associated with an increased risk of tumour development in the first 5–7 years of life, the risk being 7.5% in patients without hemihyperplasia and 12.5% in those with hemihyperplasia (Weksberg and Squire 1996). The commonest tumour associated with BWS is Wilms' tumour; others include hepatoblastoma, rhabdomyosarcoma, neuroblastoma, and adrenocortical carcinoma. Feinberg and others have shown that an 11p15 gene or genes (*WT2*) appears to be involved much more commonly in Wilms' tumours than *WT1*, demonstrating abnormalities such as loss of imprinting of the insulin growth factor 2 gene in approximately 70% of WTs tested (Feinberg 1996). This and other studies suggest that the great majority of Wilms' tumours involve an abnormality at either 11p13 or, more commonly, at 11p15. Unlike the *WT1* gene at 11p13, the candidate tumour-suppressor gene or genes at 11p15 remains to be defined. Neither *WT1* nor *WT2*, however, are associated with the rare but well described familial Wilms' tumour, which appears to segregate in an autosomal dominant fashion with low penetrance. The location of this further WT locus remains unknown at present.

In addition to these genes, which appear to be important in genesis of WT, several genes appear to be involved in the progression to more aggressive tumours (Grundy *et al.* 1994). LOH at 16q is seen in 15–20% and LOH 1p in 10% of Wilms' tumours, and appears to be associated with an adverse outcome (Feinberg 1996). A significant correlation between mutations of the tumour-suppressor gene *p53* and anaplastic histology has also been demonstrated, suggesting that *p53* mutations are required for progression to the anaplastic phenotype (Bardeesy *et al.* 1994). The cause of the genetic events described is unknown, but several case-control studies of WT have identified environmental exposures that may contribute to the development of Wilms' tumour. These include prenatal irradiation, penthrane anaesthesia during birth, household pesticides, (Olshan *et al.* 1993) parental occupational exposure to pesticides prior to birth (Sharpe *et al.* 1995), and maternal use of the analgesic dipyrone (Sharpe and Franco 1996).

Clinical presentation

The most common initial manifestation of Wilms' tumour is the presence of an asymptomatic abdominal mass. Other associated signs and symptoms include malaise, abdominal pain, gross or microscopic haematuria, fever, anorexia, and hypertension. Abdominal pain may be the result of local distention, spontaneous intralesional haemorrhage, or tumoural rupture into the peritoneal cavity. The incidence of hypertension is variable because of lack of adequate documentation, but has been reported in 30–63% of children. The aetiology is an increase in circulating renin or a renin-like substance either secreted by the tumour itself or secondary to impaired renal circulation from compression by the tumour mass. Differential diagnosis includes other abdominal neoplasms such as neuroblastoma or hepatoblastoma, other renal tumours such as renal sarcomas or hypernephroma, and benign processes involving the kidney such as multicystic dysplastic kidney, renal carbuncles, and hematomas. In the neonate and very young infant, the majority of renal tumours are benign, congenital, mesoblastic nephromas (CMN) rather than Wilms' tumour, although Wilms' tumours may occur. Rarely, WT may arise outside the kidney, occasionally as part of a teratoma. Most cases of extrarenal WT arise in the retroperitoneum adjacent to, but separate from, the kidney. Other sites include the inguinal region, scrotum, uterus, and vagina (Coppes *et al.* 1991). The most common sites of blood-borne metastases of WT at diagnosis are the lungs and the liver. Non-haematogenous extension includes lymph-node involvement, hepatic adhesion or invasion, and extension into the renal vein and inferior vena cava, which on rare occasions may extend up into the right atrium resulting in cardiac symptoms (Sabio 1981).

As well as hypertension, other paraneoplastic manifestations associated with WT include acquired Von Willebrand disease, tumour-induced glomerulonephritis, erythropoietin production, hyaluronidase secretion, and, very rarely, hypercalcaemia, the latter being seen more frequently in infants with rhabdoid tumours of the kidney and mesoblastic nephroma (Babyn *et al.* 1995).

Methods of diagnosis

The physical examination should note the presence of congenital anomalies (aniridia, hemihypertrophy, genitourinary anomalies), the location and size of the primary tumour, and measurement of the blood pressure. Complete blood count, urinalysis and blood chemistry (creatinine, serum glutamic-pyruvic transaminase, and alkaline phosphastase), and a screening coagulation evaluation should be done. Imaging studies should be limited to identifying intra- or extrarenal tumour, the presence of a normal functioning contralateral kidney, tumour thrombus in renal vein, inferior vena cava and heart, and the presence of pulmonary metastases. Ultrasound, computerized tomography (CT) scan, and magnetic resonance imaging (MRI) all have their particular advantages. Ultrasound has a specific advantage in assessment of blood vessels for flow and tumour thrombus, and can achieve most of the purposes defined above, although CT is superior at evaluating intra- and extrarenal involvement, and in demonstrating small lesions within the kidney and liver and the presence of anomalies such as horseshoe kidneys. MRI may possess the advantages of both, but the lesser availability, increased cost, and the requirement for sedation probably outweigh the advantages (Babyn *et al.* 1995).

Skeletal X-rays, bone scans, and brain CTs are reserved for patients with clear-cell sarcoma or rhabdoid tumour of the kidney.

Staging

Standardized tumour staging is important in allowing proper evaluation of different treatments. Staging is primarily based on the anatomical extent of disease as well as on factors that mandate treatment modification, such as diffuse peritoneal contamination before or during surgery. The staging system used by the two major cooperative groups (NWTS and SIOP) are very similar, although the NWTS system is based on staging of a previously untreated tumour, while the SIOP classification is based on nephrectomy following preoperative chemotherapy (Table 16.1). The critical importance of adequate lymph-node sampling is emphasized by both groups (Green *et al.* 1991, Tournade *et al.* 1993).

Table 16.1   Clinico pathologic staging system

Stage	NWTS	SIOP
I	Tumour limited to the kidney and completely excised.	
II	Tumour extending outside the kidney, complete excision. Invasion beyond the capsule, perirenal/perihilar.	
	No lymph node involvement	Lymph node negative Lymph node positive Invasion of the hilar and/or periaortic nodes histologically positive
III	Invasion beyond the capsule; incomplete excision. Preoperative biopsy Preoperative rupture Peritoneal metastases Invasion of para-aortic lymph nodes	
IV	Distant metastases	
V	Bilateral renal tumour	

Pathology

Nephroblastoma covers a large spectrum of special variants that differ in their morphological features and in their prognosis and natural history. Classically, it is viewed as a triphasic embryonal renal tumour, containing blastema, epithelial tubules, and stromal cells, but one element may predominate and may have prognostic relevance. A review of the histological patterns seen in NWTS-4 showed that tumours composed predominantly of epithelial cell types were usually low stage (81.3% stage I), presented at younger age (median 17 months), and were less chemoresponsive, while predominantly blastemal tumours were much more aggressive (76.3% stage III or IV), presented at older age (median 57 months), but were more chemoresponsive (Beckwith *et al.* 1996). Macroscopically, most Wilms' tumours are unicentric lesions that replace normal parenchyma, distort the renal outline, and commonly contain cystic, necrotic, and haemorrhagic areas. Compared to neuroblastoma, calcification is rare, but may be detected radiographically in 10% of cases, particularly after intratumoural haemorrhage. Multicentric lesions and bilateral disease are not infrequent. Anaplasia was first described by Beckwith and Palmer as an indicator of poor outcome (Beckwith and Palmer 1978). It is found in 5% of WT, being more common in older children, and is associated with a high degree of resistance to chemotherapy, rather than increased aggressiveness. Faria and Beckwith have developed new criteria for defining focal (FA) and diffuse anaplasia (DA). To qualify as FA, anaplastic changes must be confined to one or more clearly defined regions within the primary tumour and absent from extrarenal extension or metastatic deposits (Faria *et al.* 1996).

Clear-cell sarcoma and rhabdoid tumour are now considered to be distinct from WT by the National Wilms' Tumour Study Group (NWTS), so that the designation of unfavourable histology is confined to anaplastic tumours. In the SIOP classification, three groups are distinguished. The first group comprises renal tumours that follow a benign course after surgery, including two subtypes of favourable histology, multicystic nephroblastoma and Wilms' tumour with fibroadenomatous structures. The second group encompasses the typical non-anaplastic Wilms' tumour and special variants, and the third group includes the high-risk renal tumours, the clear-cell sarcoma, and rhabdoid tumour of the kidney (Schmidt and Beckwith 1995).

The existence of nephrogenic rests as precursor lesions of Wilms' tumour has been recognized for several decades. These may become hyperplastic or neoplastic and form multicentric or bilateral renal lesions. Nephrogenic rests are found in 25–40% of kidneys harbouring Wilms' tumour, and in all patients with bilateral Wilms' tumour. Two types of rests have been described, 'perilobar', associated with abnormalities around chromosome 11p15, the hemihypertrophy and BWS phenotypes which give rise to WT in 1–2% of cases, and 'intralobar' rests associated with lesions around 11p13 with a higher (4–5%) risk of developing WT (Beckwith *et al.* 1990). The increased likelihood of subsequent tumour development necessitates more careful follow-up of patients with nephrogenic rests.

Rhabdoid tumour is considered to be one of the most malignant tumours of childhood, comprising 2% of childhood renal cancer, and is characterized by a uniform cellular infiltrate with abundant eosinophilic cytoplasm, initially interpreted as rhabdomyoblastic or sarcomatous, but which may be of neural crest origin. Most renal rhabdoid tumours are diagnosed in the first 2 years of life, and are characterized by early widespread metastases and a poor response to therapy, with survival of 25% according to NWTS data (Green *et al.* 1997). This tumour often spreads to brain and there is also a significant association with primary brain tumours (often primitive neuroectodermal tumours) which may precede or follow the renal tumour. The response of these tumours to WT-type therapy is poor and most initial treatment regimens are platinum-based and include etoposide and iphosphamide or cyclophosphamide (Gururangan *et al.* 1993).

Clear-cell sarcoma of the kidney (CCSK), the bone metastasizing renal tumour of childhood, is a primitive mesenchymal neoplasm which comprises 4% of renal tumours in children. 23% of patients develop bone metastases compared to 0.3% of children with Wilms' tumour, and brain metastases are also more common (15%) and may occur as the first site of recurrence. The need to perform a skeletal survey, as well as a radionuclide bone scan, at the time of diagnosis has been emphasized and these patients, like those with rhabdoid tumours, should have CNS imaging before the initiation of therapy. The addition of adriamycin to vincristine and actinomycin D in NWTS-3 improved survival from 25% to 71.9%. At the same time, decreasing the radiation dose to the flank to 10.8 Gy did not increase the local relapse rate. The combination of etoposide and iphosphamide cured 4 of 6 patients with relapsed CCSK (Miser *et al.* 1993) and this combination, or the combination of etoposide and high-dose cyclophosphamide, may improve survival in newly diagnosed patients with advanced-stage CCSK (Green *et al.* 1994).

Prognostic factors

Many prognostic factors have been identified, though they may change as treatment becomes more effective. Extent of disease at diagnosis (stage) and tumour histology (see above) remain the two most significant prognostic variables. Age at diagnosis and tumour size are strongly associated with relapse and death rates (Breslow *et al.* 1991), and lymph-node involvement remains an adverse prognostic factor (Jereb *et al.* 1980). New biological prognostic factors have been identified recently. Grundy and coworkers correlated treatment outcome with the presence of specific genetic abnormalities. In a retrospective study of 232 children registered on NWTS-3–4, the loss of heterozygosity of markers at chromosome 16q and 1p was associated with a significantly poorer 2-year, relapse-free and overall survival (Grundy *et al.* 1994). Tumour-cell DNA content and prognosis of patients with Wilms' tumour is controversial. Amongst patients with favourable-histology Wilms' tumour, tetraploidy is associated with an unfavourable outcome in some series, as is aneuploidy in one study, but not in two others (Douglass *et al.* 1986, Rainwater *et al.* 1987, Gururangan *et al.* 1992. Aneuploidy occurs more frequently in anaplastic histology tumours, and progression to anaplasia appears to correlate with development of abnormalities of the *p53* gene within the tumour cells.

Treatment

Combined-modality strategies using surgery, radiotherapy, and chemotherapy are the key to success in Wilms' tumour. The efforts of cooperative groups (NWTS, SIOP, UKCCSG) have been aimed at intensifying treatment for patients with poor prognostic features, while reducing interventions for those at standard risk, with a result that over 80% of patients with Wilms' tumour can be cured with modern multimodal therapy tailored to specific risk-groups. The

Brazilian experience has shown that adopting a modern combined-modality treatment approach can improve survival rates significantly (de Camargo *et al.* 1987). The best way of utilizing the different treatment strategies remains a continuing challenge. Successive studies have slowly reduced the amount of therapy. Early detection is crucial for cure with minimal therapy and minimal side-effects. The Brazilian experience shows that by educating paediatricians and the target public about early detection of paediatric tumours, it is possible to increase the proportion of early-stage Wilms' tumour at diagnosis (de Camargo *et al.* 1987).

Surgery

Surgical excision of the tumour is of major importance in the clinical management. A transabdominal, transperitoneal, large incision is recommended for adequate exposure. The surgeon's responsibility is not only to undertake a complete excision without spillage, but also to precisely ascertain the degree of tumour spread, so that accurate staging is followed by the correct treatment strategy. Adequate lymph-node sampling should be performed, but radical lymph-node dissection is unnecessary. The renal vein and inferior vena cava should be palpated carefully before ligation to rule out extension of the tumour into the wall or lumen of the vein. A detailed exploration of abdominal organs should be done and all suspicious lesions must be resected.

Radiotherapy

Nephroblastoma is one of the particularly radioresponsive human neoplasms. The addition of postnephrectomy radiotherapy increased the survival of WT patients to around 50%. NWTS and SIOP trials have studied the interrelationship of chemotherapy and radiotherapy, and have been able to reduce the indications for radiotherapy and the doses used without apparent deleterious effect on the ultimate survival rates. Radiation therapy is still uniformly recommended for all stage III favourable histology Wilms' tumours, stage I–IV clear-cell sarcomas, and stage II–IV diffusely anaplastic Wilms' tumours. For favourable-histology stage IV disease, SIOP showed that lung irradiation can be limited to those children who do not achieve a complete remission of lung metastases with chemotherapy, with or without surgery. In the NWTS-3 study, half the deaths in the stage IV patients were due to interstitial pneumonitis after radiation, but with pneumocystis carinii prophylaxis and reduction of chemotherapy doses immediately post radiation, there were no deaths from interstitial pneumonitis in NWTS-4. The recommendation for low-dose radiation therapy to pulmonary metastases visible on chest radiographs, but not those visible only on CT, has been retained in the NWTS studies (Thomas *et al.* 1988). In all stage IV patients, the decision with regard to abdominal irradiation is based on the stage of the abdominal tumour. The timing of postoperative irradiation is important, as initiation of treatment more than 10 days following surgery has been related to increased risk of abdominal recurrence. The NWTS showed that a radiation dose of approximately 10 Gy was sufficient for local control of both favourable-histology WT and clear-cell sarcoma, if adriamycin was added to the vincristine and actinomycin D. A dose-response for anaplastic tumours has not been identified and an age-modulated dose scheme is recommended: < 12 m: 12–18 Gy; 12–18 m: 18–24 Gy; 19–30 m: 24–30 Gy; 31–40 m: 30–35 Gy; > 41m: 35–40 Gy. The long-term side-effects of radiation, especially on the growth of bones and soft tissues, have been well documented.

Chemotherapy

Nephroblastoma was the first paediatric, malignant, solid tumour found to be responsive to the systemic chemotherapeutic agent actinomycin D (ACT). Other agents such as vincristine (VCR), adriamycin (DOX), cyclophosphamide, and later cisplatin, iphosphamide, etoposide, and carboplatin have since been identified as being effective in WT (Tournade *et al.* 1988, Miser *et al.* 1993; de Camargo *et al.* 1994*a*). The cooperative groups, the NWTS, SIOP, UKCCSG, and the BWTSG, have done randomized trials to evaluate the use of adjuvant single or multiple agent chemotherapy in the treatment of WT. The BWTSG as well as the NWTS has demonstrated that a single-dose schedule of ACT is as effective as that of the standard divided-dose regimen, and is less myelosuppressive, as well as reducing the length of hospital stays for children and their parents (de Camargo *et al.* 1994*b*, Green *et al.* 1995). A syndrome of hepatopathy-thrombocytopaenia, thought to be due to ACT-induced veno-occlusive disease, occurs in 3.5% of unirradiated WT patients, usually during the first 10 weeks of ACT therapy. This is not seen in other studies. It is not usually fatal, and ACT therapy at a decreased dose can be reintroduced without recurrence of the problem when liver function has recovered.

Other lessons learned from the cooperative study groups about WT chemotherapy include the following: limited courses of two (NWTS, SIOP) or even single drug (UKCCSG) regimens are sufficient to cure Stage I favourable- and unfavourable-histology patients. Ten weeks of VCR and ACT gave an event-free survival (EFS) of 89% and an overall survival (OS) of 95.6% at 4 years (D' Angio *et al.* 1989).

For stage II disease, the cure rate remains excellent with limited two-drug therapy. The addition of adriamycin and radiotherapy did not add to survival in patients with this stage at diagnosis, but for patients who are still stage II after preoperative therapy, an additional drug is required. Stage III patients were shown to benefit from the addition to the standard VCR and ACT regimen of either 20 Gy of radiation, or of DOX and 10 Gy of radiation, giving a 4-year EFS of 82%, and 90.9% OS.

In stage IV FH patients, the addition of adriamycin to vincristine and dactinomycin improved survival, but cyclophosphamide, at least in the doses utilized, did not. The primary tumour is irradiated according to the local tumour stage. The question of lung irradiation is discussed previously in the section dealing with radiotherapy. EFS for stage IV FH was 79% in the NWTS-3 study and 83% in the SIOP-6 study.

The adverse outcome associated with anaplastic histology is limited to patients with stage II–IV disease and those with diffuse anaplasia, indicating that anaplasia is a marker for chemoresistance. The addition of cyclophosphamide to vincristine and actinomycin improved survival significantly for stage II–III diffuse anaplastic tumours, but had no effect on stage IV diffuse anaplastic tumours, with only 16.7% of patients treated on four-drug therapy surviving. The addition of dose-intensified cyclophosphamide/iphosphamide and/or etoposide may improve results in these patients.

Preoperative strategies

The benefit of preoperative tumour shrinkage to facilitate complete surgical removal is well known. The WT protocols of SIOP have placed major emphasis on the role of preoperative treatment since their first study in 1971 (Lemerle *et al.* 1983). The UKCCSG is addressing the question of whether preoperative chemotherapy results in improvement in staging and an overall reduction in treatment, randomizing patients with resectable, unilateral tumours over 6 months of age at diagnosis to immediate surgery or six once-weekly injections of VCR and two three-weekly injections of ACT. In 1984, investigators at the Hospital for Sick Children, Toronto (HSC), adopted a protocol that included preoperative chemotherapy. Of the first 96 consecutive patients admitted to HSC, 72 underwent preoperative chemotherapy following percutaneous biopsy. OS and EFS were 93% and 82%, respectively, at a median of 56 months. Eight patients underwent partial nephrectomy, four bilateral and four with unilateral disease. It appears that even after preoperative therapy, partial nephrectomy is possible only in a minority of patients with localized unilateral disease (Greenberg *et al.* 1991).

All groups using preoperative therapy have found significant reduction in tumour size in the majority of patients. Many patients who did not have a reduction in size were nonetheless found to have significant tumour necrosis. Invariably, it was found that once surgeons had experience of doing nephrectomies following preoperative therapy, they became enthusiastic supporters of this strategy. While mortality is very low with both the immediate nephrectomy and preoperative therapy approaches, there is a significant decrease in surgical morbidity after preoperative therapy. SIOP reports a 7% incidence of surgical complications, compared to 19% documented after NWTS-3. In the SIOP studies, after preoperative therapy, 52% of patients can be staged as I, and only 16% of non-metastatic WT patients require radiation therapy. Disadvantages of this approach are the possibility of understaging patients and of missing anaplasia. Indeed, in both the SIOP and HSC studies, there has been a higher local abdominal relapse rate, which, since it is found in both studies, appears to be unrelated to the percutaneous needle biopsy which is carried out solely at HSC. AT HSC, there has been a concomitant lowering of the pulmonary relapse rate, attributed to decreased delay in starting chemotherapy, so that the overall EFS for all stages is similar to that of the NWTS, and the OS at least as good (de Kraker *et al.* 1995). SIOP investigators believe that the response to preoperative therapy selects lower- and higher-risk patients, and that postsurgical therapy should be tailored to the risk group. Accordingly, they are testing the addition of epirubicin for stage II patients, as well as radiation therapy for stage II with positive nodes and stage III patients. Support for this hypothesis comes from the NWTS studies, where preoperative chemotherapy is limited to patients with inoperable tumours and those with synchronous bilateral tumours at diagnosis. NWTS investigators found that staging based on the extent of *viable* tumour cells after preoperative chemotherapy was directly related to outcome, and that tumours with viable cells limited to the kidney (viable stage I) experienced excellent outcomes, even if there was evidence of necrotic tumour in sites beyond the limit of stage I.

It would appear that both the immediate nephrectomy and upfront staging approach of the NWTS, and the preoperative chemotherapy approach of the SIOP, offer equivalent cure-rates for these young patients. Both approaches have advantages and disadvantages and the choice should perhaps be made by local factors.

Neonatal kidney tumours

Nearly two-thirds of abdominal masses in the newborn arise in the kidney. The majority are non-neoplastic and are due to conditions giving rise to hydronephrosis and polycystic disease. The commonest tumour arising in the kidney is the congenital mesoblastic nephroma (CMN) which comprises 78% of neonatal renal neoplasms. CMN usually presents as an asymptomatic mass, although maternal polyhydramnios, neonatal hypertension, and hypercalcaemia have been described. Neonatal Wilms' tumour is treated with surgery and chemotherapy given at 50% of the standard dose.

Recurrence of Wilms' tumour

The overall relapse rate for all patients, irrespective of stage and histology, registered on NWTS-3 was 17%. Relapse predominantly occurs during the first 3 years after diagnosis, although very late relapse of WT has been reported. Anaplastic tumours typically recur earlier than do favourable-histology tumours. The most important prognostic factors for outcome following relapse are site of recurrence, initial stage of disease, tumour histology, duration of first remission, and prior therapy (Grundy *et al.* 1989). Tumour histology is probably the single most important prognostic factor for recurrent Wilms' tumour. Post-relapse survival was 50–60% for favourable histology and 20–30% for unfavourable-histology patients. Abdominal local recurrence has a worse outlook than extra-abdominal relapse, and liver metastases after original diagnosis have a particularly poor outcome. The vast majority of extra-abdominal relapse occurs in the lung and is associated with a better prognosis. In some series, extent of pulmonary disease at relapse has also been an important prognostic factor, with recurrence limited to one lung being better than bilateral metastases. Stage at diagnosis is also important, with patients who are stage I and II initially have a significantly better survival rate after relapse than those with more advanced disease. Early relapse (between 0 and 5 months after nephrectomy) is worse than late relapse (> 12 months). Prior treatment is confounded as a prognosticator by the fact that the initial treatment is stage specific. Patients who have received prior adriamycin have a worse prognosis after relapse, as do patients who have been previously irradiated.

These patients are often responsive to retreatment and cure is possible in many. Treatment strategies are based on assessment of the risk factors outlined above. For those patients who have not previously received adriamycin (or an analogue) and radiation therapy, the addition of these agents to the therapy is suggested. For children at higher risk, studies have been limited largely to phase II trials of new agents or combinations of older agents. A reasonable approach includes a combination of two or more drugs including adriamycin, iphosphamide, etoposide, cyclophosphamide, and carboplatin (Tournade *et al.* 1988; Miser *et al.* 1993; de Camargo *et al.* 1994*a*). It has been suggested that the use of dose-intensive cyclophosphamide will avoid the increased nephrotoxicity of iphosphamide seen in patients with a single kidney. In addition to two-four-drug combination-chemotherapy, surgery and radiation therapy have an important role in relapse therapy.

High-dose therapy followed by autologous bone marrow reinfusion has been used successfully (Garaventa *et al.* 1994), and it has been suggested that this strategy be employed for all patients with adverse prognostic factors at the time of relapse, as well as refractory patients.

Synchronous, bilateral Wilms' tumour

Patients with synchronous, bilateral Wilms' tumour at diagnosis account for approximately 5% of children with WT. The median age at diagnosis is lower than that of patients with unilateral disease, and the incidence of associated congenital anomalies is higher. Nephrogenic rests are found in nearly 100% of patients. Therapeutic approaches include initial bilateral partial nephrectomies with gross removal of each tumour area only if sufficient functioning renal tissue can be preserved. Subsequent chemotherapy is indicated, with irradiation dependent upon intrarenal and abdominal extent of both tumours. In the majority of patients, who will have at least one large tumour present, initial surgery is limited to bilateral biopsies, remembering that 10% of bilateral WTs are anaplastic on one or both sides. Biopsy is followed by delayed second- or even third-look surgery to attempt resection of residual tumour, always aiming for maximal preservation of functioning renal tissue. Radical excision of the tumour(s) should never be performed at the initial operation. Radiation therapy is limited to those who have residual tumour despite chemotherapy and surgery, and bilateral nephrectomies, dialysis, and delayed renal transplantation are indicated only in patients in whom tumour cannot be eradicated by other methods. Reviews of the outcome of these children have indicated that they have an excellent prognosis, with survival rates for those having favourable-histology tumours exceeding 80% at 2 years (Blute *et al.* 1987; Alfer *et al.* 1993).

Late effects

All treatment modalities are associated with toxic effects, some of which occur early, while others occur months or years later. Long-term, deleterious effects of radiation in Wilms' tumour patients have been reported in the musculoskeletal system, the gastrointestinal tract, the urinary tract, the endocrine system, and the lungs. In long-term follow-up studies of Wilms' tumour survivors, scoliosis and musculoskeletal abnormalities have been found more frequently in irradiated patients, particularly those treated with orthovoltage radiotherapy. With modern megavoltage techniques and the significant dose reductions that have occurred, late orthopaedic effects are expected to be significantly less common. Renal insufficiency is uncommon in unilateral WT treated on standard protocols. The cumulative frequency of adriamycin cardiomyopathy was 1.7% at 15 years after diagnosis among all patients on NWTS-2-3 who received adriamycin. The gonads are the most commonly affected endocrine organ, although scatter to the thyroid may occur with lung irradiation. A variety of fertility problems, from sterility to fetal loss and premature delivery, have been reported in female patients who received whole-abdominal irradiation. In the NWTS studies, the relative risk of a second malignant neoplasm (SMN) is 10.8% among the irradiated patients and 5% among the non-irradiated patients (Evans *et al.* 1991). Of 55 SMNs occurring in survivors of WT diagnosed between 1970 and 1982, 13 were soft-tissue sarcomas, 11 leukaemia/lymphoma, and eight bone sarcomas. Long-term follow-up of all patients treated for WT is mandatory.

Future considerations

New insights are increasingly being made into the biology of Wilms' tumour, and the clinical application of these is at present being tested in the cooperative study groups. Therapeutic research is focusing on minimizing therapy to reduce long-term effects, including nephrectomy alone for patients who are under 2 years of age at diagnosis with favourable-histology tumours weighing < 550 g, reducing radiotherapy for patients with pulmonary metastases, partial nephrectomy for a small group of selected patients with unilateral disease, and finding the best combination of drugs with the least long-term toxicity (Green *et al.* 1991). In high-risk and relapsed patients, new and effective drugs and drug combinations are being sought, including the use of ultra-high dose therapy with stem-cell rescue. The exact place of these in the WT armamentarium needs to be defined.

A major outstanding problem is the identification of children at risk of developing Wilms' tumour and the definition of the role of screening in early diagnosis. The required follow-up 'surveillance' imaging after diagnosis is also controversial. These studies account for the majority of the imaging costs in the management of WT, yet the role of imaging in improving prognosis in WT relapse is unknown and requires investigation.

While outlook continues to improve for children with nephroblastoma, many questions remain as yet unanswered and clinical trials will need to continue.

References

Alfer, W. Jr, de Camargo, B., and Assuncao, M.C. (1993). Management of synchronous bilateral Wilms' tumour: Brazilian Wilms' Tumour Study Group: experience with 14 cases. *Journal of Urology*, 150: 1456.

Babyn, P., Owens, C., Gyepes, M., and D'Angio, G.J. (1995). Imaging patients with Wilms'Tumour. *Hematology, Oncology Clin N Amer*, 9, 1217–1252.

Bardeesy, N., Falkoff, D., Petruzzi, M.J., Nowak, N., Zabel, B., Adam, M., *et al.* (1994). Anaplastic Wilms'Tumour, a subtype displaying poor prognosis, harbours p53 gene mutations. *Nature Genetics*, 7, 91–97.

Beckwith, J. (1969). Macroglossia, omphalocele, adrenal cytomegaly, gigantism and hyperplastic visceromegaly. *Birth Defects*, 5, 188–196.

Beckwith, J.B. and Palmer, N.F. (1978). Histopathology and prognosis of Wilms' tumour. Results from the first National Wilms' Tumour Study. *Cancer*, 41, 1937–1948.

Beckwith, J.B., Kiviat, N.B., and Bonadio, J.F. (1990). Nephrogenic rests, nephroblastomatosis, and the pathogenesis of Wilms' tumour. *Persp Pediatr Pathol*, 10, 1–36.

Beckwith, J.B., Zuppan, C.E., Browning, N.G., Moskness, J., and Breslow, N.E. (1996). Histologic analysis of agressiveness and responsiveness in Wilms' tumour. *Medical Pediatric Oncology*, 27, 422–428.

Blute, M.L., Kelalis, P.P., Offord, K.P., Breslow, K.P., Beckwith, J.B., and D'Angio, G.J. (1987). Bilateral Wilms' tumour. *Journal of Urology*, 138, 968–973.

Breslow, N., Sharples, K., Beckwith, J.B., Takashima, J., Kelalis, P.P. Green, D.M., *et al.* (1991). Prognostic factors in nonmetastatic, favourable histology Wilms' Tumour: results of the Third National Wilms' Tumour Study. *Cancer*, 68, 2345–2353.

Clericuzio, C.L. and Johnson, C. (1995). Screening for Wilms' tumour in high-risk individuals. In: *Hematology/Oncology Clinics of North America- Wilms' tumour*, vol 9 (6) pg.1253–1265.

Coppes, M.J., Wilson, P.C.G., and Weitzman, S. (1991). Extrarenal Wilms'Tumour: Staging, Treatment and Prognosis. *Journal of Clinical Oncology*, 9, 167–274.

Coppes, M.J., Haber, D.A., and Grundy, P.E. (1994). Genetic events in the development of Wilms' Tumour. *New England Journal of Medicine*, 331, 586–590.

D'Angio, G.J., Breslow, N., Beckwith, J.B., Evans, A., Baum, E., De Lorimier, A., *et al.* (1989). The treatment of Wilms' tumour: results of the third National Wilms' Tumour Study. *Cancer*, 64, 349–360.

de Camargo, B., Andrea, M.L., and Franco, E. (1987). Catching up with history: Treatment of Wilms' tumour in a developing country *Medical Pediatric Oncology*, 15, 270–276.

de Camargo, B., Melaragno, R., Saba e Silva, N., Mendonça, N., Alvares, M.N., Morinaka, E., *et al.* (1994*a*). Phase II study of carboplatin as a single drug for relapsed Wilms' tumour: experience of the Brazilian Wilms' Tumour Study Group. *Medical Pediatric Oncology*, 22, 258–260.

de Camargo, B., Franco, E. for the Brazilian Wilms' Tumour Study Group. (1994*b*). A Randomized Clinical Trial of Single-Dose versus Fractionated-Dose Dactinomycin in the Treatment of Wilms' Tumour. Results after Extended Follow-up. *Cancer*, 73, 3081–3086.

de Kraker, J., Weitzman, S., and Voute, P.A. (1995). Preoperative strategies in the management of Wilms' tumour. In: Coppes, M.J., Ritchey, M.L., D'Angio, G.J. *Hematology/Oncology Clinics of North America-Wilms' tumour*, 9(6) pg. 1275–1285.

Douglass, E.C., Look, A.T., Webber, B., Parham, D., Wilimas, J.A., Green, A.A., *et al.* (1986). Hyperdiploidy and chromosomal rearrangement define the anaplastic variant of Wilms' tumour. *Journal of Clinical Oncology*, 4, 975–981.

Evans, A.E., Norkool, P., Evans, I., Breslow, N., and D'Angio, G.J. (1991). Late effects of treatment for Wilms' tumour: a report from the National Wilms' Tumour Study Group. *Cancer*, 67, 331–336.

Faria, P., Beckwith, B.J., Mishra, K., Zuppan, C., Weeks, D.A., Breslow, N., *et al.* (1996). Focal versus diffuse anaplasia in Wilms' tumour-new definitions with prognostic significance from the National Wilms' Tumor Study Group, *The American Journal of Surgical Pathology*, 20(8), 909–920.

Feinberg, A.P. (1996). Multiple genetic abnormalities of 11p15 in Wilms'Tumour, *Medical Pediatric Oncology*, 27, 484–489.

Garaventa, A., Hartman, O., Bernard, J.L., Zucker, J.M., Pardo, N., Castel, V., *et al.* (1994). Autologous bone marrow transplantation for pediatric Wilms' tumour: the experience of the European Bone Marrow Transplantation Solid Tumour Registry. *Medical Pediatric Oncology*, 22, 11–14.

Green, D.M., Finklestein, J.Z., Breslow, N.E., and Beckwith, J.B. (1991). Remaining problems in the treatment of patients with Wilms' tumour. *Pediatric Clin North America*, 38, 475–488.

Green, D.M., Breslow, N.E., Beckwith, J.B., Mokness, J., Finkelstein, J.Z., and D'Angio, G.J. (1994). Treatment of children with clear cell sarcoma of the kidney: a report from the National Wilms Tumour Group. *Journal of Clinical Oncology*, 12, 2131–2137.

Green, D.M., Breslow, N.E., Evans, I., Moskness, J., Finkelstein, J.Z., Evans, A.E., *et al.* (1995). Relationship between dose schedule and charges for treatment on the National Wilms' tumour Study-4: a report from the National Wilms' tumour Study Group. *Monogr Natl Cancer Inst*, 19, 21–25.

Green, D.M., Coppes, M.J., Breslow, N.E., Grundy, P.E., Ritchey, M.L., Beckwith, B., *et al.* (1997). Wilms' tumour (Nephroblastoma, renal embryonal). In: Pizzo P.A. and Poplack D.G. (eds): *Principles and Practice of Pediatric Oncology*. Philadelphia: J.B. Lippincott Company, 733–759.

Greenberg, M., Burnweit, C., Filler, R., Weitzman, S., Sohl, H., Chan, H., *et al.* (1991). Preoperative chemotherapy for children with Wilms' tumour. *Journal of Pediatric Surgery*, 26, 949–956.

Grundy, P.E., Breslow, N., Green, D.M., Sharples, K., Evans, A., and D' Angio, G.J. (1989). Prognostic factors for children with recurrent Wilms' tumour: results from the second and third National Wilms' Tumour Study. *Journal of Clinical Oncology*, 7, 638–647.

Grundy, P.E., Telzerow, P.E., Breslow, N., Mokness, J., Huff, V., and Paterson, M.C.(1994). Loss of heterozygosity for chromosomes 16q and 1p in Wilms' tumour predicts an adverse outcome. *Cancer Research*, 94, 2331–2333.

Gururangan, S., Dorman, A., Ball, R., Curran, B., Leader, M., Breatnach, F., *et al.* (1992). DNA quantitation of Wilms' tumour (nephroblastoma) using flow cytometry and image analysis. *Journal of Clinical Pathology*, 45, 498–501.

Gururangan, S., Bowman, L., Parham, D.M. Wilimans, J.A., Rao, B., Pratt, C.B., *et al.* (1993). Primary extracranial rhabdoid tumours. Clinicopathologic features and response to iphosphamide. *Cancer*, 71, 2653–2659.

Jadresic, L., Leake, J., Gordon, I., Dillon, M.J., Grant, D.B., Pritchard, J., *et al.* (1990). Clinicopathologic review of twelve children with nephropathy, Wilms' tumour, and genital abnormalities (Drash syndrome). *Journal of Pediatrics*, 117, 717–725.

Jereb, B., Tournade, M.F., Lemerle, J., Voute, P.A., Delemarre, J.F., Ahstrom, L., *et al.* (1980). Lymph node invasion and prognosis in nephroblastoma. *Cancer*, 45, 1632–1636.

Knudson, A.G. and Strong, L.C. (1972). Mutation and cancer: a model for Wilms' tumour of the kidney. *Journal of National Cancer Institute*, 48, 313–324.

Lemerle, J., Voute, P.A., Tournade, M.F., Rodary, C., Delemarre, F.M., Sarrazin, D., *et al.* (1983). Effectiveness of preoperative chemotherapy in Wilms' tumour: results of an International Society of Pediatric Oncology (SIOP) clinical trial. *Journal of Clinical Oncology*, 1, 604.

Madden, S.L., Cook, D.M., Morris, J.F., Gashler, A., Sukhtatme, V.P., and Rauscher, F.J. III (1991). Transcriptional repression mediated by the WT1 Wilms' tumour gene product. *Science*, 253, 1550–1553.

Miller, R.W., Fraumeni, J.F., and Manning, M.D. (1964). Association of Wilms' tumour with aniridia, hemihypertrophy and other congenital malformations. *New England Journal of Medicine*, 270, 922–927.

Miser, J., Krailo, M., and Hammond, G.D. (1993). The combination of iphosphamide, etoposide, and mesna: A very active regimen in the treatment of recurrent Wilms' tumour [abstract] *Proceedings of the American Society of Clinical Oncology*, 12, 417.

Olshan, A.F., Breslow, N.E., Falletta, J.M., Grufferman, S., Pendergrass, T., Robison, L.L., *et al.* (1993). Risk factors for Wilms' tumour. *Cancer*, 72, 938–944.

Parkin, D.M., Stiller, C.A., Draper, G.J., and Bieber, C.A., (1988). The international incidence of childhood cancer. *International Journal of Cancer*, 42, 511–520.

Rainwater, L.M., Hosaka, Y., Farrow, G.M., Kramer, G.M., Kelalis, P.P., and Lieber, M.M. (1987). Wilms' tumour: relationship of nuclear deoxyribonucleic acid ploidy to patient survival. *Journal of Urology*, 138, 974–977.

Sabio, H.(1981). Intracardiac extension of Wilms' tumour. *Clinical Pediatrics*, 20, 359–361.

Schmidt, D. and Beckwith, J.B. (1995). Histopathology of childhood renal tumours. In:Coppes M.J., Ritchey M.L. D'Angio G.J. *Hematology/Oncology Clinics of North America- Wilms' tumour*, 9(6)pp. 1179–1200.

Sharpe, C.R. and Franco, E.L. (1996). Use of dipyrone during pregnancy and risk of Wilms' tumour. *Epidemiology*, 7, 533–535.

Sharpe, C.R., Franco, E.L., de Camargo, B., Lopes, L., Barreto, J., Johnson, R., *et al.* (1995). Parental exposures to pesticides and risk of Wilms' tumour in Brazil. *American Journal of Epidemiology*, 141, 210–217.

Thomas, P.R.M., Tefft, M., D'Angio, G.J., and Norkool, P. (1988). Validation of radiation dose reductions used in the Third National Wilms' Tumour Study (NWTS-3) *Proceedings of the American Society of Clinical Oncology*, 29, 227.

Tournade, M.F., Lemerle, J., Brunat-Mentigny, M., Bachelot, C., Roche, H., Taboureau, O., *et al.* (1988). Iphosphamide is an active drug in Wilms' tumour: a phase II study conducted by the French Society of Pediatric Oncology. *Journal of Clinical Oncology*, 6, 792–796.

Tournade, M.F., Com-Nougue, C., Voute, P.A., Lemerle, J., De Kraker, J., Delemarre, J.F.M., *et al.* (1993). Results of the sixth international Society of Pediatric Oncology Wilms' tumour trial and study: a risk-adapted therapy approach in Wilms' tumour. *Journal of Clinical Oncology*, 11, 1014–1023.

Weksberg, R. and Squire, J. (1996). Molecular biology of Beckwith-Wiedemann syndrome. *Medical Pediatric Oncology*, 27, 462–469.

17 Neuroblastoma

H. Caron and A. Pearson

Introduction

Neuroblastoma, ganglioneuroblastoma, and ganglioneuroma are embryonal tumours of the sympathetic nervous system, derived from the primitive neural crest.

Neuroblastoma has the greatest diversity in clinical behaviour of all childhood solid tumours, with some tumours regressing spontaneously, some being chemo-curable, whilst others are resistant to intensive chemotherapy. Metastatic neuroblastoma in children over the age of 1 year is associated with the worst prognosis of all malignancies in childhood. Although initially responding to chemotherapy, relapse with drug-resistant disease occurs in the majority of children.

More is known about the molecular pathology and genetics of neuroblastoma than probably any other adult or childhood malignancy. This knowledge is already guiding therapy so that children can receive individualized treatment, thereby minimizing toxicity in good-prognosis patients and allowing intensive and novel therapy to be delivered only to those children in whom conventional treatment is unsuccessful. A therapeutic classification is at present being developed, which is based on patient characteristics and molecular tumour features, for example, *MYCN* gene amplification.

Epidemiology

The incidence of neuroblastoma per year is 10.5 per million children less than 15 years of age (Stiller and Parkin 1992). There appears to be no significant geographical variation in the incidence between North America and Europe, and similarly there are no differences between races. Neuroblastoma occurs slightly more frequently in males than females (ratio 1.2:1). The peak age of incidence is between 0 and 4 years, with a median age of 23 months (Fig. 17.1). 40% of patients clinically presenting with neuroblastoma are under 1 year of age, and less than 5% are over the age of 10 years. Cases of familial neuroblastoma have been reported (Kushner *et al.* 1986).

There are a number of features of neuroblastoma which suggest that screening might be of value in reducing mortality from the malignancy by detecting poor-prognosis disease prior to clinical presentation. Infants presenting under the age of one tend to have localized, good-prognosis disease, with favourable molecular features. In contrast, children who are diagnosed over the age

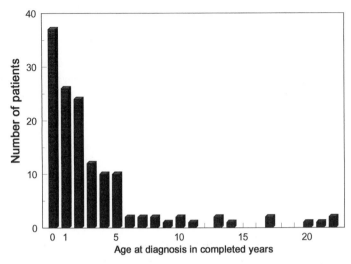

Fig. 17.1 Age distribution of patients with neuroblastoma (data from the Northern Region Young Persons' Malignancy Registry of the United Kingdom—Courtesy of Mr S. Cotterill and Mrs L. More).

of one have a significantly worse outcome, and usually have metastatic disease with genetic features indicative of an aggressive course. Screening for neuroblastoma was pioneered by Japanese investigators who demonstrated that asymptomatic tumours could be detected in infants by measurement of urinary catecholamine metabolites. Although the outlook for the children with the detected tumours was excellent, these studies were not population based and did not demonstrate a resultant reduction in neuroblastoma mortality rates. However, in regions where there were screening programmes, the incidence doubled to 20.1 per million children (Yamamoto *et al.* 1995) and the tumours detected all possessed favourable biological characteristics, i.e. triploidy, lack of MYCN amplification, and no allelic loss of 1p (Kaneko *et al.* 1990). The Quebec Neuroblastoma Screening Project was designed to answer definitively the question whether screening a large cohort of infants for neuroblastoma, at the ages of 3 weeks and 6 months, could reduce the population-based incidence of advanced disease and mortality. The initial findings indicate that screening increases the incidence of localized neuroblastoma in infants without decreasing the incidence of metastatic disease in older children (Woods *et al.* 1996). The general consensus is that screening for neuroblastoma at 6 months of age identifies tumours with a good prognosis and molecular pathology, doubles the incidence, and fails to detect the poor-prognosis disease which presents clinically at an older age. It is highly questionable whether screening at a later age will be of any therapeutic benefit. However, investigators are carefully considering this option.

Embryology, pathology, and genetics

Embryology

The neural crest is the embryonic structure which gives rise to the sympathetic nervous system. In the third gestational week, the neural plate is formed in the ectodermal germlayer. At the time of the fusion of the neural ridges into the neural tube, the neural crest is formed dorsally of the neural tube. Neural crest cells develop into a large number of mature cell types and structures. They not only form the sympathetic peripheral nervous system, but also part of the facial skeleton, the thymus, parathyroids, the enteric nervous system, and skin melanocytes. Segmentation and migration are characteristic phenomena in neural crest development. The primitive neural crest cells migrate to a position lateral to the neural tube, forming (segmented) primitive ganglia on both sides of it. From these primitive ganglia neuroblasts migrate along the dorsal pathway to form melanocytes in the skin and dorsal root sympathetic neurons. Neuroblasts migrating through a ventrolateral pathway will eventually form the side-chain (ventrolateral to the spine), the paraganglia (ventral to the spine), visceral sympathetic ganglia (abdominal organs) and the adrenal medulla. The adrenal medulla is formed by neuroblasts from the embryonal side-chain invading the primitive adrenal cortex (endodermal germlayer). The mature sympathetic nervous system consists of a neuronal part (dorsal root ganglia and side-chain) and a hormonal part (paraganglia and adrenal medulla). Both parts produce catecholamines, respectively, as a neurotransmittor and as a hormone. In the first years of life, the majority of systemic catecholamine is produced in the abdominal paraganglia. The adrenal medulla contains very few chromaffin cells at birth and enlarges and matures during the early years of life. It is thought that neuroblastoma develops in immature neuroblasts, ganglioneuroma in more differentiated sympathetic cells (ganglion cells), and pheochromocytoma in differentiated hormone-producing cells (chromaffin cells).

Pathology

Histologically, neuroblastomas are very heterogeneous and are composed of two predominant cell types: the neuroblast/ganglion cell and the Schwann cell. Schwann cells are responsible for the stromal element of the tumour. As the neuroblast is an embryonal cell, it can differentiate and mature into a ganglion cell. Recent evidence suggests that Schwann cells in neuroblastomas are reactive cells arising from non-neoplastic tissues, and are recruited into the tumour (Ambros *et al.* 1996). The typical histological appearance of an undifferentiated neuroblastoma is 'a small, round, blue cell tumour' (Fig. 2a). The cells are uniformly sized containing dense, hyperchromatic nuclei and scant cytoplasm. Homer-Wright pseudorosettes, neuroblasts surrounding eosinophil neurophil (neuritic processes), are frequently present. Ultimately, a neuroblastoma may differentiate into a mature ganglioneuroma, which is the other end of the spectrum and has three components: mature ganglion cells, Schwann cells, and neurophils (Fig. 2b). Some neuroblastomas, particularly those that are undergoing regression, have a degree of calcification. In the past, a number of histopathological classification systems of neuroblastoma have been proposed by Shimada and Joshi. The Shimada system is age linked, and the tumours are classified according to the amount of Schwann cell stroma (poor or rich) and the number of cells in mitosis or karyorrhexis. Recently, an International Neuroblastoma Pathology Classification (INPC) has been proposed (Roald *et al.*). All these classification are only applicable to tumours prior to therapy. In the INPC, the four morphological features which form the basis for the classification are:

(1) the degree of differentiation of the neuroblasts;

(2) the presence or absence of Schwann-cell stroma;

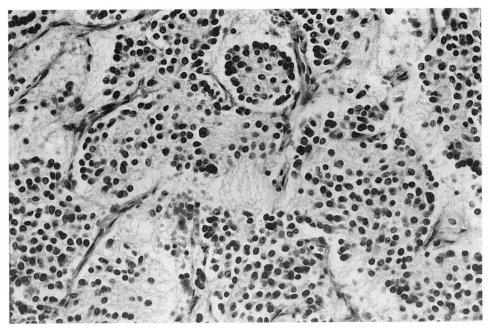

Fig. 17.2a Nest of neuroblastoma cells with poorly formed Homer-Wright pseudorosettes and eosinophil neurophils (neuritic processes). Haematoxylin and eosin, 130× magnification (courtesy of Dr A. J. Malcolm).

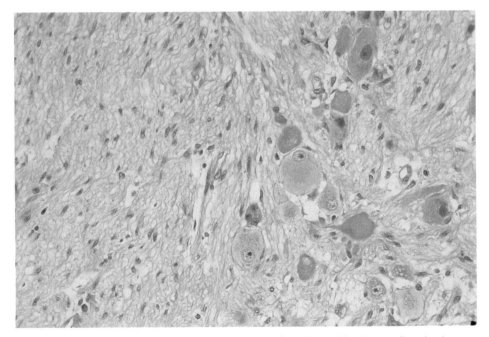

Fig. 17.2b Ganglioneuroma with mature ganglion cells, Schwann cells, and neurophils. Haemotoxylin and eosin, 280× magnification (courtesy of Dr. A. J. Malcolm).

(3) the presence or absence of neuroblastic nodules arising in a mature Schwann-cell-stroma-rich tumour;

(4) an index of tumour-cell aggressiveness (indicated by the mitotic-karyorrhexis index — MKI).

From these features the following tumours can be defined: neuroblastoma (undifferentiated, poorly differentiated, or differentiating), ganglioneuroblastoma (intermixed or nodular), and ganglioneuroma. Distinction of the two types of ganglioneuroblastomas is of major importance. Intermixed ganglioneuroblastomas are good-prognosis tumours where there is progressive differentiation, with only small nests of neuroblasts. However, with the nodular variant, there are usually macroscopic, often haemorrhagic, nodules of neuroblasts, and the associated prognosis is worse.

Genetics

Genetic predisposition

There are very few reported pedigrees of familial neuroblastoma (Kushner *et al.* 1986). In those families, the median age at diagnosis is 9 months, as opposed to 2–3 years in sporadic cases. An increased incidence of multiple primary tumours is also apparent. Together, these data suggest that a genetic predisposition for neuroblastoma development exists in these families. Cytogenetic studies and linkage analyses have not yet revealed a neuroblastoma predisposition locus.

Genetic aberrations in neuroblastoma

In neuroblastoma, several genetic abnormalities have been described with an increased frequency. Genetic studies on neuroblastoma tumour samples have focused firstly on the amplification of oncogenes or chromosomal regions, and secondly on chromosomal losses, which are thought to reflect the inactivation of tumour suppressor genes.

N-myc oncogene

The N-*myc* oncogene is present in an increased copy number in 25–35% of neuroblastomas (Fig. 17.3). It has been shown, both in cell lines and in tumour samples, that N-*myc* amplification gives rise to a strong overexpression of N-*myc* mRNA and protein. N-*myc* amplification is found in 30–40% of stage 3/4 neuroblastomas and in only 5% of localized or stage 4s neuroblastomas. N-*myc* amplified neuroblastomas are characterized by a highly aggressive behaviour with an unfavourable clinical outcome (Seeger *et al.* 1985). In N-*myc*-amplified neuroblastomas, loss of chromosome 1p is almost invariably present.

Tumour suppressor genes

Loss of tumour suppressor regions is reported in neuroblastomas for chromosome 1p (30–40%), 4p (20%), 11q (25%), and 14q (25%). For chromosome 4p, 11q, and 14q, the clinical analyses are not very extensive and no clear patterns have arisen.

Chromosome 1p loss (Fig. 17.3) occurs more frequently in older children with stage 3/4 neuroblastoma and is correlated with increased serum ferritin and LDH. In almost all samples with N-*myc* amplification, concomitant 1p loss is demonstrated, but loss of chromosome 1p also occurs in N-*myc* single-copy cases. A multivariate prognostic factor analysis showed that 1p loss was the strongest predictor of outcome of all clinical and genetic factors tested, including N-*myc*

LOH 1p36   N-myc amplification

D1S96/TaqI   NB-1 / TaqI

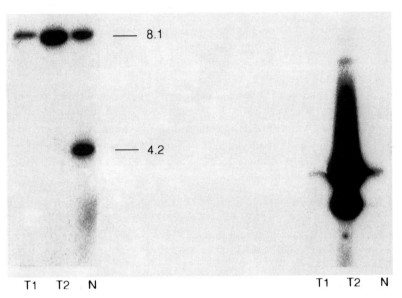

Fig. 17.3 Southern blot analysis showing N-*myc* amplification and allelic loss of chromosome 1p in the same tumour sample.

amplification (Caron *et al.* 1996). Chromosome 1p loss added considerable prognostic information to the strongest clinical factors. Other studies also report a negative prognostic impact for 1p loss (Fong *et al.* 1992; Gehring *et al.* 1995).

The expression level of several genes has been shown to correlate with prognosis, e.g. *trk-A* (Kogner *et al.* 1993; Nagakawara *et al.* 1993), *MRP* (Norris *et al.* 1996), and *CD44* (Favrot *et al.* 1994; Gross *et al.* 1994). As those genes show no structural abnormalities, it is unknown whether they are involved in tumourogenesis or whether those differences in expression levels merely reflect the differentiation status of the tumour cells.

Clinical presentation

The clinical manifestations of neuroblastoma are very varied, depending on the site of the primary tumour and whether there is metastatic disease. The classical presentation in a 3–4-year old is a pale, irritable child with a limp and periorbital ecchymoses (Fig. 17.4), whilst an infant may present with a grossly enlarged liver with subcutaneous nodules. The symptoms of neuroblastoma can be attributed either to the primary tumour, metastases, or a paraneoplastic phenomenon.

Primary tumour

Neuroblastoma primary tumours can arise at any localization coinciding with normal sympathetic nervous system structures, for example the adrenals, the sympathetic chain, or abdominal paraganglia. About 25% of primaries are found in the neck or the thorax, 70% in the abdomen, and 5% in the pelvis.

A hard, fixed, abdominal mass causing only mild abdominal discomfort is a frequent presentation. Hypertension can result from compression of the renal vessels by the tumour. Gastrointestinal symptoms are rare, except from pelvic tumours which may cause constipation and difficulties with micturition.

Primaries in the cervical region may manifest themselves only as a mass, which is mistaken for cervical lymph nodes. Horner's syndrome with unilateral ptosis, constricted pupil, and absence of sweating may occur either with cervical or thoracic lesions. Although a thoracic primary can cause signs of mediastinal pressure with cough and superior mediastinal obstruction, most commonly these are detected coincidentally on a chest radiograph carried out for other reasons.

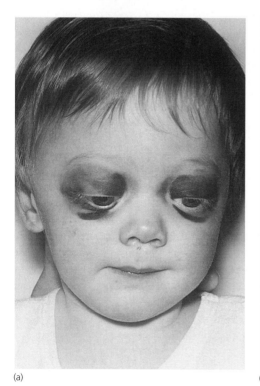 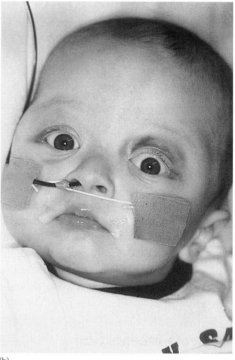

(a) (b)

Fig. 17.4(a + b) Children with stage 4 neuroblastoma with bilateral periorbital ecchymoses.

Thoracic, abdominal, and pelvic tumours can extend into the neural foramina and compress nerve roots and the spinal cord, resulting in radicular pain, paraplegia, and bowel and bladder symptoms.

Metastatic disease

The commonest metastatic sites are bone, lymph nodes, and bone marrow. Metastases to the bone are often the presenting symptom, and manifest as painful lesions which produce an irritable, unwell child. Frequently, a limp, whose cause is difficult to diagnose, is the predominant feature either at initial presentation or at relapse. Bone marrow involvement generally presents with anaemia and, later, thrombocytopaenia. The blood film may show a leucoerythroblastic picture. Lymphadenopathy is not usually generalized, nor massive. Retro-orbital and orbital metastases produce a characteristic appearance of proptosis and periorbital ecchymoses. An infant with stage 4s neuroblastoma can present with significant respiratory distress from a massively enlarged liver, as well as having non-tender, bluish-tinged subcutaneous nodules.

Paraneoplastic symptoms

Rarely, in 4% of patients, opsomyoclonus can be a presentation of neuroblastoma. This syndrome comprises myoclonic, irregular, jerking, random eye movements often associated with cerebellar ataxia. The symptoms generally tend to occur with good-prognosis tumours and mostly resolve with regression of the disease (Altman and Baehneer 1976).

An intractable, secretory diarrhoea, probably mediated by vasoactive intestinal polypeptide (VIP), can cause hypokalaemic dehydration—Kerner Morrison syndrome. Like opsomyoclonus, this entity usually occurs with ganglioneuromas or ganglioneuroblastomas (Kaplan *et al.* 1980).

Unlike the presentation in pheochromocytoma, hypertension, tachycardia, and episodes of sweating are less common in neuroblastoma.

Diagnosis and staging

Diagnostic criteria

The diagnostic criteria for neuroblastoma have been clearly defined by the International Neuroblastoma Staging System (INSS) working party (Brodeur *et al.* 1993). Neuroblastoma can be diagnosed either by a tissue biopsy, with a histological appearance of neuroblastoma, or by the presence of a non-haemopoietic tumour in the bone marrow, together with raised urinary cate-cholamines. In the bone marrow, neuroblastoma often has the appearance of pseudorosettes with increased reticulin and fibrous tissue. The presence of neuroectodermal antigens on the surface of the malignant cells, detected by monoclonal antibodies, further confirms the diagnosis.

Staging system

Before 1988, neuroblastoma was staged according to a number of different systems (Evans, Paediatric Oncology Group (POG), St Jude's Children's Research Hospital (SJCRH), and TNM).

However, following the publication of the INSS, there is now an international consensus that the INSS should be used exclusively.

Details are shown in Table 17.1. It is essentially a postsurgical staging system with major dependence on the assessment of resectability and surgical examination of lymph-node involvement. The central feature of stage 3 disease is invasion across the midline by the tumour, with often a main blood vessel being encased. A number of investigations are required to delineate the extent of spread of the disease, and have been defined by the INSS (Table 17.2).

Radiodiagnostics

Either CT scan or MRI imaging can delineate the extent of the primary tumour and associated lymph-node masses, as well as other metastatic disease. Within the abdomen, detection of liver metastases can be carried out by CT scanning, whilst the extent of lymph-node involvement and the margins of the primary tumour can be visualized equally well by either technique. Abdominal ultrasound can replace CT or MRI when carried out by an experienced paediatric radiologist. MRI is the optimal technique to demonstrate intraspinal extension through neural foramina.

MIBG scanning

Meta-iodobenzylguanidine (MIBG) is taken up preferentially into cells of the sympathetic nervous system involved in catecholamine synthesis. Therefore, if the compound is radiolabelled it can localize primary and metastatic neuroblastomas (Fig. 17.5) with a sensitivity of > 90% and a specificity of > 98%. To prevent uptake of radioactive iodine in the thyroid, the organ is specifically blocked by Lugol's iodine prior to administration of the isotope.

Between 5 and 10% of neuroblastomas do not take up MIBG and therefore if there is no positivity in the primary tumour, metastases cannot be detected. It is widely recognized that MIBG is the most sensitive technique and surpasses 99m Tc-diphosphonate scintigraphy of bones or skeletal survey. However, if there is no uptake of MIBG into the primary tumour, it is recommended that a 99m Tc bone scan is carried out.

Tumour markers

There is a large number of urinary catecholamines which can be elevated in the urine in patients with neuroblastoma. The most frequently measured metabolites are vanilglycolic acid (VGA = vanillylmandelic acid = VMA), vanilglycol (VG), cathechol acetic acid (CAA), vanilacetic acid (VAA = homovanillic acid = HVA), and vanilactic acid (VLA); in addition, concentrations of dopamine may be assessed. Approximately 90–95% of all patients with neuroblastoma will have increased urinary secretion of these metabolites. A simplified schema depicting catecholamine metabolism is shown in Fig. 17.6. Measurement of the ratio of the urinary concentration of catecholamine metabolite to creatinine in a urine sample gives the most reliable results. The serum concentrations of lactate dehydrogenase (LDH), ferritin, and neurone-specific enolase are useful prognostic markers (Silber *et al.* 1991).

Table 17.1 INSS International Staging System for Neuroblastoma (from Brodeur *et al.* 1993)

Stage 1	Localized tumour with complete gross excision, with or without microscopic residual disease; representative ipsilateral and contralateral lymph nodes negative for tumour microscopically (nodes attached to and removed with the primary tumour may be positive).
Stage 2a	Localized tumour with incomplete gross excision; representative ipsilateral and non-adherent lymph nodes negative for tumour microscopically.
Stage 2b	Localized tumour with complete or incomplete gross excision; with ipsilateral non-adherent lymph nodes positive for tumour. Enlarged contralateral lymph nodes must be negative microscopically.
Stage 3	Unresectable unilateral tumour infiltrating across the midline[2] with or without regional lymph node involvement; *or*, localized unilateral tumour with contralateral regional lymph node involvement; or mid-line tumour with bilateral extension by infiltration (unresectable) or by lymph node involvement.
Stage 4	Any primary tumour with dissemination to distant lymph nodes, bone, bone marrow, liver skin and/or other organs (except as defined in Stage 4S).
Stage 4S	Localized primary tumour (as defined for Stage 1, 2a, or 2b) with dissemination limited to skin, liver and/or bone marrow[3] (limited to infants < 1 year).

[1] Multifocal primary tumours (e.g. adrenal primary tumours) should be staged according to the greatest extent of the disease, as defined above, and followed by $_M$, e.g. 3_M.

[2] The mid-line is defined as the vertebral column. Tumours originating on one side and 'crossing the mid-line' must infiltrate to or beyond the opposite side of the vertebral column.

[3] Marrow involvement of Stage 4S should be minimal; i.e. less than 10% of total nucleated cells identified as malignant on bone marrow biopsy or on marrow aspirates. More extensive marrow involvement will be considered to be Stage 4. The MIBG scan (if done) should be negative in marrow.

Table 17.2 Assessment of extent of disease (from Brodeur *et al.* 1993)

Tumor site	Recommended tests
Primary tumor	CT and/or MRI scan* with 3D measurements; MIBG scan, if available.[φ]
Metastatic sites[φ] Bone marrow	Bilateral posterior iliac crest marrow aspirates and trephine (core) bone marrow biopsies required to exclude marrow involvement. A single positive site documents marrow involvement. Core biopsies must contain at least 1 cm of marrow (excluding cartilage) to be considered adequate.
Bone	MIBG scan; ^{99}Tc scan required if MIBG scan negative or unavailable, and plain radiographs of positive lesions are recommended.
Lymph nodes	Clinical examination (palpable nodes), confirmed histologically. CT scan for non-palpable nodes (3D measurements).
Abdomen/liver Chest	CT and/or MRI scan* with 3D measurements. AP and lateral chest radiographs. CT/MRI necessary if chest radiograph positive, or if abdominal mass/nodes extend into chest

AP, anteroposterior.

* Ultrasound considered suboptimal for accurate 3D measurements.

[φ] The MIBG scan is applicable to all sites of disease.

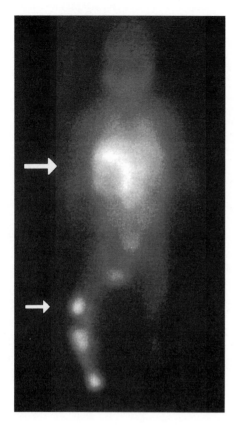

Fig. 17.5 MIBG scan showing a right-sided adrenal primary tumour (large arrow) and multiple bone metastasis (small arrow) (courtesy of Dr C. Hoefnagel).

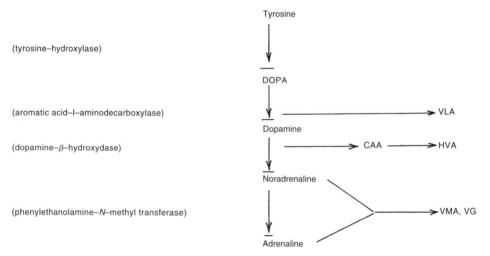

Fig 17.6 Simplified scheme of catecholamine metabolism. Enzymes are in brackets.

Bone marrow examination

Metastatic disease to the bone marrow is one of the commonest occurrences in poor-prognosis neuroblastoma. Studies in the past have documented that metastatic disease may be present in the bone marrow, but it may not be easy to detect by examination of a bone marrow aspirate. Therefore, the international consensus, as specified by the INSS, is that all patients should have histological examinations of bone marrow aspirate and trephine carried out from two different sites. In this way, the likelihood of detecting 'patchy' bone marrow involvement is increased. Bone marrow aspirate examinations can be assessed using conventional microscopy and usually, if there is involvement, multiple clumps of a non-haemopoietic malignancy are observed. The non-haemopoietic cells tend to cluster and form pseudorosettes. International guidelines suggest that for a bone marrow histological examination to be adequate, at least 1 cm of haemopoietic tissue should be examined.

Treatment strategies

Current therapy

Stage 1 and 2 tumours

The present consensus is that stage 1 and 2 tumours should be resected with no acute or long-term sequelae. Even if there is residual disease, no chemotherapy or radiation treatment should be given (DeBernardi *et al.* 1995; Kushner *et al.* 1996). Currently, the Localised Neuroblastoma European Study Group (LNESG) recommends therapy for recurrent localized tumours by further resection only and it is possible that a recurrent tumour may eventually regress spontaneously.

Stage 3 tumours

In the past, infants with stage 3 tumours have received postoperative chemotherapy. This has been associated with acute and long-term sequelae from chemotherapy, and there may be significant surgical morbidity and, indeed, mortality. Furthermore, in some reports there are more deaths resulting from the effects of therapy than from disease (Berthold *et al.* 1996). It is now recommended that, after surgery, careful observation with measurement of urinary catecholamine concentrations and radiological imaging only is required. A residual, persisting mass associated with some elevation of urinary catecholamines, may be a mature ganglioneuroma. Only a definite increase in tumour size should be evidence of progression.

Children over the age of 1 year with stage 3 neuroblastoma have been treated with surgical resection of the primary tumour, chemotherapy, 'second look' surgery, followed by radiotherapy and/or further chemotherapy (Castleberry *et al.* 1991). Stage 3 neuroblastomas are now being subclassified according to *MYCN* gene copy number, and only those with amplification and/or 1p deletions treated with intensive chemotherapy.

Stage 4 tumours in children over the age of 1 year

The therapeutic approach adopted by most cooperative groups for stage 4 disease over the age of one is to administer initial chemotherapy, followed by surgical resection of the primary tumour and consolidation with myeloablative therapy (MAT) with haemopoetic stem-cell support (Philip *et al.*

1987; Pole *et al.* 1991). Immune modulation or differentiation therapy, i.e. 13 cis retinoic acid, GD2 antibody, or Interleukin 2, is often given at the time of minimal residual disease, i.e. following MAT. Permutations of the active cytotoxic drugs have been used in induction chemotherapy. However, a platinum compound, either cisplatin or carboplatin, etoposide, and cyclophosphamide are most commonly used (Kushner *et al.* 1994). Whether there is a benefit in the inclusion of doxorubicin is unknown. The VECI regimen is a good example of such a multidrug combination (vincristine 1.5 mg/m² day 1, carboplatin 400 mg/m² day 3, teniposide 150 mg/m² day 4, iphosphamide 3000 mg/m² day 1 and 2). Recently, there has been a trend for higher doses of agents to be given in intensive schedules. A randomized, ongoing study (ENSG5) examines the benefits of increased dose intensity following a pilot study (Pearson *et al.* 1992).

Infants with stage 4s and 4 neuroblastoma

The majority of infants with stage 4s neuroblastoma require no therapy, as their disease regresses spontaneously. Only life-threatening symptoms, such as the need for respiratory support due to a rapidly enlarging liver, are indications for therapy. A number of therapeutic options have been utilized in this situation, including low-dose radiotherapy to the liver and low-intensity chemotherapy. It is essential that the smallest amount of effective therapy is administered, and frequently only one course is needed to induce regression. With this approach, 85% of children with the disease will be cured.

In the past, patients with stage 4 neuroblastoma under the age of one, who did not fit the criteria for 4s disease, received conventional chemotherapy but without MAT, due to the superior prognosis in babies and the toxicity of MAT (DeBernardi *et al.* 1992).

MIBG as anti-cancer agent

The adrenaline analogue, MIBG, is actively taken up and stored in more than 90% of neuroblastoma tumours. Incorporation of the ^{131}I-radioisotope in MIBG makes it possible to use this for targeted radiotherapy. Currently, ^{131}I-MIBG is used in three groups of neuroblastoma patients:

(1) those with unresectable, localized tumours;

(2) for initial treatment of unresectable stage 3 and stage 4 patients;

(3) in patients with recurrence.

In cases of unresectable, mainly abdominal or pelvic neuroblastoma,[131] I-MIBG treatment has been used to render these tumours operable, or even to circumvent surgery.

Efforts are underway to use ^{131}I-MIBG as the only initial anticancer agent in unresectable stage 3 and stage 4 patients. The administration of multiple courses of ^{131}I-MIBG results in a rapid and high response rate with very little toxicity. Following initial MIBG treatment, surgical resection of the primary tumour, intensive combination chemotherapy, and myeloablative therapy for stage 4 cases is given (De Kraker *et al.* 1995).

Future developments in therapy

Individualization of therapy according to molecular pathological features

As there are many molecular pathological features of neuroblastoma which are of prognostic importance, it is anticipated that in the future a therapeutic classification can be developed based on patient's age, tumour stage, and molecular pathological features. To this end the INSS working group is developing International Neuroblastoma Risk Groups (INRG).

Of all the molecular, pathological, prognostic features, amplification of the *MYCN* gene is the most extensively studied marker, although markers like loss of chromosome 1p might identify a larger group of poor-prognosis patients than *MYCN* amplification alone. At present, therapy for stage 3 neuroblastoma is determined by *MYCN* gene copy number. In stage 3 patients with tumours with a single copy of *MYCN* and especially those of favourable histology, surgery and a short course of chemotherapy are now being recommended, with survival rates of 85% without intensive chemotherapy or radiation. Tumours with *MYCN* amplification progress rapidly and are associated with a 5-year survival of only 20%. In view of this, the consensus is that these tumours should be treated in the same way as stage 4 neuroblastomas over the age of one.

Amplification of *MYCN* may also identify infants with metastatic neuroblastoma (stage 4 and 4s) who have a very poor prognosis. These patients should be treated with an intensive chemotherapy regimen and MAT. Those infants with metastatic disease with single-copy *MYCN* tumours should be treated with less intensive treatment. For the subgroup of infants with hyper-diploid tumours, without allelic loss of chromosome 1p or *MYCN* amplification, the outcome is excellent, and whether any therapy is required is very debatable (Look *et al.* 1991).

Although the overall prognosis for *MYCN*-amplified stage 1 and 2 tumours is worse, with a 50% survival (DeBernardi *et al.* 1995), there is no international consensus about the appropriate treatment for these rare cases. As there is no convincing evidence that patients who are treated at recurrence have a worse survival than those who have intensive chemotherapy at presentation, an observational policy is appropriate.

Defining the optimum chemotherapy agents, dose, and schedule

There is no shortage of active chemotherapeutic agents in neuroblastoma; the therapeutic challenge is to determine the optimum combination, dose, and schedule. There are no current randomized studies comparing different combinations and dose; however, there is one ongoing randomized study (ENSG5) examining the benefit of increased dose intensity. In this study, the same agents are given in the same cumulative doses in both arms, but the dose intensity is 1.8 times greater in the rapid-schedule arm (Pearson *et al.* 1992).

The role of myeloablative therapy (MAT) with autologous bone marrow rescue (ABMR)

Based on a randomized study showing a slight survival advantage for high-dose melphalan and ABMR as consolidation therapy (ENSG1) (Pinkerton *et al.* 1987), MAT has been widely used. There is no convincing evidence that any of the more complex multi-agent MAT regimens results in a better 2-year, event-free survival (EFS) rate than 40%, despite toxic death rates ranging from 1–22% (Gordon *et al.* 1992). Recently, results with the combination melphalan and busulphan have been promising and further evaluation is needed. The role of consolidation with MAT is, at present, being evaluated by the Children's Cancer Group of North America. Patients at the end of treatment are randomized either to receive further chemotherapy or consolidation MAT with ABMR (Matthay *et al.* 1995). There is no convincing evidence to suggest that allogeneic is superior to autologous bone marrow (Matthay *et al.* 1994), nor that there is a benefit in purging the marrow.

Treatment results

Stage 1 and 2

An excellent EFS and overall survival is expected for these patients following surgery alone, with a > 90% EFS for stage 1 and 85% for stage 2 disease. Stage 2 tumours with *MYCN* amplification have survival rates of 50%.

Stage 3

65% of all patients with stage 3 tumours are long-term survivors. *MYCN* amplification identifies a group with only a 20% probability of EFS, whilst 85% of those with favourable histology without *MYCN* amplification survive.

Stage 4 in children over the age of one

Children with stage 4 neuroblastoma over the age of one have one of the worst prognoses of all childhood malignancies. In the majority, the malignancy is initially chemosensitive, then drug-resistant disease recurs. The results of the strategy described above are internationally consistent, and if an intensive chemotherapy regimen is employed, a 5-year survival rate of 25% can be expected.

Stage 4 and 4s in infants under the age of one

The EFS for stage 4s is 85%, with some infants dying due to large tumour masses, and a minority progressing to overt, aggressive stage 4 disease. For infants with stage 4 disease, a 60% survival can be expected, with *MYCN* amplification identifying the poor-prognosis group.

Clinicobiological entities

Clinical observations suggest that the entire spectrum of neuroblastomas is, in fact, more like a syndrome which is made up of several distinct subsets of disease. Specific clinical behaviour is observed for disseminated stage 4s neuroblastoma with a high likelihood of spontaneous regression, as opposed to the more frequent stage 4 neuroblastoma of which most cases have an unfavourable clinical course despite intensive multimodality therapy. Localized neuroblastomas (stage 1/2) have a very good prognosis after resection. Data from neuroblastoma screening areas show that the incidence of stage 1/2 neuroblastoma rises sharply without a significant decrease of stage 3/4 neuroblastoma at a later age. This implies that a fair proportion of localized neuroblastoma regresses spontaneously, before clinical detection.

These observations suggest at least three different neuroblastoma entities, i.e. 'disseminated, prone to regression', 'disseminated, aggressive', and 'localized, favourable'. Most likely, these different clinical entities have different biological abnormalities driving the malignant transformation. Clinical parameters like stage, age, serum ferritin and LDH reflect the biological factors determining the neuroblastoma category. As such they are useful prognostic factors. However, they are not fully reliable in predicting the clinical course. Stage 4s neuroblastoma can show tumour progression or recurrence with 'disseminated, aggressive' characteristics and an unfavourable outcome in 10–20% of the cases, some localized cases suffer from incurable tumour recurrence, and 15–25% of the stage 4 cases can be cured with intensive therapy.

Several genetic abnormalities strongly correlated to a 'disseminated, aggressive' phenotype have been reported. N-*myc* amplification and loss of chromosome 1p identify high-risk patients, independently of age, stage, and other clinical characteristics.

The identification of the different biological abnormalities characteristic of each of the disease entities encompassing the neuroblastoma syndrome will eventually allow an optimal choice of treatment for each patient. In future, specific treatment modalities targeting the biological aberration might become feasible.

References

Altman, A.J. and Baehneer, R.L. (1976). Favourable prognosis for survival in children with coincident opsomyoclonus and neuroblastoma. *Cancer*, 37, 846.

Ambros, I.M., Zellner, A., Roald, B., Amann, G., Ladenstein, R., Printz, D., *et al.* (1996). Role of ploidy, chromosome 1p, and Schwann cells in the maturation of neuroblastoma. *New England Journal of Medicine*, 334, 1505–1511.

Berthold, F., Hero, B., Breu, H., Christiansen, H., Erttmann, R., Gnekow, A., *et al.* (1996). The recurrence patterns of stages I, II and III neuroblastoma: experience with 77 relapsing patients. *Annals of Oncology*, 7, 183–187.

Brodeur, G.M., Pritchard, J., Berthold, F., Carlsen, N.L., Castel, V., Castleberry, R.P., *et al.* (1993). Revisions of international criteria for neuroblastoma diagnosis, staging and response to treatment. *Journal of Clinical Oncology*, 11, 1466–1477.

Caron, H., Van Sluis, P., De Kraker, J., Bokkerink, J., Egeler, M., Laureys, G., *et al.* (1996). Allelic loss of chromosome 1p as a predictor of unfavourable outcome in patients with neuroblastoma. *New England Journal of Medicine*, 334, 225–30.

Castleberry, R.P., Kun, L.E., Shuster, J.J., Altshuler, G., Smith, I.E., Nitschke, R., *et al.* (1991). Radiotherapy improves the outlook for patients older than 1 year with POG stage C neuroblastoma. *Journal of Clinical Oncology*, 9, 789.

DeBernardi, B., Pianca, C., Boni, L., Brisigotti, M., Carli, M., Bagnulo, S., *et al.* (1992). Disseminated neuroblastoma (stage IV and IV-S) in the first year of life. Outcome related to age and stage. Italian Cooperative Group on Neuroblastoma. *Cancer*, 70, 1625–1633.

DeBernardi, B., Conte, M., Mancini, A., Donfrancesco, A., Alvisi, P., Toma, P., *et al.* (1995). Localized resectable neuroblastoma: results of the second study of the Italian Cooperative Group for Neuroblastoma. *Journal of Clinical Oncology*, 13, 884–893.

De Kraker, J., Hoefnagel, C.A., Caron, H., Valdes Olmos, R.A., Zsiros, J., Heij, H.A., *et al.* (1995). First line targeted radiotherapy, a new concept in the treatment of advanced stage neuroblastoma. *European Journal of Cancer*, 31A (4), 600–602.

Favrot, M.C., Combaret, V., and Lasset, C. (1994). CD44, a new prognostic marker for neuroblastoma. *Lancet*, 329, 1965.

Fong, C.T., White, P.S., Peterson, K., Sapienza, C., Cavenee, W.K., Kern, S.E., *et al.* (1992). Loss of heterozygosity for chromosome 1 or 14 defines subsets of advanced neuroblastomas. *Cancer Research*, 69, 1780–1785.

Gehring, T., Berthold, F., Edler, L., Schwab, M., and Amler, L.C. (1995). Chromosome 1p loss is not a reliable prognostic marker in neuroblastoma. *Cancer Research*, 55, 5366–5369.

Gordon, S.J., Pearson, A.D.J., Reid, M.M., and Craft, A.W. (1992). Toxicity of single-day high-dose vincristine, melphalan, etoposide and carboplatin consolidation with autologous bone marrow rescue in advanced neuroblastoma. *European Journal of Cancer*, 28A, 1319–1323.

Gross, N., Beretta, C., Peruisseau, G., Jackson, D., Simmons, D., and Beck, D. (1994). CD44-H expression by human neuroblastoma cells: relation to MYCN amplification and lineage differentiation. *Cancer Research*, 54, 4238–4242.

Kaneko, Y., Kanda, N., Maseki, N., Nakachi, K., Takeda, T., Okabe, I., *et al.* (1990). Current urinary mass screening for catecholamine metabolites at 6 months of age may be detecting only a small portion of high-risk neuroblastomas: A chromosome and N-myc amplification study, *Journal of Clinical Oncology*, 8, 2005–2013.

Kaplan, S., Holbrook, C., McDaniel, H.G., Buntain, W.L., and Crist, W.M. (1980). Vasoactive intestinal peptide secreting tumors of childhood. *American Journal of Dis Child*, 134, 21.

Kogner, P., Barbany, G., Dominici, C., Castello, M.A., Raschella, G., and Persson, H. (1993). Coexpression of mRNA for TRK protooncogene and low affinity nerve growth factor receptor in neuroblastoma with favourable prognosis. *Cancer Research*, 53, 2044–2050.

Kushner, B.H., Gilbert, F., and Helson, L. (1986). Familial neuroblastoma: Case reports, literature review, and etiologic considerations. *Cancer*, 57, 1887.

Kushner, B.H., LaQuaglia, M.P., Bonilla, M.A., Lindsley, K., Rosenfield, N., Yeh, S., *et al.* (1994). Highly effective induction therapy for stage 4 neuroblastoma in children over 1 year of age. *Journal of Clinical Oncology*, 12, 2607–2613.

Kushner, B.H., Cheung, N-K.V., LaQuaglia, M.P., Ambros, P.F., Ambros, I.M., Bonilla, M.A., *et al.* (1996). Survival from locally invasive or widespread neuroblastoma without cytotoxic therapy. *Journal of Clinical Oncology*, 14, 373–381.

Look, A.T., Hayes, F.A., Schuster, J.J., Douglass, E.C., Castleberry, R.P., Bowman, L.C., *et al.* (1991). Clinical relevance of tumour cell ploidy and N-myc gene amplification in childhood neuroblastoma. *Journal of Clinical Oncology*, 9, 581–591.

Matthay, K.K., Seeger, R.C., Reynolds, C.P., Stram, D.O., O'Leary, M.C., Harris, R.E., *et al.* (1994). Allogeneic versus autologous purged bone marrow transplantation for neuroblastoma: A report from the Children's Cancer Group. *Journal of Clinical Oncology*, 12, 2382–2386.

Matthay, K.K., O'Leary, M.C., Ramsay, N.K., Villablanca, J., Reynolds, C.P., Atkinson, J.B., *et al.* (1995). Role of myeloablative therapy in improved outcome for high risk neuroblastoma: reviews of recent Children's Cancer Group results. *European Journal of Cancer*, 31A (4), 572–575.

Nagakawara, A., Arima-Nagakawara, M., Scavarda, N.J., Azar, C.G., Cantor, A.B., and Brodeur, G.M. (1993). Association between high levels of expression of the TRK gene and favourable outcome in human neuroblastoma, *New England Journal of Medicine*, 328, 847–854.

Norris, M., Sharon, B., Bordow, B., Marshall, G.M., Haber, P.S., Cohn, S.L., *et al.* (1996). Expression of the gene for multidrug resistance-associated protein and outcome in patients with neuroblastoma. *New England Journal of Medicine*, 334, 231–237.

Pearson, A.D.J., Craft, A.W., Pinkerton, C.R., Meller, S.T., and Reid, M.M. (1992). High dose rapid schedule chemotherapy for disseminated neuroblastoma. *European Journal of Cancer*, 28A, 1654–1659.

Philip, T., Bernard, J.L., Zucker, J.M., Pinkerton, R., Lutz, P., Bordigoni, P., *et al.* (1987). High dose chemoradiotherapy with bone marrow transplantation as consolidation treatment in neuroblastoma: an unselected group of stage 4 patients over 1 year of age. *Journal of Clinical Oncology*, 5, 266–271.

Pinkerton, C.R., Pritchard, J., and de Kraker, J. (1987). ENSG 1. Randomized study of high dose melphalan in neuroblastoma. In: Dicke KA, Spitzer G, Japannath S, eds Autologous Bone Marrow Transplantation. Texas, University of Texas Press, 401–406.

Pole, J.G., Casper, J., Elfenbein, G., Gee, A., Gross, S., Janssen, W., *et al.* (1991). High dose chemoradiotherapy supported by marrow infusions for advanced neuroblastoma: a Paediatric Oncology Group study. *Journal of Clinical Oncology*, 9, 152–158.

Seeger, R.C., Brodeur, G.M., Sather, H., Dalton, A., Siegel, S.E., Wong, K.Y., *et al.* (1985). Association of multiple copies of the N-myc oncogene with rapid progression of neuroblastomas. *New England Journal of Medicine*, 313, 1111–6.

Silber, J.H., Evans, A.E., and Friedman, M., (1991). Models to predict outcome from childhood neuroblastoma: the role of serum ferritin and tumor histology. *Cancer Research*, 51, 1426–33.

Stiller, C.A. and Parkin, D.M. (1992). International variations in the incidence of neuroblastoma. *International Journal of Cancer*, 52, 538–43.

Woods, W.G., Tuchman, M., Robison, L.L., Bernstein, M., Leclerc, J.M., Brisson, L.C., *et al.* (1996). A population-based study of the usefulness of screening for neuroblastoma. *Lancet*, 348, 1682–87.

Yamamoto, K., Hayashi, Y., Handada, R., Kikuchi, A., Ichikawa, M., Tanimura, M., *et al.* (1995). Mass screening and age-specific incidence of neuroblastoma in Saitama Prefecture, Japan. *Journal of Clinical Oncology*, 13, 2033–2038.

18   Germ-cell tumours

A. Barrett

Incidence

These are rare tumours with an incidence of 3–4 per million per year, comprising up to about 3% of cases in childhood cancer registries. Because of the many different histological subtypes and the variation with age of different presentations and sites, the true population-based incidence is difficult to determine, as most published papers are concerned with small personal series. It is clear, however, that the incidence of germ-cell tumours (GCT) has been rising in recent years. In the German paediatric cancer registry, a rise from 0.22/100,000 in 1980 to 0.60 in 1992 has been noted (Göbel *et al.* 1993), and Mann and Stiller (1994) in the UK have reported rises in the age-standardized rate per 1,000,000 of 1.9 to 2.8 for males and 2.2 to 2.8 for females for the years 1962–76 and 1977–91, respectively. Over the same time period, there has been a reduction in mortality due to the introduction of effective chemotherapy and standardized surgical approaches.

About 50% of germ-cell tumours are benign. Approximately 50% arise in the gonads, 25% in the coccyx, and 20% in the brain. The rest occur in miscellaneous extragonadal sites, including the retroperitoneum, face, maxilla, oropharynx, mouth, neck, heart, stomach, bladder, liver, spinal cord, posterior fossa, thyroid, vagina, and vulva. This differs from the situation in adults, where extragonadal tumours are much less common, representing only 2–5% of all GCT.

Epidemiology and aetiology

Two main groups of GCT can be recognized—those arising in infancy and those in adolescence, at or after puberty. These differ in a number of characteristics. Pure yolk sac tumours are common in infancy, seminoma is extremely rare, extragonadal sites are commoner, and infantile tumours lack the isochromosome 12p (duplication of the short-arm chromosome 12) seen in tumours of adults and adolescents (Hawkins and Perlman 1996).

All GCT appear to arise from primitive germ cells which have undergone malignant transformation. During the development of the embryo, primordial germ cells migrate from the yolk sac endoderm, around the hind gut to the genital ridge in the retroperitoneum. The gonad develops in this position and subsequently descends to the scrotum or pelvis. Extragonadal tumours can arise from misplaced primordial germ cells, either because of aberrant migration or arrested descent (Chaganti *et al.* 1994) (Fig. 18.1).

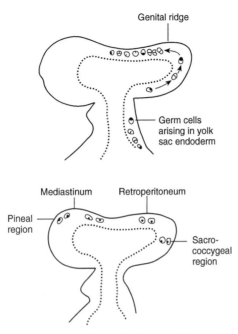

Fig. 18.1 Diagrammatic representation of origin and migration of germ cells from yolk sac to the genital ridge. Aberrant migration can lead to tumour development in extragonadal sites.

Factors such as maldescent and disorders of sexual differentiation may predispose to germ-cell tumours, possibly partly because of associated gonadal atrophy. There may also be a relationship to chemical or environmental factors or viral infection. About 10% of unilateral and 45% of bilateral GCT of the testis are associated with maldescent. This suggests a 10–50-fold excess risk. About 20% have an inguinal hernia, and hydrocoele at the time of presentation is also common (Giwercman *et al.* 1987).

There are data to suggest an association with exposure to herbicides. An increased incidence of GCT in clams off the coast of Maine appears to correlate with increasing aquatic toxicant levels (van Beneden 1994) and there is a high rate of human ovarian cancer in the same geographical area. Deletion of a possible tumour-suppressor gene on the long arm of chromosome 12 has been postulated as a mechanism for tumour induction, and in mice deletion of the inhibin gene is known to lead to the development of gonadal tumours (Samaniego *et al.* 1990; Hoffner *et al.* 1994).

Germ-cell tumours are found in dysgenetic gonads in a number of conditions with chromosomal abnormalities, associated most often with a Y chromosome in a phenotypic female. Early removal of the gonads is needed to avoid the development of malignancy (Krasna *et al.* 1992). Speculation about an association of GCT with mumps orchitis has not been confirmed.

Familial cases have been rarely reported, but no single, significant, linkage group has been identified. Bilateral or multifocal tumours occur very rarely. GCT may be seen in association with some family cancer syndromes (Li and Fraumeni 1972; Heimdal *et al.* 1993).

Other congenital anomalies appear to be associated with GCT in children—inguinal hernia, cardiovascular malformations, and genitourinary system aberrations are the commonest with

Table 18.1   Factors associated with germ-cell tumours

1. Atrophy
      ? chemical
      ? viral
      associated with maldescent

2. Disorders of sexual differentiation with dysgenetic gonads
      mixed gonadal dysgenesis
      pure gonadal dysgenesis (Sywer syndrome)
      Turners syndrome with mosaicism (45X/46XX)
      testicular feminization
      pseudohermaphroditism
      persistant mullerian duct syndrome
      Kleinfelters (47 XXY) (usually associated with mediastinal GCT)

3. Familial—cause unknown
      father/son pairs
      brother/sister
      sister/sister

4. Other tumours
      AML (myelodysplasia (especially with mediastinal GCT)
      Li Fraumeni syndrome/Lynch

gonadal tumours, and musculoskeletal and CNS defects with sacro-coccygeal lesions (Mann *et al.* 1989) (Table 18.1).

Histology

A number of different classifications are in use and some tumours have several synonyms. The WHO classification (which broadly corresponds with the British system and is based on Teilum's original scheme) is shown in Fig. 18.2. Tumours are divided into those arising from totipotent germ cells (germinoma, seminoma) and those from undifferentiated cells with consequent differentiation into embryonic and extra-embryonic structures. For completeness, a list of gonadal non-germ-cell tumours is given in Table 18.2.

Germinomas are characterized by monotonous, uniformly large cells with abundant clear cytoplasm arranged in lobules, separated by fibrovascular stroma. Scattered, syncytiotrophoblastic, giant cells may be seen. These produce human chorionic gonadotrophin (HCG) which may be detected in serum or by immunocytochemical staining. Their presence does not seem to infer a worse prognosis. Tumours associated with elevated alpha-fetoprotein (AFP) produced by yolk sac elements are always classified as non-seminomatous germ-cell tumours, even if histological examination suggests pure seminoma.

Mature teratomas are composed of tissues from all three germ layers—ectoderm, mesoderm, and endoderm. They contain recognizable tissue elements such as bone, hair, and teeth, and are encapsulated, multicystic tumours. Immature teratomas appear macroscopically like mature tera-

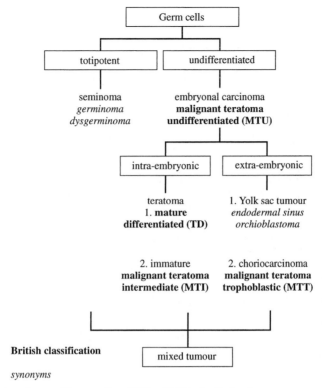

Fig. 18.2 Classification of germ-cell tumours (from WHO and British classifications).

tomas and are seen up to the age of about seven. These show immature tissues, in particular neuroepithelial elements, and are divided into three grades from grade 1, which shows immature elements in one low power field per slide, up to grade 3 where more than four low power fields per slide show neuroepithelium or other immature tissue.

Yolk sac tumours are the most common pure malignant GCT in children. Histologically, the tumour consists of a loose network of spaces and microcysts lined by flat or cuboidal cells. Four patterns are recognized—pseudopapillary, microcystic, solid, and polyvesicular vitelline. Characteristic Schiller-Duval bodies may be found, with a central blood vessel core surrounded by two layers of tumour cells with appearances similar to a primitive glomerulus. Eosinophilic PAS-positive hyaline globules are seen frequently.

Choriocarcinoma is extremely rare, and in adolescence is usually seen as part of a mixed tumour. It may be associated with gynaecomastia and raised serum HCG. These tumours are haemorrhagic and friable, and are composed histologically of syncytiotrophoblasts which stain for HCG, and cytotrophoblasts which are arranged in solid sheets and nests in a villus-like structure.

Presentation of GCT

GCT in many sites present with asymptomatic masses. Specific site-related symptoms and histological types by site and age are shown in Table 18.3.

Table 18.2 Non-germ-cell tumours of the gonads

Leydig—cell (interstitial cell tumours)
    associated with precocious puberty
    virilization/gynaecomastia
    most are benign

Sertoli—cell (androblastoma)
    any age including infancy
    most are benign

granulosa—theca cell (ovary)
    5% before puberty
    majority produce oestrogens
    associated with precocious puberty
    may be non-secreting or androgen producing
    may be associated with undescended testes or gonadal dysgenesis

gonadoblastoma
    found in dysgenetic gonads
    phenotypic females in 80%
    XY or XY/mosaic chromosomes
    often very small
    nests of germ and immature sex cord stromal cells
    collagenous stroma
    calcification common
    benign but up to 60% become malignant (usually to dysgerminoma)

lymphomas/leukaemias

Investigation and staging

Testicular tumours are commonly classified in Europe using the Royal Marsden Hospital system or a modification of it, and ovarian tumours with the FIGO classification (Table 18.4). In other sites, the presence or absence of metastatic disease is the most important prognostic factor, with stage I indicating tumour which can be completely excised, and stage IV metastatic disease. Stage, histology, and completeness of surgical excision are of prognostic significance. Absolute levels of marker elevation are of lesser importance than the rate of fall with appropriate treatment, which should be within the half-life (5–7 days for AFP, 24–36 hours for HCG) (Bartlett *et al.* 1991) (Fig. 18.3).

In infants, AFP levels are normally elevated, falling to adult levels by about 8 months. Tables of normal values with age must therefore be consulted to determine the significance of elevated values in this age-group. Liver damage or tumour lysis following treatment can also lead to elevated levels. The β subunit of human chorionic gonadotrophin (HCG) indicates the presence of syncytiotrophoblastic elements, while AFP is produced by yolk sac elements. An isoenzyme of LDH (LDH-1), the gene for which is found on chromosome 12p, and placental alkaline phosphatase, a fetal isoenzyme found in the sera of 30% of patients with dysgerminoma, may also be useful markers. Estimation of serum levels of AFP and HCG should be obtained preoperatively where possible, with cerebrospinal fluid (CSF) measurements in the case of intracranial germ-cell tumours. If AFP or HCG levels remain high after surgery, or do not fall with a rate consistent with the half-life, further treatment with chemotherapy is indicated.

Table 18.3 Specific site-related symptoms and histological patterns by site and age

Site	Symptom	Age	Histology
testis	painless testicular mass	0–5 years adolescence and post pubertal	yolk sac/teratoma (85% are stage I) mixed germ-cell tumour/teratoma
ovary	abdominal pain or distention, palpable mass, vaginal bleeding, amenorrhoea, precocious puberty, ascites, constipation	infancy adolescence	mature teratoma mature (10% bilateral), immature, dysgerminoma, mixed cell tumours, gonadoblastoma in streak or dysgenetic ovaries
anterior mediastinum	incidental finding, cough, dyspnoea, chest pain	mostly occurs in males	teratoma/mixed cell yolk sac
sacro-coccygeal	prenatal, obstructed labour dermal pit, mass, constipation, urinary disturbance	prognosis better with young age	mature teratoma (80%) immature teratoma, yolk sac tumours
intracranial pineal (62%)	↑ ICP, Parinaud's syndrome		mixed cell, teratoma, yolk sac tumour, embryonal carcinoma
suprasellar (31%) basal ganglia	DI, visual disturbance, hypopituitarism hemiparesis, precocious puberty DI, occulomotor palsy, speech disturbance, hemianopsia	adolescence	predominantly germinoma mixed

↑ ICP raised intracranial pressure; DI diabetes insipidus

Table 18.4 Staging systems for GCT of testis and ovary

Testis (RMH system)		Ovary FIGO	
I	disease localized to testis, markers ↓ normal postop	I	disease confined to ovaries a) one ovary b) both ovaries c) tumour on surface of ovary, capsule rupture or ascites
I (poor risk)	marker elevation, vascular or lymphatic invasion		
II	abdominal nodal disease	II	pelvic extension
III	abdominal and supradiaphragmatic nodal disease	III	intra-abdominal extension outside the pelvis
IV	metastases to lung or elsewhere	IV	metastases outside the peritoneal cavity liver metastases
	POG/CCG staging differs because of surgical staging of non-marker secreting tumours		

POG/CCG Paediatric Oncology Group/Children's Cancer Group

For ovarian and testicular tumours, CT scanning of the abdomen is needed to exclude tumour involvement of the para-aortic and/or renal hilar nodes, and mesenteric disease, ascites, and liver metastases for ovarian tumours. CT scanning of the chest for all extracranial GCT will be needed to exclude lung metastases. Unless these results are abnormal, further investigations are unlikely to be positive, but a bone scan should be done for patients with stage IV disease. Bone marrow is rarely involved. MRI scanning may show different components within an abdominal, retroperitoneal, or mediastinal mass, but cannot differentiate between active and inactive tumour. For intracranial tumours, MRI scanning of the brain and spinal meninges should be undertaken if possible preoperatively, or failing that, within the first 5 days postoperatively. This is the best technique for demonstrating the extent of the primary tumour and excluding multifocal brain tumour or spinal seedlings. Where available, it has largely replaced the older techniques of myelography or CT scanning with contrast agents. For suprasellar tumours, full hormone assessment should be carried out and diabetes insipidus must be ruled out. MRI scanning may give better definition of sacro-coccygeal tumours than CT scanning, although the bony resolution of CT may better demonstrate coccygeal involvement.

Treatment

Indications for surgery

Surgical removal is curative for mature (benign) teratomas, for immature teratomas of low grade, and for stage I testicular or ovarian tumours with markers which return to normal postoperatively.

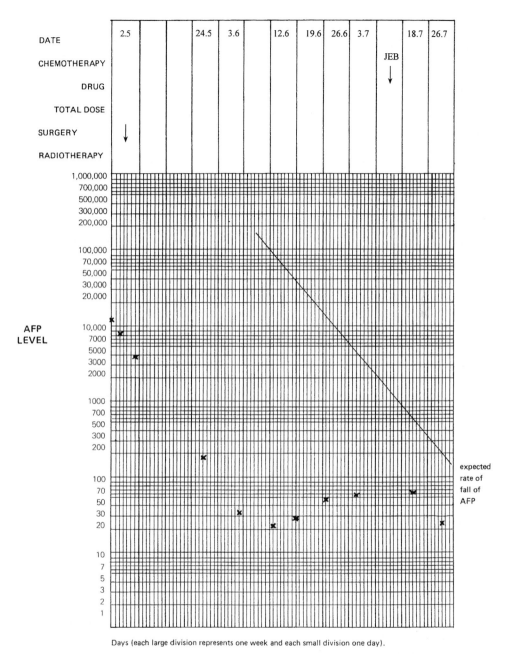

Fig. 18.3 Graph showing expected (solid line) and actual (✗) rates of fall of AFP following surgical removal of tumour. The rise after an initial fall heralded clinical relapse. JEB chemotherapy with carboplatin, etoposide, and bleomycin.

Orchidectomy should be carried out after high cord ligation through an inguinal approach. For ovarian tumours, sampling of the contralateral ovary and retroperitoneal nodes may be considered at the time of unilateral oophorectomy. For sacro-coccygeal lesions, excision must include the coccyx to prevent local recurrence. For other tumours, surgery is used to remove any residual disease following chemotherapy.

Radiotherapy

Dysgerminoma is a highly radiosensitive tumour. Radiotherapy may have a role in the management of stage II ovarian or testicular dysgerminoma, intracranial dysgerminoma, or in more advanced stage disease where residual tumour would be difficult to excise. Residual pelvic disease after surgical removal of stage II ovarian dysgerminoma will be cured in most patients by radiotherapy given with doses as low as 24–30 Gy.

In intracranial dysgerminoma, high cure rates of 80–95% can be achieved with craniospinal irradiation.

Tumours of this histological type, however, are also sensitive to chemotherapy, and the late toxicity of radiotherapy has led to an interest in investigating the role of chemotherapy. The optimum strategy is currently being sought in a SIOP randomized trial comparing standard craniospinal irradiation in one arm with chemotherapy, with local tumour radiotherapy.

For intracranial malignant teratomas and yolk sac tumours, chemotherapy alone is known to be inadequate for cure. In this situation, the role of chemotherapy added to radiotherapy is being investigated. Initial biopsy may be followed by neoadjuvant chemotherapy, surgery to remove any residual disease, and radiotherapy to the tumour bed. For patients presenting with spinal seedlings demonstrated by CSF cytology or a positive spinal MRI, chemotherapy is followed by craniospinal irradiation (see Chapter 12).

Chemotherapy

Since the first reports of the effectiveness of combination chemotherapy with platinum, vinblastine, and bleomycin by Einhorn in 1977 (Einhorn and Donohue 1977), a number of drugs have been shown to be effective in the treatment of germ-cell tumours. Drugs with single-agent activity include cisplatin, carboplatin, vinblastine, bleomycin, actinomycin, doxorubicin, methotrexate, etoposide, and iphosphamide (Loehrer et al. 1986; Pinkerton et al. 1990). Most commonly used drug combinations are shown in Table 18.5. Careful studies by German and British groups have suggested that bleomycin and etoposide may be necessary to maintain optimal control rates. Many groups use either bleomycin, etoposide with cisplatin or carboplatin (Pinkerton et al. 1991), or cisplatin, iphosphamide, and vinblastine as primary therapy (Göbel et al. 1993). Most schedules use between four and six courses of chemotherapy, and no advantage has been shown for maintenance therapy (Einhorn et al. 1989). In adult patients whose disease relapses after successful first-line chemotherapy, second remissions may be obtained using cisplatin and iphosphamide with either etoposide or vinblastine in up to 25% of patients (Loehrer et al. 1986).

There is some evidence that intensifying treatment with high-dose carboplatin and etoposide, with or without cyclophosphamide or iphosphamide, may increase the proportion of patients surviving up to 4 years after disease relapse by 15% or so (Nichols et al. 1992). These intensive approaches do not seem to have been reported yet in the treatment of relapsed disease in childhood and might be precluded by the risk of cumulative normal tissue toxicity.

Table 18.5 Chemotherapy for GCT

Drugs		Regimens
PVB	cisplatin	20 mg/m^2 iv days 1–5
	vinblastine	0.2 mg/kg iv days 1–2
	bleomycin	15 μ/m^2 days 2, 9, 16
JEB	carboplatin	600 mg/m^2 day 1
	etoposide	120 mg/m^2 days 1–3
	bleomycin	15 μ/m^2 day 2
BEP	bleomycin	15 μ/m^2 day 2
	etoposide	120 mg/m^2 days 1–3
	cisplatin	100 mg/m^2 iv day 1
CE/EI	carboplatin	600 mg/m^2 (AUC measure) day 1
	etoposide	100 mg/m^2 days 1, 2, 3
	etoposide	100 mg/m^2 3 days from day 22
	iphosphamide	1800 mg/m^2 5 days from day 22
PEI	cisplatin	20 mg/m^2 days 1–5
	etoposide	100 mg/m^2 days 1–3
	iphosphamide	1500 mg/m^2 days 1–5

(Source: Williams *et al.* 1987)

Specific sites

Testis

Germ-cell tumours of the testis commonly present as a painless unilateral swelling. Haemorrhage into a cyst, or additional trauma, may occasionally cause pain when a differential diagnosis of torsion of the testis may be considered. Backache may be a symptom if the para-aortic nodes are involved by tumour.

Staging investigations preoperatively should include measurement of serum AFP and β-HCG, and CT scanning of abdomen and chest. Initial treatment should be by orchidectomy through an inguinal incision with high cord ligation. Histological examination should include examination of the cut end of the cord for tumour, and search for vascular or lymphatic invasion, which indicate the need for further treatment.

Orchidectomy alone is curative for benign teratoma or stage I malignant tumours of any histological type, as long as there are no risk factors for relapse (see above) and any elevated markers return to normal values.

All other stages of disease should be treated with chemotherapy with a combination regimen (as shown in Table 18.5), with a minimum of two (poor-risk stage I disease) and up to six courses. Residual abdominal masses for malignant teratoma should be surgically removed because of the potential risk of dedifferentiation or metastases, even from apparently completely mature elements. Similarly, thoracotomy should be considered for residual lung metastases.

Ovary

Tumours in the ovary often present around puberty with abdominal distension with or without pain. Ascites may be present. There may be bowel or bladder symptoms from direct compression by a large mass or with hormonal disturbance such as precocious puberty, vaginal bleeding, or amenorrhoea. Most tumours are unilateral, and surgery should remove one ovary and one tube only, except in the rare cases of bilateral mature teratoma where partial excision is not possible, or streak ovaries where both should be removed to avoid subsequent development of gonadoblastoma (Scully 1970; Krasna *et al.* 1992). Surgery for an established, unilateral gonadoblastoma should also remove the contralateral ovary. Surgical staging, including removal or biopsy of para-aortic nodes and examination of the liver, such as may be undertaken for carcinoma of the ovary, is not appropriate.

No additional therapy is needed for true stage Ia disease, whatever the histology. For other stages, subsequent treatment depends on histology.

Dsygerminoma is sensitive to radiotherapy, and local pelvic irradiation to doses of 30 Gy for stage II disease will result in high cure rates. However, because of the late sequelae of radiotherapy, chemotherapy may be preferred in the younger girl and may be equally effective (Teinturier *et al.* 1994). Radiotherapy may be more appropriate than surgery for residual disease which may be densely fibrotic.

It is not yet clear when chemotherapy should be given for immature teratoma, but it may be considered postoperatively for patients with grade III histology.

All yolk sac tumours and malignant teratomas, except stage I, should receive chemotherapy with one of the regimens shown in Table 18.5.

Sacro-coccygeal region

These tumours, which are commoner in girls than boys, may be obvious prenatally on ultrasound or may present at birth with a large protruding mass. Lesser degrees of external abnormality, such as sacral pitting, may be associated with a large presacral mass which will cause disturbance of bowel or bladder function. In these cases, CT scanning will demonstrate the presacral mass. At birth or in early infancy these tumours are mostly mature teratoma with normal serum markers and, after biopsy to exclude malignant elements, should be excised together with the coccyx to prevent local recurrence. If there is raised serum AFP indicating yolk sac tumour or there are malignant elements on biopsy of the tumour, primary chemotherapy should be given followed by resection including the coccyx. Delay in excision of benign tumours may predispose to malignant change, so early surgery is advised (Schroppe *et al.* 1992).

Mediastinum

Mediastinal germ-cell tumours arise in the anterior mediastinum where they may be mistaken for normal thymus. The differential diagnosis includes T-cell leukaemia and lymphoma, from which they must be differentiated by marker or bone marrow studies or open biopsy. They are often diagnosed incidentally from chest X-ray, although they may cause cough, shortness of breath, or chest pain. They are commoner in males than females, may be associated with Klinefelters syndrome (Lachman *et al.* 1986), and have a poorer outcome to treatment than gonadal germ-cell tumours (Lack *et al.* 1985; Lakhoo *et al.* 1993). Secondary leukaemias have been reported, particularly in association with mediastinal GCT. In infants, yolk sac tumours or mature teratoma are most frequent (Orazi *et al.* 1993), whereas in older children, mixed-cell tumours are commoner. Primary surgical excision is usually not feasible, but residual tumour should be removed after appropriate chemotherapy has produced good regression.

Intracranial tumours

These are dealt with in Chapter 12 and their treatment summarized with that of other sites in Table 18.6.

Outcome of treatment

High cure rates can be expected from the treatment of these tumours, as is shown in the survival curves from the UKCCSG data (Fig. 18.4), which are similar to those obtained from other cooperative groups (Göbel *et al.* 1990; Albin *et al.* 1991). Care must be taken to minimize long-term sequelae. Renal toxicity from cisplatin and iphosphamide is of major concern, and ototoxicity with high-tone hearing loss occurs after cisplatin administration. Bleomycin may produce lung fibrosis, which can be precipitated by exposure to high oxygen concentrations, so that care must be taken with any anaesthetics given after this chemotherapy.

Etoposide has been associated with an increased risk of second tumour induction. In a series of adult patients from the Royal Marsden Hospital, 42 out of 859 patients with germ-cell tumours treated with chemotherapy containing etoposide developed leukaemia, giving a relative risk of 6.2 (Horwich and Bell 1994). There were no excess deaths from other causes in that series. Second malignancies resulting from etoposide administration must be distinguished from those arising from germ cells which are predominantly associated with mediastinal disease (Ladanyi *et al.* 1990; Orazi *et al.* 1993).

Fertility is preserved and pregnancy and delivery are unaffected by treatment, unless there is pituitary damage or iphosphamide is used. Children born to survivors have been normal.

Craniospinal irradiation will produce long-term problems of spinal growth with reduction in sitting height. Pituitary functional impairment (though less severe than may be produced by the primary tumour itself) and intellectual impairment may occur. The severity of the damage is inversely proportional to the age of the child at the time of treatment. Spinal irradiation may affect gonadal function because of scattered radiation.

Future improvements in outcome of these tumours are likely to come from tailoring treatment according to our growing understanding of prognostic risk factors, use of preoperative chemotherapy to increase operability, reduction in radiotherapy where appropriate, and intensification of therapy only for those patients at highest risk of relapse.

Table 18.6 Treatment recommendations

Stage	Histology and site	Treatment
any stage	mature teratoma (any site)	surgical excision
stage I	any malignant germ-cell tumour	surgical excision (unilateral for ovary and testis) with inguinal orchidectomy and surgical staging for ovarian tumours
poor-risk stage I	any malignant germ-cell tumour	chemotherapy after local excision
stage II–IV	malignant teratoma, gonads, retroperitoneum, mediastinum	chemotherapy and surgical excision of residual disease
stage III	grade III immature	surgery and chemotherapy
stage II–IV	dysgerminoma	chemotherapy radiotherapy for residual disease
IC GCT	mature	biopsy and excision
	malignant teratoma and yolk sac	biopsy, chemotherapy PEI + R/T tumour bed (54 Gy) CSF seeding CS R/T (30 Gy + 24 boost)
	germinoma	trial CS R/T (24 + boost 16 Gy) vv chemo + focal R/T (40 Gy) CE/IE × 2 SIOP study
	immature	as malignant if high-grade, incomplete excision, otherwise as benign
gonadoblastoma		bilateral excision
sacro-coccygeal tumours (benign)	AFP normal no evidence of metastatic disease, distinct capsule	primary surgical excision (including coccyx)
malignant		primary chemotherapy followed by surgical excision including the coccyx

IC GCT Intracranial germ cell tumours; PEI; CE/IE see table 18.5

MALIGNANT EXTRA-GONADAL GERM-CELL

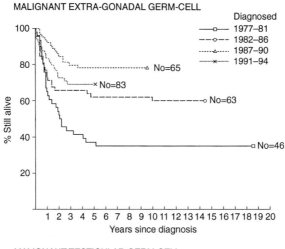

MALIGNANT TESTICULAR GERM-CELL

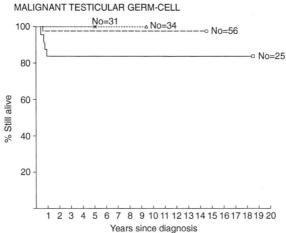

MALIGNANT OVARIAN GERM-CELL

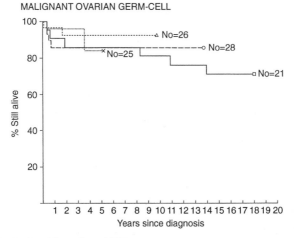

Fig. 18.4 Survival after treatment for malignant GCT.

References

Albin, A., Krailo, M., Ramsey, N.K.C., Malogolowkin, M.H., Isaacs, H., Raney, R.B., *et al.* (1991). Results of treatment of malignant germ cell tumors in 93 children: a report from the Children's Cancer Study Group. *Journal of Clinical Oncology*, 9, 1782.

Bartlett, N.L., Freiha, F.S., and Torto, F.M. (1991). Serum markers in germ cell neoplasms. *Haematology Oncology Clin North Am*, 5, 1245.

Chaganti, R.S.K., Rodriguez, E., and Matthew, S. (1994). Origin of adult male mediastinal germ cell tumours. *Lancet*, 343, 1130.

Einhorn, L.H. and Donohue, J.P. (1977). Cis-diaminedichloroplatinum, vinblastine and bleomycin combination chemotherapy in disseminated testicular cancer. *Annals of Internal Medicine*, 87, 293.

Einhorn, L.H., Williams, S.D., Loehrer, P.J., Birch, R., Drasga, R., Omura, G., *et al.* (1989). Evaluation of optimal duration of chemotherapy in favorable prognosis disseminated germ cell tumors: a Southeastern Cancer Study Group protocol. *Journal of Clinical Oncology*, 7, 387–391.

Giwercman, A., Grindsted, J., Hansen, B., Jensen, O.M., and Skakkebaek, N.E. (1987). Testicular cancer risk in boys with maldescended testes: a cohort study. *Journal of Urology*, 138, 1214.

Göbel, U., Haas, R.J., Calaminus, G., Bamberg, M., Bokkerink, E.B., Engert, J., *et al.* (1990). Treatment of germ cell tumors in children: results of European trials for testicular and non-testicular primary sites. *Crit Review of Oncology & Hematology*, 10, 89–98.

Göbel, U., Galaminus, G., Teske, C., Bamberg, M., Bokkerink, J.P., Haas, R.J., *et al.* (1993). BEP/VIP in children and adolescents with malignant non-testicular germ cell tumours. A comparison of the results of treatment in therapy studies MAKEI 83/86 and 89P/89. *Klin Padiatr*, 205, 231–40.

Hawkins, E. and Perlman, E. (1996). Germ cell tumors in childhood, morphology and biology. In Parham D.M., ed. Pediatric neoplasia: morphology and biology. New York: Raven Press, 297.

Heimdal, K., Lothe, R.A., Lystad, S., Holm R., Fossa, S.D., and Berresen, A. (1993). No germline TP53 mutations detected in familial and bilateral testicular cancer. *Genes Chromosomes Cancer*, 6, 92.

Hoffner, L., Deka, R., and Chakravarti, A. (1994). Cytogenetics and origins of pediatric germ cell tumors. *Cancer Genetics and Cytogenetics*, 74, 54.

Horwich, A. and Bell, J. (1994). Mortality and cancer incidence following radiotherapy for seminoma of the testis. *Radiotherapy and Oncology*, 30(3), 193–198.

Krasna, I.H., Lee, M.L., Smilow, P., Sciorra, L., and Eierman, L. (1992). Risk of malignancy in bilateral streak gonads: the role of the Y chromosome. *Journal of Pediatric Surgery*, 27, 1376.

Lachman, M.F., Kim, K., and Koo, B. (1986). Mediastinal teratoma associated with Klinefelter's syndrome. *Arch Pathol Lab Med*, 119, 1067.

Lack, E.E., Weinstein, H.J., and Welch, K.J. (1985). Mediastinal germ cell tumors in childhood: a clinical and pathologic study of 21 cases. *Journal of Thoracic Cardiovascular Surgery*, 89, 826.

Ladanyi, M., Samaniego, F., Reuter, V.E., Motzer, R.J., Jhanwar, S.C., Bosl, G.J., *et al.* (1990). Cytogenetic and immunohistochemical evidence for the germ cell origin of a subset of acute leukemias associated with mediastinal germ cell tumors. *Journal of the National Cancer Institute*, 82, 221.

Lakhoo, K., Boyle, M., and Drake, D.P. (1993). Mediastinal teratomas: review of 15 pediatric cases. *Journal of Pediatric Surgery*, 28, 1161.

Li, F.P. and Fraumeni, J.F. Jr. (1972). Testicular cancers in children. *Journal of the National Cancer Institute*, 44, 1575.

Loehrer, P.J., Einhorn, L.H., and Williams, S.D. (1986). VP-16 plus ifosfamide plus cisplatin as salvage therapy in refractory germ cell cancer. *Journal of Clinical Oncology*, 4, 528.

Mann, J.R. and Stiller, C.A. (1994). Changing pattern of incidence and survival in children with germ cell tumours (GCTs). *Advances in the Bioscience*, 92, 59–64.

Mann, J.R., Pearson, D, and Barrett, A. (1989). Results of the United Kingdom Children's Cancer Study Group's malignant germ cell tumor studies. *Cancer*, 54, 1687.

Nichols, C.R., Anderson, J., Lazarus, H.M., Fisher, H., Greer, J., Stadtmauer, E.A., *et al.* (1992). High dose carboplatin and etoposide with autologous bone marrow transplantation in refractory germ cell cancer: an Eastern Co-operative Oncology Group protocol. *Journal of Clinical Oncology*, 10, 558–63.

Orazi, A., Neiman, R., Ulbright, T., Heereman, N., John, K., and Nichols, C. (1993). Hematopoietic precursor cells within the yolk sac tumor component are the source of secondary hematopoietic malignancies in patients with mediastinal germ cell tumors. *Cancer*, 71, 3873.

Pinkerton, C.R., Broadbent, V., Horwich, A., Levitt, J., McElwain, T.J., Meller, S.T., *et al.* (1990). 'JEB': a carboplatin based regimen for malignant germ cell tumors in children. *British Journal of Cancer*, 62, 257–62.

Pinkerton, C.R., Levitt, J., Oakhill, A. *et al.* (1991). Carboplatin, etoposide, bleomycin regimen for advanced germ cell tumors in children. *Journal of Clinical Oncology*, 8, 14.

Samaniego, F., Rodriguez, E., Houldsworth, J., Murty, V.V., Ladanyi, M., Lele, K.P., *et al.* (1990). Cytogenetic and molecular analysis of human male germ cell tumors: chromosome 12 abnormalities and gene amplification. *Gene Chromosomes Cancer*, 1, 289.

Schroppe, K.P, Lobe, T., Rao, B., Mutabagani, K., Kay, G.A., Gilchrist, B.F., *et al.* (1992). Sacrococcygeal teratoma: the experience of four decades. *Journal of Pediatric Surgery*, 27, 1075.

Scully, R.E. (1970). Gonadoblastoma: a review of 74 cases. *Cancer*, 25, 1340.

Teinturier, C., Gelez, J., Flamant, F., Habrand, J.L., and Lemerle, J. (1994). Pure dysgerminoma of the ovary in childhood: treatment results and sequelae. *Medical and Pediatric Oncology*, 23, 1.

van Beneden, R.J. (1994). Molecular analysis of bivalve tumours: models for environmental/genetic interactions. *Environmental Health Perspectives*, 102, 81–83

Williams, S.D., Birch, R., Einhorn, L., Irwin, L., Greco, F.A., and Loehrer, P.J. (1987). Treatment of disseminated germ cell tumours with cisplatin, bleomycin and either vinblastine or etoposide. *N Engl J Med*, 316, 1435.

19 Hepatic tumours

Y. Tsuchida and H. Ikeda

When a child presents with a mass in the upper quadrant of the abdomen, the differential diagnosis includes hepatic malignancy which must be distinguished from a benign hepatic tumour, non-neoplastic hepatomegaly, and other abdominal tumours such as neuroblastoma or Wilms' tumour. According to published descriptions of cases of hepatic tumours, two-thirds of hepatic neoplasms were malignant (55–65%) and approximately 90% of the malignant tumours were epithelial tumours, hepatoblastoma, or hepatocellular carcinoma. Benign vascular tumours and malignant mesenchymal tumours account for the rest. The ratio of hepatoblastoma to hepatocellular carcinoma is approximately 1.8:1 in Western countries, but the incidence of hepatoblastoma is 5–6 times higher than that of hepatocellular carcinoma in Japan. Each tumour has its own specific age-group in which the majority of patients are seen, and associated congenital anomalies or underlying disorders are seen in some patients.

Hepatoblastoma

Hepatoblastoma is the most common malignant hepatic tumour in children in any part of the world, except areas where hepatocellular carcinoma is more common due to endemic hepatitis B infection with its vertical transmission (Chen *et al.* 1988). Approximately 1–2% of all malignant tumours in children are hepatoblastoma. The incidence of hepatoblastoma in children younger than 15 years is less than 1 per 1, 000, 000 in North America (Young and Miller 1975). In Japan, the incidence appears to be higher than in Western countries and the ratio of males to females is 1.2:1. Although hepatoblastoma occurs at any age under 15 years, more than 80% of the tumours are seen in children 3 years of age or younger, and 45% of the patients are diagnosed during the first year of life.

Genetics and biology

Hepatoblastoma may occur in association with a variety of congenital anomalies, disorders, and environmental factors. Beckwith-Wiedemann syndrome and hemihypertrophy carry an increased risk of this tumour as well as Wilms' tumour, rhabdomyosarcoma, and adrenocortical tumours. Abnormalities on the short arm of chromosome 11 have been shown in both Beckwith-Wiedemann syndrome and hepatoblastoma, and loss of heterozygosity of 11p15 has frequently been observed (Albrecht *et al.* 1994). A tumour-suppressor gene or a growth factor gene which is located in the 11p15.5 region may be responsible for the development of the tumour. Hepato-blastoma is a specific malignant tumour in children from families with familial adenomatous poly-posis. Inactivation of the adenomatous polyposis coli gene, which is a putatively mutated tumour-suppressor gene in familial adenomatous polyposis, may be responsible for the tumouri-genesis (Kurahashi *et al.* 1995; Giardiello *et al.* 1996). Rare occurrence of the tumour in children with trisomy 18 syndrome or Prader-Willi syndrome has been reported, but the relationship between the syndrome and development of hepatoblastoma is unclear (Hashizume *et al.* 1991; Tanaka *et al.* 1992). Some possible connections between contraceptive intake, alcohol abuse during pregnancy, and hormonal treatment for sterility and the occurrence of hepatoblastoma have been reported (Otten *et al.* 1977; Khan *et al.* 1979; Melamed *et al.* 1982). Maternal occupational exposure to metals, petroleum products, and paints or pigments, and paternal exposure to metals appear to be risk factors (Buckley *et al.* 1989). It was also reported that a patient's extremely low birth weight (< 1000 g) was associated with the development of hepatoblastoma, although the reason for the association is unknown (Ikeda *et al.* 1997). These clinical and epidemiological analyses suggest that hepatoblastoma is an embryonal tumour which results from developmental disturbances during organogenesis due to a number of aetiological factors.

Cytogenetic studies of tumour cells have shown that trisomy of chromosomes 2 and 20 is frequently observed in hepatoblastoma (Soukup and Lampkin 1991; Swarts *et al.* 1996). Overexpression of p53 protein has been demonstrated with a variable incidence by immunohisto-chemistry, but the mutation of the *p53* gene is infrequent (Kennedy *et al.* 1994; Chen *et al.* 1995). Abnormalities of p53 may not be as important as in adult hepatocellular carcinomas.

DNA content analyses have shown that patients with diploid hepatoblastoma have a better prognosis than those with aneuploid tumour. Tumours with a low-proliferation index are also prognostically favourable (Hata *et al.* 1991; Schmidt *et al.* 1993).

Pathology

Hepatoblastoma is usually solitary, and 20% of tumours extend multifocally or infiltrate diffusely into the liver. The cut surface has a lobulated appearance due to fibrous septa. Multiple varie-gated nodules with haemorrhage and necrosis are surrounded by a pseudocapsule. The adjacent liver is not cirrhotic. Microscopically, pure epithelial hepatoblastoma is distinguished from mixed hepatoblastoma, which contains mesenchymal tissue in addition to epithelial elements (Weinberg and Finegold 1983; Haas *et al.* 1989). The epithelial components exhibit a range of differentia-tion represented by fetal, embryonal, and anaplastic cells. Well-differentiated 'fetal' cells are smaller than normal hepatocytes and have a low nucleocytoplasmic ratio, minimal nuclear pleo-morphism, and small nucleoli. Mitoses are infrequent. The cells are arranged in slender cords, usually two cell layers thick, which often contain canaliculi with or without bile. Sinusoids and vessels resembling central veins are present. Foci of extramedullary haematopoiesis are common (Fig. 19.1). Poorly differentiated 'embryonal' cells have a higher nucleocytoplasmic ratio and mitoses are seen more frequently than in fetal areas. The embryonal cells grow in sheets assum-ing a tubular configuration, or rosettes which recapitulate some features of the embryonic liver (Fig. 19.2). 'Anaplastic' type hepatoblastoma consists of sheets of cells with scant cytoplasm and a high mitotic rate, which are small, undifferentiated, round-to-oval or spindle in shape, and mono-typic. The term 'macrotrabecular' is used to indicate foci of tumour cells which are repetitively

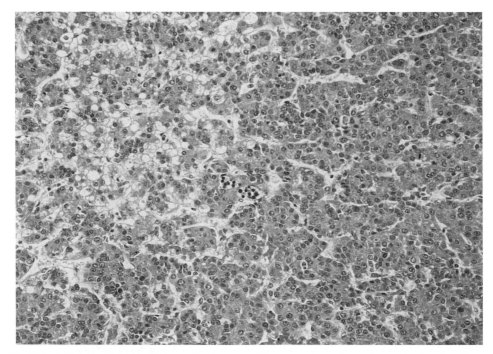

Fig. 19.1 Fetal hepatoblastoma. Cells are smaller than normal hepatocytes, have a low nucleocytoplasmic ratio, and are arranged in slender cords. A cluster of haematopoietic cells is seen.

arranged in trabeculae, 10 or more cells thick. The tumour cells may be fetal or embryonal in appearance or indistinguishable from the cells of adult hepatocellular carcinoma. Immature mesenchymal components in mixed hepatoblastoma include osteoid, chondroid, or rarely rhabdomyoblastic tissues in addition to blood vessels or haematopoietic tissues which are an integral part of the tumour. The epithelial differentiation occasionally yields squamous pearls or mucus-secreting glands, and neuronal differentiation is rarely seen in hepatoblastoma.

Although available data are limited, epithelial components of hepatoblastoma are associated with improved prognosis, and the pure fetal type is prognostically favourable when completely resected (Haas *et al.* 1989). It is not yet conclusive that the presence of macrotrabecular foci predicts a poor prognosis. The prognostic importance of mesenchymal components has not been determined.

Diagnosis

Since a child with advanced disease occasionally presents with anorexia, weight loss, or anaemia, the general condition of the patient should be carefully examined. Necessary supportive management is given when the general condition has deteriorated, while diagnostic studies are done for suspected hepatoblastoma.

Alpha-fetoprotein (AFP) is a glycoprotein synthesized in the yolk sac and the liver at an early stage of fetal life. The production of AFP stops at birth and the serum AFP concentration

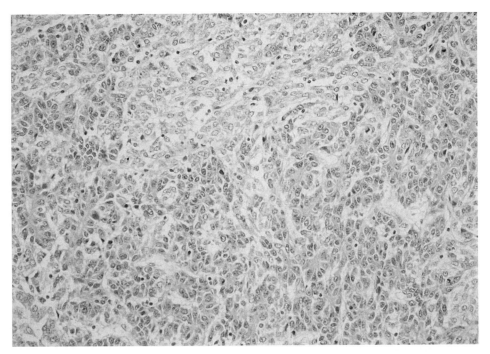

Fig. 19.2 Embryonal hepatoblastoma. Cells grow in sheets assuming a tubular configuration or rosettes which recapitulate some features of the embryonic liver.

decreases exponentially from a mean of approximately 50, 000 ng ml^{-1} to a level of less than 20 ng ml^{-1} at 6–8 months of age. The serum AFP concentration is raised above the upper limit of the normal ranges for the patient's age in more than 98% of patients. Although the AFP concentration is relatively higher in hepatoblastomas with embryonal histology than in tumours with fetal histology, this is not prognostically significant. Fractionation of AFP by lectin-affinity immunoelectrophoresis differentiates hepatic malignant tumours from yolk sac tumour and benign hepatic disease, such as hepatitis or cirrhosis (Tsuchida *et al.* 1989; Ishiguro and Tsuchida 1994). AFP derived from hepatoblastoma or hepatocellular carcinoma includes a subfraction which binds to *Lens culinaris* haemagglutinin (LCH), but AFP from a benign hepatic disease does not react with LCH. The presence of a greater amount (> 25%) of AFP fraction which is not reactive to concanavalin A (Con A) differentiates AFP derived from a yolk sac tumour from that of hepatic origin (Fig. 19.3a and b). Since serum AFP concentrations are expected to decline exponentially after complete tumour resection, and remain within the normal limits unless recurrence occurs, the measurement of AFP is useful practically in monitoring the disease course, as well as in making a diagnosis.

Isosexual precocious puberty may develop in patients with hepatoblastoma secreting human chorionic gonadotropin (β-HCG). Virilization in male children with testicular and penile enlargement and growth of pubic hair has been reported (Murthy *et al.* 1980).

Thrombocytosis may be seen in some patients, but mild normochromic normocytic anaemia is usual. Interleukin-6, which seems to be produced in stromal cells in response to local secretion of

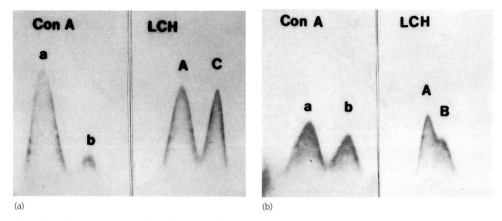

Fig. 19.3 Alpha-fetoprotein (AFP) subfraction profile in (a) hepatoblastoma, and (b) yolk sac tumour. AFP derived from hepatoblastoma includes a subfraction which binds to *Lens culinaris* haemagglutinin (LCH). The presence of a greater amount (> 25%) of fraction non-reactive to concanavalin A (Con A) differentiates AFP derived from a yolk sac tumour from AFP of hepatic origin. a: reactive; b: non-reactive; A: strongly reactive; B: weakly reactive; C: non-reactive.

cytokines from tumour cells, has been shown to mediate thrombocytosis and acute reactions including fever (von Schweinitz *et al.* 1993). Routine work-up occasionally demonstrates hypercholesterolaemia or osteoporosis. The latter may be complicated by pathological fracture.

Pretreatment imaging studies include plain radiography, ultrasonography, and computed tomography (CT) or magnetic resonance imaging (MRI). Plain films of the abdomen occasionally demonstrate the presence of calcifications. On ultrasonography, the echogenicity of the tumour is minimally increased and usually inhomogeneous. Hypoechoic or anechoic areas, which reflect necrosis or haemorrhage within the tumour, may be seen. The unenhanced CT demonstrates the tumour with decreased attenuation in respect to the surrounding liver parenchyma, which is emphasized with intravenous contrast infusion. T1-weighted images of MRI show decreased signal intensity of the tumour, but T2-weighted images show increased signal intensity. In addition to the qualitative evaluation, the surgical resectability of the tumour is determined. Tumours involving both lobes of the liver or vascular structures such as the portal veins or the inferior vena cava are usually unresectable. The presence or absence of portal and para-aortic lymphadenopathy and lung metastases are evaluated by either CT or MRI. With modern MRI techniques, adequate information for treatment is obtained. Surgeons, however, prefer to have an angiogram performed to define the relationship of the tumour to major hepatic vessels. Anatomical variation of hepatic arteries should be identified. Hepatic angiography may also be combined with tumour embolization or intra-arterial infusional chemotherapy.

Bone scan should be done to investigate metastatic spread. Bone marrow aspirates are unnecessary.

Staging

There is no universally accepted system of staging in hepatoblastoma. In the staging system of the Children's Cancer Group and the Paediatric Oncology Group in the US, stage I tumour is defined as a tumour resected completely at initial laparotomy, stage II as a tumour with micro-scopic residue, stage III as a tumour with gross residual tumour. Children with distant metastases have stage IV disease (Ortega *et al.* 1991; Douglass *et al.* 1993). The staging system used in the German Cooperative Paediatric Liver Tumour Study HB-89 was identical to the system in the US (von Schweinitz *et al.* 1994). The International Society of Paediatric Oncology (SIOP) has devel-oped a pretreatment staging system to classify the tumour by identifying the number of liver seg-ments involved (Vos 1995). Staging laparotomy is unnecessary in this system, and stage can be determined from the results of imaging studies. A classification is adopted in Japan which is based on the number of liver segments involved, the extent of local invasion, the regional lymph-node involvement, and the presence of distant metastases.

Surgical treatment

Complete surgical resection has been the most effective treatment for children with hepatoblas-toma, but less than 50% of tumours are resectable at the time of diagnosis. Tumours involving both lobes of the liver or invading the porta hepatis are usually unresectable, and preoperative chemotherapy is indicated to render the tumour resectable. Histological diagnosis prior to chemotherapy may be made on specimens obtained by fine-needle biopsy. A wedge biopsy of the tumour through a small laparotomy incision is preferred to obtain a specimen large enough for the investigation of biological characteristics of the tumour.

The tumour is deemed resectable if it is localized in one or two segments of the liver. Complete resection is achieved by performing a segmentectomy or a standard lobectomy. Left or right trisegmentectomy may be done when the tumour occupies three segments of the liver. The abdomen is entered through a large transverse incision above the umbilicus. The liver is mobilized by dividing the ligaments which attach the liver to the abdominal wall and the diaphragm to facilitate access to the hepatic veins and the inferior vena cava. Sudden circulatory deterioration may occur if the inferior vena cava is angulated by an excess displacement of the liver. Dissection begins in the porta hepatis, and the branches of the hepatic artery, portal vein, and bile duct are isolated and divided according to the part of the liver to be excised. The hepatic vein should be carefully identified, ligated, and divided, because haemorrhage from an injured hepatic vein is difficult to control and may be fatal in some cases. After ligation of the hepatic vessels, an ischaemic colour change on the surface of the liver demarcates the lobe to be resected. Many surgeons prefer to use an ultrasonic surgical aspirator (CUSA) in dissection. A narrow margin between the tumour and the dissection line is acceptable in some fetal-type hepa-toblastoma. The raw surface of the remaining liver is checked for bleeding and bile leakage, and covered with fibrin glue if necessary. Postoperative chemotherapy is withheld for one or two weeks.

Pulmonary recurrence, which is probably the late appearance of metastatic deposits present at the time of diagnosis or initial operation, may develop usually within 12 months after diagnosis. Intensive chemotherapy should be given prior to resection of the pulmonary metastases, and patients with pulmonary metastases are usually treated primarily with an aggressive surgical approach, as long as the number and location of metastatic nodules is precisely known by means of radiological evaluation (Black *et al.* 1991). Patients may survive disease-free after several thoracotomies (Fig. 19.4).

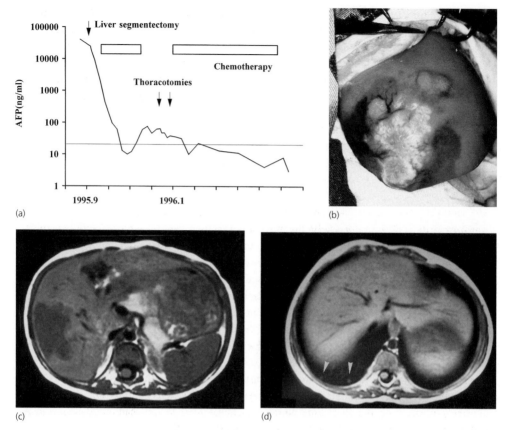

Fig. 19.4 Serum AFP levels became normal after nine courses of chemotherapy with cisplatin and THP-adriamycin, and the resection of pulmonary metastases. (b) Gross appearance of hepatoblastoma which originated in the right lobe of the liver. (c) T1-weighted MR images showed decreased signal intensity of the tumour. (d) MR was useful in evaluating the number and location of metastatic nodules (arrowed) ranging from 3–5 mm in diameter.

Chemotherapy and clinical trials

In late 1980s, the Paediatric Oncology Group of the US conducted a study to evaluate the survival rate in children with grossly resected hepatoblastoma treated with cisplatin, vincristine, and fluorouracil, and to assess the response rate and survival rate in children with initially unresectable tumours treated with the combination (Douglass *et al.* 1993). Patients with completely resected tumours whose histology was purely fetal were monitored without further treatment. Patients with completely resected tumours with other histology or patients with microscopic residual disease received five courses of chemotherapy postoperatively. The first course was cisplatin alone, and the four subsequent courses consisted of cisplatin, vincristine, and fluorouracil. Actuarial survival at 5 years was 90%. Patients with unresectable or metastatic disease received the same initial five courses. Two more courses were given after tumour resection, and radiotherapy in addition to chemotherapy was given to those whose tumour remained unresectable. Twenty-four of 31 patients with unresectable disease achieved a complete remission after chemotherapy and surgery, and actuarial survival at 4 years was 67%. Only one of eight patients with metastatic disease achieved remission and survived.

During the same period, the Children's Cancer Group of the US undertook a study to test the feasibility of administering adriamycin by continuous infusion, and cisplatin to patients with unresectable or incompletely resected hepatoblastoma and hepatocellular carcinoma (Ortega *et al.* 1991). A second-look operation was performed after four courses of chemotherapy. Out of the 33 patients with hepatoblastoma, there was no evidence of residual disease in nine (27%) patients, and complete resection of the remaining tumour was possible in seven (21%). Four additional courses of chemotherapy were given to those patients with total tumour resection at the second-look operation, while patients with residual disease received chemotherapy and radiation. The overall response rate of hepatoblastoma patients was 76% and the survival at 2 years was 67%.

The German Cooperative Paediatric Liver Tumour Study HB-89 was started in 1989 (von Schweinitz *et al.* 1995). In this study, all children had initial laparotomy, except infants under 1 year of age with high serum AFP and distant metastases. Tumours confined to one lobe of the liver were resected by a conventional lobectomy. In tumours involving both lobes, or those with distant metastases, a biopsy was taken and followed by chemotherapy. A second-look operation was carried out after two to four courses of chemotherapy. Chemotherapy consisted of a combination of iphosphamide, cisplatin, and adriamycin, and in cases of complete tumour regression, high-dose cisplatin and adriamycin as a continuous infusion were added. In their study, complete tumour resection was achieved in 76% of patients with advanced or metastatic disease and was significantly related to disease-free survival.

SIOP has been conducting a study which adopted a regimen of continuous infusion of cisplatin and adriamycin, assuming that it is less toxic than a regimen of bolus administration (Plaschkes *et al.* 1994). Preliminary results showed that more than 80% of patients had complete resection and that the overall survival at 18 months was also more than 80%.

In Japan, a study conducted by the Japanese Study Group for Paediatric Liver Tumours is now in progress (Hata *et al.* 1994). A chemotherapeutic regimen for unresectable tumours is similar to the one used in the SIOP study, but adriamycin is replaced by THP-adriamycin to reduce the cardiac toxicity of the regimen. The effectiveness of intra-arterial infusion chemotherapy, compared with that of systemic intravenous chemotherapy, is also being investigated. Conclusive results have not yet been reported.

A combination of etoposide, iphosphamide, and cisplatin for relapsed, refractory, solid tumours has been tested by POG (van Hoff *et al.* 1995). Daily doses of cisplatin 20 mg m^{-2}, etoposide 100 mg m^{-2}, and iphosphamide 1.5 g m^{-2} are administered for 3 days. All of the evaluable 10 patients responded to the treatment, and six of them had a complete response with a duration ranging from 4–48 months (see Table 19.1).

Experimental treatment

The systemic infusion of chemotherapeutic agents has been advocated, and acceptable results have been reported, as already mentioned. Despite aggressive chemotherapeutic regimens, however, approximately 30% of unresectable tumours are still resistant to treatment, which is the reason why an alternative treatment has to be sought. Intra-arterial infusion of chemotherapeutic

Table 19.1 Chemotherapy regimens in clinical trials for hepatoblastoma

1. *Paediatric Oncology Group*

   Stage I, favourable histology: no further treatment

   Stage I, unfavourable histology and stage II:
   Course 1: cisplatin 90 mg/m^2 alone
   Course 2–5: cisplatin 90 mg/m^2 on day 1, and vincristine 1.5 mg/m^2, and fluorouracil 600 mg/m^2 on day 3, every 3 weeks
   (Cisplatin dose was modified to 3 mg/kg[1] for children weighing less than 10 kg)

   Stages III and IV:
   Course 1–5 same as stages I and II
   After tumour resection, two courses of cisplatin, vincristine, and fluorouracil are added.
   If still unresectable, two courses of chemotherapy and radiotherapy are given.

2. *Children's Cancer Group*

   Unresectable or incompletely resected HB:
   Cisplatin 100 mg/m^2 on day 1 and adriamycin 20 mg/m^2 per day continuously infused on days 1–4, every 3–4 weeks

3. *German Cooperative Paediatric Liver Tumour Study HB-89*

   Unresectable or incompletely resected HB:
   Iphosphamide 0.5 g/m^2 bolus and 3.0 g/m^2 over 72 hours on days 1–3, cisplatin 20 mg/m^2 5 times on days 4–8, and adriamycin 60 mg/m^2 over 48 hours on days 9–10, two to four courses every 3 weeks
   Two courses of chemotherapy are administered in patients with unresectable tumour at second-look operation.
   If tumour involution is insufficient, cisplatin 90 mg/m^2 over 4 hours on day 1 and adriamycin 80 mg/m^2 over 96 hours on days 2–5 are administered.

4. *International Society of Paediatric Oncology (SIOPEL)*

   Cisplatin 80 mg/m^2 over 24 hours on day 1 and adriamycin 60 mg/m^2 over 48 hours on days 2–3, every 3 weeks

5. *Japanese Study Group for Paediatric Liver Tumour (J-PLT)*

   Resectable HB:
   Cisplatin 40 mg/m^2 and THP-adriamycin 30 mg/m^2 on day 1, six courses every 4 weeks
   Unresectable HB:
   Cisplatin 80 mg/m^2 over 24 hours on day 1, and THP-adriamycin 60 mg/m^2 over 48 hours on days 2–3, six courses every 4 weeks

agents via the hepatic artery, with the intention of increasing the antitumour effect of the agents, may yield promising results (Tsuchida *et al.* 1990).

Ligation of the hepatic artery or tumour embolization with materials such as gelfoam in combination with chemotherapy may be effective in decreasing tumour volume. Immunotargeting chemotherapy with an anti-AFP monoclonal antibody conjugated with adriamycin or cisplatin is still experimental (Hata *et al.* 1992).

Liver transplantation has been done as a final approach to the treatment of refractory hepatoblastomas (Tagge *et al.* 1992). Although only a limited number of patients have undergone the procedure, the results were successful in some patients. The shortage of donors continues to be one of the major problems in the transplant programme.

Hepatocellular carcinoma

Hepatocellular carcinoma accounts for 10–30% of primary, malignant, hepatic tumours in Western countries and Japan, but is more prevalent and outnumbers hepatoblastoma in areas where hepatitis B virus infection is endemic. In Taiwan, 80% of primary, malignant, hepatic tumours in children are hepatocellular carcinoma (Chen *et al.* 1988). The tumour usually occurs in children older than 5 years of age. Male predominance is more prominent than it is in hepatoblastoma.

Hepatitis B virus infection is causally associated with the development of hepatocellular carcinoma. A study from Taiwan demonstrated a high positive rate of hepatitis B surface antigen (HBsAg) in Taiwanese children with the tumour (Chen *et al.* 1988). A method using the polymerase chain reaction demonstrated the integration of DNA sequences of the virus in tumours of children who were serologically negative for hepatitis B (Pontisso *et al.* 1992). This finding supports the idea that hepatitis B virus may play a role in the development of this tumour in children from non-endemic areas, and without overt infection. In adult hepatocellular carcinoma, the sequence of nucleic acids of the hepatitis C virus was detected by the same method in tumour tissues (Gerber *et al.* 1992), but no association between hepatitis C virus infection and childhood hepatocellular carcinoma has been demonstrated.

The tumour is recognized to be associated with a number of underlying chronic liver diseases, including tyrosinaemia, biliary atresia, idiopathic neonatal hepatitis, and α_1-antitrypsin deficiency. Children with the chronic form of hereditary tyrosinaemia develop cirrhosis and eventually hepatocellular carcinoma (Salt *et al.* 1992). The incidence of the tumour exceeds 35% if the children survive for more than 2 years (Weinberg and Feingold 1983). Patients with biliary atresia who survive more than 3 years after portal-jejunostomy are at high risk for the tumour. Patients with α_1-antitrypsin deficiency are also at high risk, but the tumour usually develops in adult life (Eriksson *et al.* 1986). Glucose-6-phosphatase deficiency (type 1 glycogen storage disease), Fanconi's anaemia, and Wilson's disease are among the associated disorders. Long-term parenteral nutrition and resultant biliary cirrhosis is also an underlying cause of hepatocellular carcinoma (Vileisis *et al.* 1982).

Pathology

The gross and microscopic features of hepatocellular carcinoma in children are similar to those seen in adults, except for the lower incidence of underlying cirrhosis. Pre-existing cirrhosis is present in 5–30% of children, whereas 50–85% of adult hepatocellular carcinomas occur in cirrhotic liver. The tumour occurs as multiple nodules or a diffusely infiltrating mass involving both lobes of the liver. The cut surface is often bile-stained, and haemorrhage and necrosis within the tumour are seen more often than in hepatoblastoma. Pseudoencapsulation is less conspicuous. Tumour cells are larger than normal hepatocytes. Histological features distinguishing hepatocellular carcinoma from hepatoblastoma include broad trabeculae, nuclear pleomorphism, nucleolar prominence, and the presence of tumour giant cells. Extramedullary haematopoiesis is not seen in hepatocellular carcinoma.

Diagnosis

Abdominal pain and a palpable mass are the most common initial manifestations and hepato-splenomegaly is the sign most frequently observed in hepatocellular carcinoma. Fever, weight loss, and jaundice are occasionally observed. Shock due to tumour rupture and intra-abdominal bleeding may be the initial manifestation. Anaemia and mild hyperbilirubinaemia are the principal laboratory abnormalities, and the serum AFP concentration is high in 50–80% of patients. Serological evaluation should be done to examine for the possible presence of hepatitis B infection.

The sonographic findings of hepatocellular carcinoma are much like those of hepatoblastoma. The tumour has typically lower attenuation than normal tissue on unenhanced CT, and lower signal intensity on T1-weighted images and higher signal intensity on T2-weighted images than the surrounding liver on MR. Calcification is seen in up to 10% of cases. As these are the same findings as those in hepatoblastoma, differentiation of the two may be difficult by radiological studies. Occasionally, however, the growth patterns of the tumours may be useful in differentiating them. Tumours with smaller satellite lesions and those invading the portal vein or metastasizing are more often hepatocellular carcinomas. Metastatic spread is to the lungs, regional lymph nodes, and rarely to the bone.

Treatment

It is true that complete resection is the basis of successful treatment in hepatocellular carcinoma as in hepatoblastoma, but the resectability of the tumour remains as low as 10–20%. The unresectability and the presence of jaundice at presentation seem to be factors indicating unfavourable prognosis. Most children with the tumour die within 12 months of diagnosis. Although the intensive chemotherapy regimens of the several cooperative studies have been used, the results so far have generally been dismal.

The Children's Cancer Group reported that cisplatin and continuous infusion of adriamycin had been administered to 14 patients with unresectable or metastatic hepatocellular carcinomas, and only two of the patients were alive without evidence of the disease at the time of the report (Ortega *et al.* 1991). In the German Cooperative Paediatric Liver Tumour Study HB-89, in which unresectable or incompletely resected tumours were treated with the combination of iphosphamide, cisplatin, and adriamycin, only three of 10 patients were free from the tumour (von Schweinitz *et al.* 1994). A preliminary result from the SIOP liver tumour study group has shown that nine of 43 patients (21%) treated with cisplatin and adriamycin are alive, with no evidence of the disease at intervals ranging from 4–39 months (Plaschkes *et al.* 1994).

Total hepatectomy and orthotopic liver transplantation appears to be an effective method for the treatment of hepatocellular carcinoma (Tagge *et al.* 1992). An aggressive treatment with liver transplantation, including upper abdominal exenteration followed by multiple organ transplantation, has been performed. Four (44%) out of the nine patients who underwent the procedures were alive with no evidence of disease, with a mean duration of 2.3 years. Other experience with liver transplantation in children with tyrosinaemia showed that pulmonary metastases might develop from the occult tumour present at the time of transplantation (Salt *et al.* 1992).

Fibrolamellar carcinoma (fibrolamellar variant of hepatocellular carcinoma)

Fibrolamellar carcinoma, a distinctive variant of hepatocellular carcinoma, occurs in the non-cirrhotic livers of older children and young adults, without sex preference. The tumour is not associated with underlying liver disease, viral infection, or metabolic abnormality. The serum AFP is not high in the majority of patients. A specific abnormality of the vitamin B_{12}-binding protein has been documented (Paradinas *et al.* 1982). The level of unsaturated vitamin B_{12}-binding protein is significantly high in fibrolamellar carcinoma and rises with disease progression. The imaging characteristics are generally similar to those described for hepatocellular carcinoma. The gross appearance of the tumour most often consists of single, well-circumscribed, pseudoencapsulated rather than diffusely infiltrating masses, which may be similar to those of focal nodular hyperplasia. The differentiation between these two lesions requires microscopic evaluation. Microscopically, fibrolamellar carcinoma is characterized by large, plump, and polygonal cells encompassed by fibrous bands. The cytoplasm is granular and deeply eosinophilic, and is ultrastructurally abundant in mitochondria.

Fibrolamellar carcinoma differs from the ordinary hepatocellular carcinoma in clinical presentation and biological behaviour, as well as in histological features (Farhi *et al.* 1983). The former is characterized by a longer duration of symptoms prior to diagnosis and increased frequency of resectability (60%). Histologically, mitoses are less frequent in fibrolamellar carcinoma. Importantly, prolonged disease-free survival compared to that usual for hepatocellular carcinoma is expected if the tumour is completely resected, although the prognostic difference between the tumours was reported to be insignificant after adjustment for disease stage (Haas *et al.* 1989).

Biological investigation of fibrolamellar carcinoma has been rare except for one study which showed the non-diploid DNA content of the tumour.

Undifferentiated (embryonal) sarcoma of the liver

Undifferentiated (embryonal) sarcoma of the liver is a highly aggressive tumour most often presenting in late childhood as an abdominal mass, pain, or fever. There is no sex preponderance. The levels of serum AFP have been reported to be always within the normal range. The gross findings of the tumour are relatively consistent and show cystic areas and gelatinous tissues with extensive necrosis and haemorrhage. Demarcation from the surrounding liver appears sharp, but there may be microscopic infiltration and permeation to the veins. Histologically, the tumour shows a proliferation of spindle cells, with occasional polygonal or round cells loosely or densely arranged in a myxomatous background. Bizarre and multinucleated giant cells and PAS (periodic acid-Schiff)-positive hyaline globules of various sizes are frequently observed. Entrapped bile ducts, together with non-neoplastic hepatocytes, are observed at the periphery of the tumour. Positive immunostaining for histiocytic markers (α_1-antitrypsin, α_1-antichymotrypsin), muscle markers (desmin and muscle-specific actin), and vimentin is fairly consistent (Aoyama *et al.* 1991). Along with the electron microscopic findings, a mesenchymal origin of the tumour, presumably from a very primitive precursor cell, is suggested.

Radiological evaluation by ultrasonography and computerized tomography (CT) typically reveals a large intrahepatic mass with a wide range of solid and cystic components, which correlate with areas of haemorrhage, necrosis, and cystic degeneration. Complete excision and adjuvant multiagent chemotherapy appear to be essential in achieving long-term survival. No rationally invented adjuvant treatment, however, is known, due to the lack of large-scale clinical studies. Although a literature review showed that more than a third of the patients had survived without evidence of the disease for an average of 3 years, it seems too early to be optimistic about prognosis (Leuschner *et al.* 1990).

Other liver tumours

The other primary, malignant, mesenchymal tumours of the liver include rhabdomyosarcoma, leiomyosarcoma, angiosarcoma, fibrosarcoma, yolk sac tumour, and rhabdoid tumour. Embryonal rhabdomyosarcomas are rare, malignant tumours of the biliary tract, and may be found anywhere from the ampulla of Vater to the liver proper. Tumours with evidence of striated muscle differentiation are diagnosed as rhabdomyosarcomas, but a histological distinction between undifferentiated sarcoma and rhabdomyosarcoma may sometimes be difficult. Rhabdomyosarcomas are detected in patients usually less than 4 years of age, and tend to present with obstructive jaundice. A dismal prognosis with an average survival of less than 6 months has been reported, but aggressive surgery, combined with multiagent chemotherapy and radiotherapy, may provide the best chance for longer survival.

Yolk sac tumour and choriocarcinoma, though extremely rare, may arise in the liver. The presence of aberrant germ cells is thought to explain the development of yolk sac tumour in the liver.

A variety of paediatric solid tumours, including neuroblastoma, Wilms' tumour, rhabdomyosarcoma, and yolk sac tumour, metastasize to the liver. Details are discussed in the chapters describing these tumours.

References

Albrecht, S., von Schweinitz, D., Waha, A., Kraus, J.A., von Deimling, A., and Pietsch, T. (1994). Loss of maternal alleles on chromosome arm 11p in hepatoblastoma. *Cancer Research*, 54, 5041–4.

Aoyama, C., Hachitanda, Y., Sato, J.K., Said, J.W., and Shimada, H. (1991). Undifferentiated (embryonal) sarcoma of the liver. *American Journal of Surgical Pathology*, 15, 615–24.

Black, C.T., Luck, S.R., Musemeche, C.A., and Andrassy, R.J. (1991). Aggressive excision of pulmonary metastases is warranted in the management of childhood hepatic tumours. *Journal of Paediatric Surgery*, 26, 1082–6.

Buckley, J.D., Sather, H., Ruccione, K., Rogers, P.C., Haas, J.E., Henderson, B.E., *et al.* (1989). A case-control study of risk factors for hepatoblastoma. *Cancer*, 64, 1169–76.

Chen, T., Hsieh, L.L., and Kuo, T. (1995). Absence of p53 gene mutation and infrequent overexpression of p53 protein in hepatoblastoma. *Journal of Pathology*, 176, 243–7.

Chen, W.J., Lee, J.C., and Hung, W.T. (1988). Primary malignant tumours of liver in infants and children in Taiwan. *Journal of Paediatric Surgery*, 23, 457–61.

Douglass, E.C., Reynolds, M., Finegold, M., Cantor, A.B., and Glicksman, A. (1993). Cisplatin, vincristine, and fluorouracil therapy for hepatoblastoma: a Paediatric Oncology Group Study. *Journal of Clinical Oncology*, 11, 96–9.

Eriksson, S., Carlson, J., and Velez, R. (1986). Risk of cirrhosis and primary liver cancer in alpha-1-antitrypsin deficiency. *New England Journal of Medicine*, 314, 736–9.

Farhi, D.C., Shikes, R.H., Murari, P.J., and Silverberg, S.G., (1983). Hepatocellular carcinoma in young people. *Cancer*, 52, 1516–25.

Gerber, M.A., Carol-Shieh, Y.S., Shim, K.S., Thung, S.N., Demetris, A.J., Schwartz, M., *et al.* (1992). Detection of replicative hepatitis C virus sequences in hepatocellular carcinoma. *American Journal of Pathology*, 141, 1271–7.

Giardiello, F.M., Petersen, G.M., Brensinger, J.D., Luce, M.C., Cayonette, M.C., Bacon, J., *et al.* (1996). Hepatoblastoma and APC gene mutation in familial adenomatous polyposis. *Gut*, 39, 867–9.

Haas, J.E., Muczynski, K.A., Krailo, M., Ablin, A., Land, V., Vietti, T.J., *et al.* (1989). Histopathology and prognosis is childhood hepatoblastoma and hepatocarcinoma. *Cancer*, 64, 1082–95.

Hashizume, K., Nakajo, T., Kawarasaki, H., Iwanaka, T., Kanamori, Y., Tanaka, K., *et al.* (1991). Prader-Willi syndrome with del(15)(q11,q13) associated with hepatoblastoma. *Acta Paediatrica Japonica*, 33, 718–22.

Hata, Y., Ishizu, H., Ohmori, K., Hamada, H., Sasaki, F., Uchino, J., *et al.* (1991). Flow cytometric analysis of the nuclear DNA content of hepatoblastoma. *Cancer*, 68, 2566–70.

Hata, Y., Takada, N., Sasaki, F., Abe, T., Hamada, H., Takahashi, H., *et al.* (1992). Immunotargeting chemotherapy for AFP-producing paediatric liver cancer using the conjugates of anti-AFP antibody and anti-tumour agents. *Journal of Paediatric Surgery*, 27, 724–7.

Hata, Y., Uchino, J., Iwafuchi, M., Ohi, R., Ohnuma, N., Okabe, I., *et al.* (1994). Treatment of advanced hepatoblastoma: a report of the Japanese Study Group for Paediatric Liver Tumour (JPLT). *Medical and Paediatric Oncology*, 23, 287.

Ikeda, H., Matsuyama, S., and Tanimura, M. (1997). Association between hepatoblastoma and very low birth weight: a trend or a chance? *Journal of Paediatrics*, 130, 557–60.

Ishiguro, T., and Tsuchida, Y. (1994). Clinical significance of serum alpha-fetoprotein subfractionation in paediatric diseases. *Acta Paediatrica*, 83, 709–13.

Kennedy, S.M., Macgeogh, C., Jaffe, R., and Spurr, N.K. (1994). Overexpression of the oncoprotein p53 in primary hepatic tumours of childhood does not correlate with gene mutations. *Human Pathology*, 25, 438–42.

Khan, A., Bader, J.L., Hoy, G.R., and Sinks, L.F. (1979). Hepatoblastoma in child with foetal alcohol syndrome. *Lancet*, i, 1403–4.

Kurahashi, H., Takami, K., Oue, T., Kusafuka, T., Okada, A., Tawa, A., *et al.* (1995). Biallelic inactivation of the APC gene in hepatoblastoma. *Cancer Research*, 55, 5007–11.

Leuschner, I., Schmidt, D., and Harms, D. (1990). Undifferentiated sarcoma of the liver in childhood: morphology, flow cytometry, and literature review. *Human Pathology*, 21, 68–76.

Melamed, I., Bujanover, Y., Hammer, J., and Spirer, Z. (1982). Hepatoblastoma in an infant born to a mother after hormonal treatment for sterility. *New England Journal of Medicine*, 307, 820.

Murthy, A.S.K., Vawter, G.F., Lee, A.B. Jockin, H., and Filler, R.M. (1980). Hormonal bioassay of gonadotropin-producing hepatoblastoma. *Archives of Pathology and Laboratory Medicine*, 104, 513–7.

Ortega, J.A., Krailo, M.D., Haas, J.E., King, D.R., Ablin, A.R., Quinn, J.J., *et al.* (1991). Effective treatment of unresectable or metastatic hepatoblastoma with cisplatin and continuous infusion doxorubicin chemotherapy: a report from the Children's Cancer Study Group. *Journal of Clinical Oncology*, 9, 2167–76.

Otten, J., Smets, R., De Jager, M., Gerard, A., and Maurus, R. (1977). Hepatoblastoma in an infant after contraceptive intake during pregnancy. *New England Journal of Medicine*, 297, 222.

Paradinas, F.J., Melia, W.M., Wilkinson, M.L., Portmann, B., Johnson, P.J., Murray-Lyon, I.M., *et al.* (1982). High serum vitamin B_{12} binding capacity as a marker of the fibrolamellar variant of hepatocellular carcinoma. *British Medical Journal*, 285, 840–2.

Plaschkes, J., Perilongo, G., Shafford, E., Brock, P., Brown, J., Dicks-Mireaux, C., *et al.* (1994). SIOP trial report: childhood hepatocellular carcinoma: preliminary results of the SIOPEL-1 study of preoperative chemotherapy: continuous infusion of cisplatin and doxorubicin (PLADO). *Medical and Paediatric Oncology*, 23, 287.

Pontisso, P., Morsica, G., Ruvoletto, M.G., Barzon, M., Perilongo, G., Basso, G., *et al.* (1992). Latent hepatitis B virus infection in childhood hepatocellular carcinoma. *Cancer*, 69, 2731–5.

Salt, A., Barnes, N.D., Rolles, K., Calne, R.Y., Clayton, P.T., and Leonard, J.V. (1992). Liver transplantation in tyrosinaemia type 1: the dilemma of timing the operation. *Acta Paediatrica*, 81, 449–52.

Schmidt, D., Wischmeyer, P., Leuschner, I., Sprenger, E., Langenau, E., von Schweinitz, D., *et al.* (1993). DNA analysis in hepatoblastoma by flow and image cytometry. *Cancer*, 72, 2914–9.

Soukup, S.W., and Lampkin, B.L. (1991). Trisomy 2 and 20 in two hepatoblastomas. *Genes and Chromosomes in Cancer*, 3, 231–4.

Tagge, E.P., Tagge, D.U., Reyes, J., Tzakis, A., Iwatsuki, S., Starzl, T.E., *et al.* (1992). Resection, including transplantation, for hepatoblastoma and hepatocellular carcinoma: impact on survival. *Journal of Paediatric Surgery*, 27, 292–7.

Tanaka, K, Uemoto, S., Asonuma, K., Katayama, T., Utsunomiya, H., Akiyama, Y., *et al.* (1992). Hepatoblastoma in a 2-year-old girl with trisomy 18. *European Journal of Paediatric Surgery*, 2, 298–300.

Tsuchida, Y., Honna, T., Fukui, M., Sakaguchi, H., and Ishiguro, T. (1989). The ratio of fucosylation of alpha-fetoprotein in hepatoblastoma. *Cancer*, 63, 2174–6.

Tsuchida, Y., Bastos, J.C., Honna, T., Kamii, Y., Hori, T., and Mochida, Y. (1990). Treatment of disseminated hepatoblastoma involving bilateral lobes. *Journal of Paediatric Surgery*, 25, 1253–5.

van Hoff, J., Grier, H.E., Douglass, E.C., and Green, D.M. (1995). Etoposide, ifosphamide, and cisplatin therapy for refractory childhood solid tumours. *Cancer*, 75, 2966–70.

Vileisis, R.A., Sorensen, K., Gonzalez-Crussi, F., and Hunt, C.E. (1982). Liver malignancy after parenteral nutrition. *Journal of Paediatrics*, 100, 88–90.

von Schweinitz, D., Hadam, M.R., Welke, K., Mildenberger, H., and Pietsch, T. (1993). Production of interleukin-1 and interleukin-6 in hepatoblastoma. *International Journal of Cancer*, 53, 728–34.

von Schweinitz, D., Burger, D., and Mildenberger, H. (1994). Is laparotomy the first step in treatment of childhood liver tumour?: the experience from the German Cooperative Paediatric Liver Tumour Study HB-89. *European Journal of Paediatric Surgery*, 4, 82–6.

von Schweinitz, D., Hecker, H., Harms, D., Bode, U., Weinel, P., Burger, D., *et al.* (1995). Complete resection before development of drug resistance is essential for survival from advanced hepatoblastoma: a report from the German Cooperative Paediatric Liver Tumour Study HB-89. *Journal of Paediatric Surgery*, 30, 845–52.

Vos, A. (1995). Primary liver tumours in children. *European Journal of Surgical Pathology*, 21, 101–5.

Weinberg, A.G. and Finegold, M.J. (1983). Primary hepatic tumours of childhood. *Human Pathology*, 14, 512–37.

Young, J.L. and Miller, R.W. (1975). Incidence of malignant tumours in U.S. children. *Journal of Paediatrics*, 86, 254–8.

20 Retinoblastoma

E. Schvartzman and G. Chantada

Retinoblastoma is a malignant endo-ocular tumour of children arising in the embryonic neural retina. It is the prototypical model for hereditary cancer development. Because of its rarity, most paediatricians and paediatric oncologists see few cases of this neoplasm, and diagnosis and management have been traditionally in the scope of ophthalmologists. Thus, many health professionals fail to identify early diagnostic clues which are usually first noticed by the parents. In fact, ophthalmologists usually establish the diagnosis, decide the local treatment modalities, and monitor the response.

Although estimates vary, it occurs with a frequency of approximately 1 in 15,000–18,000 live births in developed countries (Donaldson *et al.* 1997). However, it is more frequent in some developing nations, especially in Latin America, Africa, and Asia (Magrath *et al.* 1997). In some areas of Latin America, retinoblastoma occurs more frequently than other paediatric neoplasms and is the most common solid tumour of children in some areas of Brazil, Colombia, Mexico, and Argentina. In such countries, retinoblastoma is detected late, when extraocular dissemination has already occurred, leading to more morbidity (blindness) and mortality (Erwenne and Franco 1989). Retinoblastoma may be associated with poverty (Schvartzman, unpublished thesis). The incidence of retinoblastoma has doubled in this century, probably due to the propagation of the gene by survivors of the disease, and perhaps as a result of increased exposure to mutagenic agents. The frequency of bilateral disease is higher at institutions serving as referral centres.

There seems to be no predisposition for race or sex, and no predilection for either eye. The average age of patients at diagnosis is 24 months in unilateral cases and 13 months in bilateral cases. When bilaterally occurs (30% of all cases), the tumour arises independently within each eye. Some bilateral cases present as unilateral disease, and tumours in the other eye are detected at follow-up examination (Abramson *et al.* 1994). This feature emphasizes the need for frequent examinations under anaesthesia in unilaterally affected children, especially in those younger than 1 year.

Genetics

Retinoblastoma can occur in a familial or sporadic form. Only 6–10% are familial. It can also be classified into two different subgroups: bilateral or unilateral and heritable or non-heritable. Non-heritable cases are always unilateral, whereas 90% of the heritable cases are bilateral and 10% are unilateral (usually multifocal). All bilateral cases are heritable, whether familial or sporadic.

In 1971, Knudson developed a mathematical model to explain the heredity of retinoblastoma (Knudson 1971). He suggested that 'two hits' must occur at a gene level for retinoblastoma to develop. In heritable cases, a first event or 'hit' is a germinal mutation, i.e. inherited and present in all cells of an affected individual. The second 'hit' occurs sometime during the development of the retinal cells, leading to retinoblastoma. By contrast, in the non-hereditary cases, both events occur in the retinal cells in an acquired fashion, and none is detected in the germ line. Heritable retinoblastoma is inherited as an autosomal dominant trait with 80–100% penetrance. This model revolutionized the understanding of carcinogenesis, since it was also applicable to other tumour-suppressor genes.

The retinoblastoma gene (*RB1*) was isolated at chromosome 13q14 and cloned in 1987. It is a very large gene, spanning over 200 Kb. It was subsequently discovered that the retinoblastoma gene plays a key role in the regulation of cell growth in normal cells. Mutations at the *RB1* gene have been found in other non-retinoblastoma tumours, such as osteosarcoma, small cell lung carcinoma, and breast carcinomas.

Abnormalities at chromosome 13q14 can be detected by conventional karyotyping studies in only 5% of the cases. In the remaining ones, mutations must be detected using more sophisticated molecular techniques. The mutations found in these cases vary from family to family, making molecular diagnosis very difficult and time consuming, since there are no hot spots within the retinoblastoma gene. The first 'hit' is usually a deletion or translocation at the retinoblastoma gene, occurring either in the maternal or paternal alelle. The second hit frequently involves the loss of heterozygosity of the remaining alelle, leading to neoplastic transformation.

Molecular diagnosis of retinoblastoma plays a major role in genetic counselling. If a germ-line mutation is identified in a family, other siblings can be tested and regular fundoscopic examinations (under general anaesthesia in younger children) can be avoided in those who do not carry the abnormal gene. Prenatal diagnosis is also feasible, and when a *RB1* mutation is detected in a fetus from an affected family, earlier delivery can be advised to treat the tumours as soon as possible.

Histology

Retinoblastoma is a tumour of neuroepithelial origin which may be classified as one of the primitive neuroectodermal tumours of childhood. It consists of small, undifferentiated, anaplastic cells with scanty cytoplasm and large nuclei that stain deeply with haematoxylin, arising from the nucleated layers of one or both eyes. Calcification occurs in necrotic areas and is a common feature of large tumours. Classically, two types of retinoblastoma have been described. The most common type is composed of highly undifferentiated retinoblasts; the other consists of more differentiated photo-receptor cells with neuroepithelial rosette formation. These Flexner-Wintersteiner rosettes are characteristic of retinoblastoma but they can be present in other ophthalmic tumours (medullo-epithelioma). Less commonly seen in well-differentiated tumours is a 'bouquet-like' arrangement of benign-appearing cells with abundant cytoplasm, small nuclei, and long cytoplasmic processes traversing a fenestrated membrane. Depending on the level within the retina from which the retinoblastoma arises, the tumour may grow either in an endophytic pattern into the vitreous cavity or in an exophytic form into the subretinal space. Because of their friable nature, endophytic tumours can eventually seed the vitreous cavity and simulate a severe endophthalmitis. These active seeds of retinoblastoma can remain viable for long periods and eventually reimplant in the retina, giving rise to new tumours. In addition, seeding may occur following external beam irradiation and aggressive chemotherapy, since portions of the calcified mass break away and may contain viable tumour cells. Vitreous seeding usually means that the eye cannot be salvaged, and enucleation is eventually necessary in most such cases. When the tumour grows from the retina outward into the subretinal space (exophytic pattern) it produces a retinal detachment, sometimes with no clear view of the mass, and can resemble Coat's disease or other forms of exudative retinal detachment. When the tumour grows as a mass without retinal detachment, it may be pedunculated on a relatively small supporting stalk. Both patterns may occur in the same eye. Neither type is related to prognosis or responsiveness to treatment, but may affect the ease or difficulty in diagnostic evaluation. Another uncommon type of growth pattern, diffuse infiltrating retinoblastoma, is characterized by a flat infiltration of the retina by tumour cells, and is found usually in older children (Bhatnagar and Vine 1991). In some cases, spontaneous regression of retinoblastoma has been documented. Retinoblastoma can disseminate outside the eye, following the course of the optic nerve and/or the subarachnoid space to the chiasm, the brain, and the meninges. It can also escape from the eyeball through the sclera and invade the orbit and beyond it to the surrounding structures. The tumour cells can also reach the choroid. From there, they may gain access to the systemic circulation giving rise to haematogenous metastases. Metastatic retinoblastoma usually involves the CNS either as a solitary mass or multiple lesions, or with leptomeningeal dissemination. It can also invade facial structures such as the preauricular lymph nodes and the bones of the skull. It can also give rise to haematogenous metastases involving the bone and bone marrow and, less frequently, the liver, lungs, or any other organ.

Signs and symptoms

Signs of retinoblastoma are often first noted by parents, who generally consult an ophthalmologist for one or more of these signs, which in order of frequency are leukocoria (Fig. 20.1), strabismus, red, painful eye frequently accompanied by glaucoma, and poor vision. Less common signs are rubeosis iridis (a reddish colouration of the iris), orbital cellulitis, heterochromia iridis (change in the colour of different parts of the iris), unilateral mydriasis, hyphaema (haemorrhage into the anterior chamber, which produces a visible meniscus behind the iris), nystagmus, and , in a very small proportion of children, failure to thrive and abnormal facies. The earliest visible evidence of the tumour is a white reflex known as the cats-eye reflex or leukocoria. This indicates a large tumour which has usually grown from the periphery. The whitish glow seen through the pupil is light momentarily reflected from the tumour. It is only seen when the child looks sideways or if the observer is at an oblique angle to the child's face as he looks straight ahead. When a tumour arises in the macular region, the reflex may be seen when a tumour is quite small. The parents may note this abnormal appearance in a flash photograph since it bounces light through the pupil and conjunctiva to produce a white appearance in a colour snapshot.

The second most common sign is strabismus. Testing for strabismus is recommended as part of vision screening for all young children. This occurs when the tumour arises in the macular area, leading to an inability to fixate and subsequent deviation of the involved eye. Although infants have some degree of strabismus during the first few months of life, binocular fixation should be well established by 6 months of age. Another presenting symptom that can develop secondary to a small

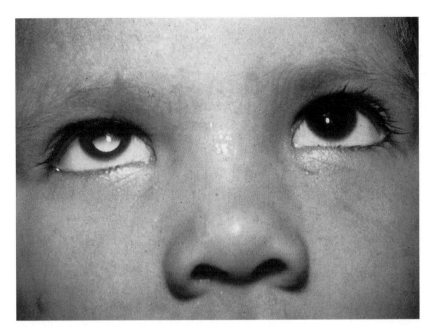

Fig. 20.1 Patient with advanced intraocular disease and leukocoria.

lesion is decreased visual acuity. Most children with retinoblastoma are too young to complain about visual impairment, but it may be the initial manifestation of the tumour in older children.

Another clinical manifestation is a red, painful eye, frequently accompanied by glaucoma. Blindness is a late sign and, if present unilaterally, is often missed by parents and paediatricians. A syndrome associated with deletion of the long arm of chromosome 13 (the 13q-deletion syndrome) has been reported with the features of microcephaly, hypertelorism, microophthalmos, epicanthal folds, micrognathia, short neck with lateral folds, low-set ears, imperforate anus, hypoplastic or absent thumbs, and psychomotor and mental retardation. Identification of these abnormalities may preceed recognition of concomitant retinoblastoma. Such children require karyotype analysis and retinal examination.

Another way in which the disease may be diagnosed early is by investigation in infants who have family history of retinoblastoma. A thorough examination of any child with a positive family history of retinoblastoma should be performed shortly after birth and periodically thereafter by an experienced ophthalmologist.

Diagnosis

The most important step in diagnosis is examination of the eye under anaesthesia through fully dilated pupils, with indirect ophthalmoscopy and scleral depression by an experienced ophthalmologist. Retinoblastoma is one of the few paediatric neoplasms that can be accurately diagnosed without histopathological confirmation. Ultrasonography (US) can be very helpful in the differential diagnosis of children with leukocoria. Two-dimensional B scan demonstrates the presence of a mass in the posterior segment in cases where the fundus may be obscured by detachment or haemorrhage, and shows a rounded or irregular intraocular mass with numerous highly reflective echoes in the orbit directly behind the tumour.

Computed tomography (CT) and magnetic resonance imaging (MRI) are useful to evaluate the optic nerve, orbital, central nervous system involvement, and the presence of intraocular calcifications (Fig. 20.2). The presence of intraocular calcification with US, CT, or MRI is suggestive of retinoblastoma, but not pathognomonic. CT and MRI are also able to detect the rare presence of an associated pineoblastoma. This synchronous tumour, an entity that has been termed trilateral retinoblastoma, occurs in 2–3% of bilateral, heritable retinoblastoma cases and it is not considered a metastasis but a separate primary tumour with universally fatal outcome (Zimmerman *et al.* 1982). However, it seems to be less frequent in developing nations such as Latin America (no cases in 181 consecutive patients in our series).

Bone marrow aspiration and biopsy and lumbar puncture for cytologic examination of the cerebrospinal fluid are mandatory when extraocular disease is evident. Its yield is insignificant in patients with localized intraocular disease (Pratt *et al.* 1989).

In the presence of symptoms suggestive of metastatic disease (bone pain), a bone scan is indicated.

Serum and aqueous lactate dehydrogenase determination has been used to differentiate retinoblastoma from lesions which stimulate it, but nowadays, intraocular biopsy to obtain tissue and aspiration of aqueous humour for enzyme studies are contraindicated.

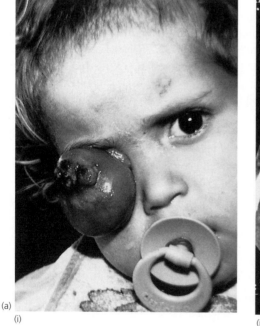

(a)

(i)

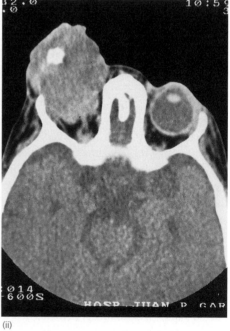

(ii)

Fig. 20.2 (a) Patient (i) and CT (ii) with orbital invasion of right-eye by unilateral retinoblastoma before treatment. Note tumour calcification and optic nerve extension. (b) The same patient (i) and CT (ii) after two cycles of chemotherapy with idarubicin (single agent).

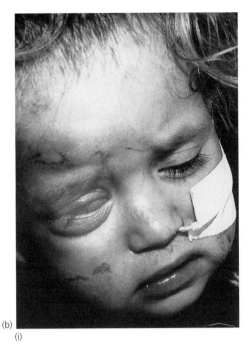
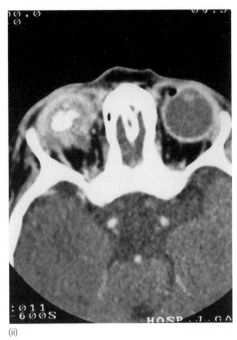

(b)

(i)   (ii)

Fig. 20.2 *Continued*

The differential diagnosis of retinoblastoma is shown in Table 20.1.

Table 20.1 Differential diagnosis of retinoblastoma

Intraocular retinoblastoma
    Coat's disease
    Persistent hyperplastic primary vitreous
    Retrolental fibroplasia
    Retinal hamartoma
    Endophthalmitis
    Toxocara infection
    Astrocytic hamartomas
    Medulloepithelioma
    Cataracts
    Uveitis

Extraocular Retinoblastoma
    Orbital cellulitis
    Metastatic neuroblastoma
    Orbital rhabdomysarcoma
    Leukaemia
    Lymphoma

Staging

The most widely used grouping system for retinoblastoma was proposed by Reese and Ellsworth (Table 20.2) and has become adopted as the standard for intraocular disease. Here, prognosis refers entirely to preservation of useful vision in the affected eye if radiation therapy is delivered via lateral portal, photon therapy, and not to long-term survival. There is no widely accepted staging system for patients with extraocular disease. The Grabowski, Abramson, and Ellsworth clinicopathological classification (Grabowski and Abramson 1987) was used at the Hospital de Pediatria JP Garrahan, Buenos Aires, Argentina (HPG), and found useful to classify patients with differing risk of relapse according to the degree of microscopical extension. This system subdivides patients into those with intraocular disease (intraretinal, prelaminar optic nerve invasion, and choroidal invasion), those with extraocular regional extension (extrascleral and retrolaminar extension), CNS invasion, and systemic metastatic disease. Nevertheless, this classification does not accurately predict outcome, since those with CNS invasion are scored as stage III, although the prognosis is not different or may even be worse than those with systemic metastases who are scored as stage IV. Other staging systems in use are based on the same features with minor differences (Howarth *et al.* 1980).

Treatment

Two aspects of treatment of retinoblastoma must be considered; firstly the local therapeutic options to treat intraocular disease, and secondly systemic therapy for patients with extraocular, regional, or metastatic disease.

In developed countries, most patients present with intraocular disease, and survival is around 95% (Donaldson *et al.* 1997). In these cases, treatment planning must consider the potential preservation of useful vision, minimizing long-term sequelae. The size, number, and location of

Table 20.2   Reese-Ellsworth staging system for intraocular retinoblastoma

Group		Description
I	(a)	Solitary tumour less than 4 dd (disc diameter), at or behind the equator
	(b)	Multiple tumours none larger than 4 dd, all at or behind the equator
II	(a)	Solitary tumour 4–10 dd, at or behind the equator
	(b)	Multiple tumours, 4–10 dd, at or behind the equator
III	(a)	Any lesion anterior to the equator
	(b)	Solitary tumour larger than 10 dd behind the equator
IV	(a)	Multiple tumours, some larger than 10 dd
	(b)	Any lesion extending anterior to the ora serrata
V	(a)	Massive tumours involving over half the retina
	(b)	Vitreous seeding

tumours, as well as the status of the remaining eye, are taken into account to choose the best therapy. Even though an increasing number of patients with unilateral retinoblastoma can avoid enucleation in developed nations, in less privileged areas, eye preservation is uncommon (3% of the HPG series). Most patients with bilateral retinoblastoma come with advanced intraocular disease in one eye, often needing enucleation, and less advanced disease in the other eye which can usually be preserved (70% in the HPG series). Only 17% of patients with bilateral retinoblastoma had both eyes preserved. This feature is more common in patients with a family history of retinoblastoma, in whom the diagnosis is made earlier. On the other hand, 13% of patients with bilateral retinoblastoma, had both eyes removed for advanced intraocular disease, either on admission or after failure of local therapy.

In developing countries, retinoblastoma is usually diagnosed after extraocular spread is evident (33% in the HPG series) (Erwenne and Franco 1989). In these cases, treatment of retinoblastoma aims to save the patient's life, since death from metastatic disease is possible (Schvartzman *et al.* 1996).

Treatment modalities

Surgery

Enucleation is the simplest and safest therapy for retinoblastoma. A prosthetic eyeball is fitted several weeks after the procedure, minimizing cosmetic effects. However, when enucleation is performed in the first 2 years of life, facial asymmetry develops because of inhibition of orbital growth. Most patients with Reese-Ellsworth group V tumours require enucleation, especially when no useful vision can be achieved after successful treatment of the tumours. However, if the contralateral eye also has advanced disease, a conservative approach may be undertaken and a few eyes can be retained. Enucleation is mandatory when glaucoma, anterior chamber invasion, or rubeosis iridis are present, and when local therapy cannot be evaluated due to a cataract or failure to follow a patient closely. A long optic nerve stump should be obtained. Enucleation can be delayed when extrascleral extension is evident at diagnosis. Orbital masses usually shrink considerably after a few courses of chemotherapy, allowing enucleation to be performed and therefore avoiding orbital exenteration (Schvartzman *et al.* 1996). (Fig. 20.2). Intraocular surgery, such as vitrectomy, is contraindicated in patients with retinoblastoma, since it can increase the risk of orbital relapse.

External beam radiotherapy (EBRT)

Retinoblastoma is a radiosensitive tumour and radiotherapy is the elective local therapy for retinoblastoma (Abramson 1989). However, long-term side-effects limit its use. EBRT is usually delivered using a linear accelerator to a dose of 40–45 Gy, with conventional fractionation involving the whole retina. Infants must be anaesthetized and immobilized during the procedure, and close cooperation between the ophthalmologist and the radiotherapist is essential for planning the fields. Most radiotherapists use a D-shaped lateral field which minimizes the risk of radiation-induced cataracts. Nevertheless, the anterior retina is underdosed with this technique, and recurrent tumours near the ora serrata are not uncommon. The success rate of EBRT with this technique depends not only on tumour size, but also on location. Ophthalmoscopic regression patterns following radiotherapy have been characterized (Abramson 1989). Local control rates range from 58–80% (Donaldson *et al.* 1997). Most recurrences after radiotherapy can be retreated successfully with cryo or photocoagulation. Long-term sequelae of radiotherapy are of great concern. Like enucleation, it causes growth inhibition of the orbital bone, leading to severe cosmetic sequelae and, more importantly, it has been associated with an increased risk of secondary malignancies (Roarty *et al.* 1988).

Plaque radiotherapy

Radioactive episcleral plaques using ^{60}Co, ^{106}Ru, or ^{125}I are being increasingly used in the treatment of retinoblastoma (Abramson 1989). They are usually prescribed for small- and medium-sized single tumours not amenable to cryo or photocoagulation which have recurred after EBRT, but recently they have also been used as primary therapy, especially after chemoreduction. There is not enough evidence yet to determine whether this modality is associated with second malignancies.

Cryo and photocoagulation

These modalities are used to treat small (usually less than 5 mm) and accessible tumours (Abramson 1989). They are widely available and can be repeated several times until local control is achieved. Cryotherapy is usually prescribed to treat anterior tumours and it is applied with a small probe placed on the conjunctiva. On the other hand, photocoagulation is generally used for posterior tumours using either argon laser or xenon are photocoagulation.

Nevertheless, photocoagulation should be avoided in tumours near the macula or the optic disc, since it may leave a scar causing severe amblyopia. Both modalities cause little or no morbidity or long-term sequelae.

Newer modalities

In recent years, some groups have used chemotherapy as primary treatment for intraocular disease in order to decrease tumour size and make the tumours suitable for local therapy (Gallie *et al.* 1996). Chemotherapy was found to be ineffective in intraocular disease in the past, but with the use of newer drugs with greater penetration of the eye, this modality has reemerged. This approach may avoid EBRT (Gallie *et al.* 1996) or enucleation in more advanced cases. Carboplatin alone or in combination with vincristine and VP16 or VM26 is used. Nevertheless, data about the value of this modality are preliminary and its relative benefit needs to be validated with longer follow-up. However, chemoreduction is now performed at most centres as the primary treatment in patients with bilateral retinoblastoma and potential for useful vision (Fig. 20.3).

Chemotherapy

The role of adjuvant chemotherapy is controversial. There are no large, prospective, randomized trials and most studies are based on a small number of patients with differing risks of relapse. In

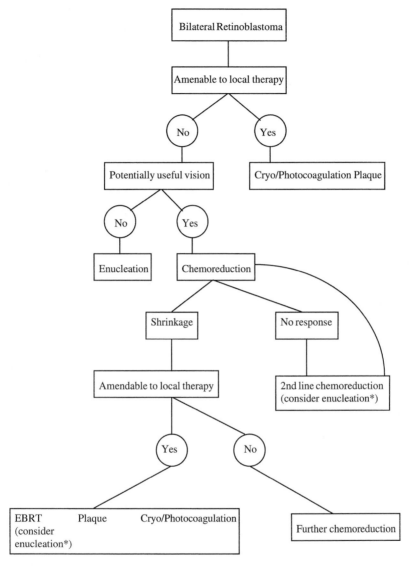

Fig. 20.3 Guidelines for local therapy in patients with bilateral retinoblastoma at the HPG. (*) In these cases, the most adequate local therapy must take into account the status of the remaining eye.

addition, the lack of a widely accepted staging system makes the comparison between various series even more difficult. Most studies are based on the determination of histopathological risk factors (Howarth *et al.* 1980, Grabowski and Abramson 1987; Zelter *et al.* 1991; Schvartzman *et al.* 1996). However, in most cases, such risk factors were based upon retrospective examination of patients treated over long periods of time with different regimens (Kopelman *et al.* 1987). Postenucleation histopathological staging is therefore essential to define groups with different risk of relapse. Some authors recommend adjuvant chemotherapy for patients with intraocular disease and potential risk factors such as short optic nerve stump (< 5 mm), undifferentiated tumours, or prelaminar optic nerve invasion (Howarth *et al.* 1980; Zelter *et al.* 1991). Nevertheless, our group prospectively treated a large number of these patients successfully without any therapy other than enucleation (Schvartzman *et al.* 1996). At the HPG, 64 such patients have been treated with no other adjuvant therapy and none have relapsed. The role of isolated choroidal invasion as a prognostic factor for relapse is more controversial. In an update of our published series, including 30 patients with isolated choroid invasion prospectively treated from 1987–1996 without adjuvant chemotherapy, event-free survival (PEFS) is 93%. Choroidal invasion may only be relevant when it is combined with post-laminar optic nerve invasion (Shields *et al.* 1993).

When the cut end of the optic nerve is free of tumour, the management is controversial. Adjuvant chemotherapy was used in most series (Grabowski and Abramson 1987; Zelter *et al.* 1991; Schvartzman *et al.* 1996) and most patients achieved a long-term survival. In our current protocol, patients with this condition receive no other therapy than enucleation, provided there is no major choroidal invasion. So far, 10 patients have been treated accordingly and none have relapsed. Those patients with optic nerve invasion beyond the surgical margin, especially when choroidal invasion is present, need adjuvant intensive chemotherapy and orbital radiotherapy involving the optic chiasm. With this therapy, approximately 80% can achieve long-term survival. Most recurrences involve the CNS. The role of intrathecal chemotherapy and cranial radiotherapy to prevent CNS dissemination in these patients is not established (Howarth *et al.* 1980; Schvartzman *et al.* 1996). When overt extraocular disease is present, pre-enucleation chemotherapy is warranted (Schvartzman *et al.* 1996) (Fig. 20.4). The agents used most commonly are carboplatin, cisplatin, etoposide, teniposide, cyclophosphamide, iphosphamide, vincristine, adriamycin, and, more recently, idarubicin used in combination (Grabowski and Abramson 1987; Zelter *et al.* 1991; Schvartzman *et al.* 1996). Even though most previous reports claimed that overt invasion of the orbit and preauricular lymph nodes was associated with a fatal outcome, most of these patients can now achieve long-term survival with a multimodal approach combining chemotherapy, surgery, and radiotherapy of the involved areas. On the other hand, even though a complete remission is usually achieved in patients with metastatic disease (haematogenous or CNS), it is usually short-lived, and ultimate survival is infrequent (Kingston *et al.* 1987; Schvartzman *et al.* 1996). This phenomenon may be caused by the overexpression of p170 glycoprotein by the retinoblastoma cells, which has been associated with multidrug resistance to chemotherapeutic agents (Chan *et al.* 1991). High-dose chemotherapy followed by autologous stem-cell rescue is a rational approach to circumvent drug resistance and may cure some of these patients. The current approach to the systemic treatment of retinoblastoma and its results at the HPG are summarized in Figs 20.4 and 20.5, respectively.

Second malignancies

The presence of a germ-line mutation at the retinoblastoma gene confers on affected individuals a high predisposition for secondary malignancies. With current therapy there are more patients with bilateral retinoblastoma dying of secondary malignancies than those who succumb from the retinoblastoma itself. The risk of developing a second malignancy among these children exists

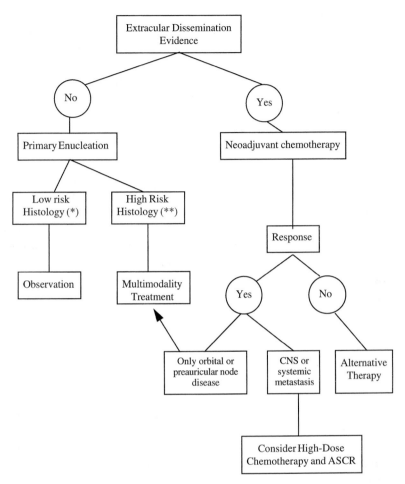

Fig. 20.4 Guidelines for the management of advanced retinoblastoma at the HPG. (*) Low-risk histology includes intraretinal extension, prelaminar optic nerve and isolated choroid invasion (or both). Patients with post-laminar optic nerve invasion and surgical margin free of tumour. (**) High-risk histology includes any degree of scleral invasion, post-laminar optic nerve (resection margin free of tumour) invasion with choroidal invasion. All patients with post-laminar optic nerve invasion beyond the cut end. ASCR: Autologous stem-cell rescue.

regardless of the therapy received. However, most second cancers seen in patients with bilateral retinoblastoma are sarcomas, usually osteosarcomas of the irradiated orbit. Radiotherapy and chemotherapy may increase the risk of a second malignancy, probably by causing a 'second hit' to mesenchymal cells already predisposed to malignancy. Sarcomas outside the orbit, melanomas, lung, and breast cancer have also been reported. The incidence of secondary malignancies increases with time, reaching 38% at 30 years (Roarty *et al.* 1988). Secondary malignancies in these patients are usually very aggressive and are frequently fatal. Therefore, a high index of suspicion is needed to allow early detection.

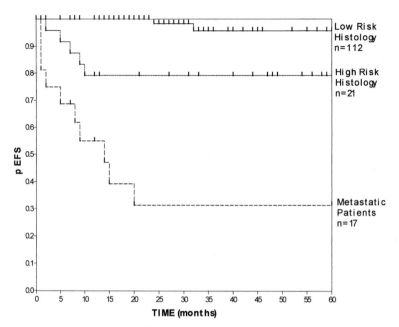

Fig. 20.5 Probability of event-free survival (PEFS) in patients with retinoblastoma treated in two successive protocols at the HPG from 1987–1996. Low- and high-risk histology definitions as for Fig. 20.4. Metastatic patients were defined as those with CNS, systemic, and/or orbital or lymph-node extension. Only the latter survived.

Acknowledgement

We would like to acknowledge the work and dedication of the multidisciplinary staff who care for patients with retinoblastoma at the Hospital de Pediatria J.P. Garrahan, Buenos Aires, Argentina: Dr Julio Manzitti and Dr Adriana Fandino (Ophthalmology), Dr Elsa Raslawski (Radiotherapy), and Dr Maria T.G. de Davila (Pathology).

References

Abramson, D.H. (1989). The focal treatment of retinoblastoma with emphasis on xenon arc photocoagulation. *Acta ophthalmologica*, 76:1–62 (suppl 194).

Abramson, D.H., Gamell, L.S., Ellsworth, R.M., Kruger, E.F., Servodidio, C.A., Turner, L., *et al.* (1994). Unilateral retinoblastoma: new intraocular tumours after treatment. *British Journal of Ophthalmology*, 78, 698–701.

Bhatnagar, R. and Vine A. (1991). Diffuse infiltrating retinoblastoma. *Ophthalmology*, 98, 1657–1661.

Chan, H.S., Thorner P.S,. Haddad, G., and Gallie, B.L. (1991). Multidrug-resistance phenotype in retinoblastoma correlates with P-glycoprotein expression. *Ophthalmology*, 98, 1245–1431.

Donaldson, S., Egbert, P., Newsham, I., Webster, K., and Kavenee, W.K. (1997). Retinoblastoma. In Pizzo P and Poplack D (eds): Principles and Practice of Pediatric Oncology (ed 3). Philadelphia. PA. Lippincott, pp. 699–716.

Ellsworth, R.M. (1969). The practical management of retinoblastoma. *Trans. Am. Opthalmol. Soc.*, 67, 462–534.

Erwenne, C. and Franco, E. (1989). Age and lateness of referral as determinants of extraocular retinoblastoma. *Ophthalmic Ped Gen*, 10: 179–184.

Gallie, B., Budning, A., DeBoer, G. *et al.* (1996). Chemotherapy with focal therapy can cure intraocular retinoblastoma without radiation *Arch Ophthalmol*, 114: 1321–1328.

Grabowski, E.F. and Abramson, D.H. (1987). Intraocular and extraocular retinoblastoma. *Hematol Oncol Clin N Am.*, 1:721–735.

Howarth, C., Meyer, D., Hustu, O., Johnson, W.W., Shanks, E., and Pratt, C. (1980). Stage-related combined modality treatment of retinoblastoma. Results of a prospective study. *Cancer*, 45, 851–858.

Kingston, J., Hungerford, J., and Plowman, N. (1987). Chemotherapy in metastatic retinoblastoma. *Ophthalmic Ped Gen*, 8:69–72.

Knudson, A.G. (1971). Mutation and cancer: statistical study of retinoblastoma. *Proc Natl Acad Sci USA*, 68, 820–823.

Kopelman, J.E., McLean, I.W., and Rosenberg, S.H. (1987). Multivariate Analysis of Risk Factors for Metastasis in Retinoblastoma Treated by Enucleation. *Ophthalmology*, 94, 371–377.

Magrath, I., Shad, A., Epelman, S., de Camargo, B., Petrilli, A.S., Gd-el-Mawla, N., *et al.* (1997). Pediatric Oncology in Countries with limited resources. In Pizzo P, Poplack D, eds. *Principles and Practice of Pediatric Oncology.* (ed 3) Philadelphia PA: Lippincott, pp. 1395–1420.

Pratt, C.B., Meyer, D., Chenaille, P., and Crom, D.B. (1989). The use of bone marrow aspirations and lumbar punctures at the time of diagnosis of retinoblastoma. *Journal of Clinical Oncology*, 7, 140–143.

Roarty, J.D., McLean, I.W., and Zimmermann, L.E. (1988). Incidence of second neoplasms in patients with bilateral retinoblastomas. *Ophthalmology*, 95:1583–1587.

Schvartzman, E., Chantada, G., Fandino, A., de Davila, M.T., Raslawski, E., and Manzitti, J. (1996). Results of a stage-based protocol for the treatment of retinoblastoma. *Journal of Clinical Oncology*, 14:1532–1536.

Shields, C., Shields, J., Baez, K., Cater, J., and De Potter, P.V. (1993). Choroidal invasion of Retinoblastoma. Metastatic potential and clinical risk factors. *British Journal of Ophthalmology*, 77, 544–548.

Zelter, M., Damel, A., Gonzalez, G., and Schwartz, L. (1991). A prospective study on the treatment of retinoblastoma in 72 patients. *Cancer*, 68, 1685–1690.

Zimmerman, L.E., Burns, R.P., Wankum, G., Tully, R., and Esterly, J.A. (1982). Trilateral Retinoblastoma associated with bilateral retinoblastoma. *J Pediatr Ophthalmol Strab*, 19, 310–315.

21 Rare tumours

P.A. Voûte

All paediatric tumours are rare but there are some which are particularly rare. The clinician is faced with the problem how to manage these unusual neoplasms. Carcinoma and especially carcinoma of the endocrine organs such as thyroid, adrenal cortex, and pancreas and nasopharyngeal carcinoma belong to this group.

Thyroid carcinoma

The incidence of thyroid cancer rises with age in childhood. Neck irradiation in infancy and childhood is a predisposing cause of its development. Most of the tumours are highly differentiated papillary or less differentiated follicular and 'mixed' tumours.

Metastases can be found in local lymph nodes and in lungs. The clinical presentation is invariable, with neck swelling in the thyroid region (Fig. 21.1). For investigation, ultrasonography and isotope scanning are important; thyroid cancers present as cold, non-cystic nodules. Needle aspiration biopsy is advocated by some as a diagnostic procedure. Thyroglobulin is a reliable tumour marker in differentiated thyroid cancers (Kirk *et al.* 1992). But a history of previous irradiation, hard consistency of the nodule, or cervical lymphadenopathy are very suspicious and are indications for immediate surgical removal.

Concerning treatment, there is no consensus regarding the optimal surgical procedure. Exelby and Frazell (1969) reported a 5-year survival rate of 92.1% in children treated for thyroid cancer. Aggressive thyroidectomy is associated with few recurrences, but causes permanent hypothyroidism and can be associated with permanent hypoparathyroidism and nerve damage. Hemithyroidectomy with isthmusectomy can be performed if the tumour is located in one lobe of the thyroid. In case of metastases in cervical lymph nodes, a cervical lymph-node dissection is advocated. If there are distant metastases, a therapeutic dose of radioiodine should be administered (Hung 1994).

Medullary carcinoma of the thyroid occurs frequently in association with polyendocrine and/or neuroectodermal neoplasia, but can also be found as a sporadic tumour.

In cases of medullary cell tumours, multiple endocrine neoplasia syndrome type II is often present in relatives. Calcitonin is a marker of medullary cell carcinoma.

Total thyroidectomy is generally recommended for medullary cell tumours because they are often multifocal.

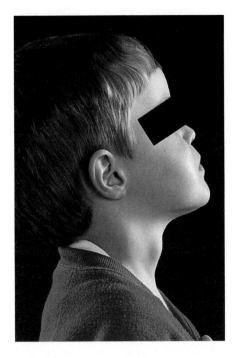

Fig. 21.1 6-year-old boy with papillary carcinoma of the thyroid.

Tumours of the adrenal cortex

As with other endocrine glands, general symptoms can result from an overproduction of hormones. In tumours of the adrenal cortex, excess secretion may be the result of hyperplasia, a benign adenoma, or—when sufficiently undifferentiated—an adenocarcinoma (Flack and Chrousos 1992).

Adenoma

Multiple minute nodes on or in the adrenal cortex are occasionally found and are usually not associated with any history of disturbance in endocrine secretion.

Large masses of cells compressing the adjacent parenchyma of the glands are true tumours, and are probably best described as adenomas. Generally they are 1–2 cm in diameter.

The clinical features of cortical adenomas are related to the excretion of steroids as in carcinoma.

Carcinoma of the adrenal cortex

This very rare tumour always arises in the adrenal gland itself, although sometimes tumours are described in ectopic cortical tissue. The clinical symptoms are primarily caused by excessive hormone production and therefore can be diagnosed relatively early when the tumour is still small. Normally, the tumour shows a considerable degree of differentiation.

The quantity and the types of substances secreted by these tumours vary considerably from tumour to tumour. They may secrete androgens, glucocorticoids, a mixture of these, or oestrogens or aldosterone. In general the steroids secreted are not only increased in amount but also disordered in proportion. They may appear in increased amounts in the plasma and urine. Even more rare are non-hormonal cortical tumours.

An abdominal mass cannot always be palpated, but the symptoms and signs of virilization and Cushingoid features, feminization and/or hyperaldosteronism, and/or mixed syndromes can be found (Fig. 21.2).

This situation must be differentiated from adrenal cortical hyperplasia and/or secondary hypercorticosteroidism resulting from hypothalamic lesions and Cushing's syndrome.

Treatment consists of surgical removal of the tumour, after which supportive and postoperative substitution therapy are of importance. Metastases may be found, but these are often also highly differentiated tumours, in which case surgical removal is advocated. Other treatment such as chemotherapy and radiotherapy gives disappointing results.

Tumours of the pancreas

Tumours of the pancreas in children present a clinical picture which depends on the type of cell from which they arise. Pancreatic adenomas and adenocarcinomas may arise in either the exocrine or endocrine cells.

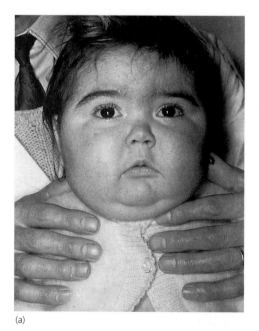

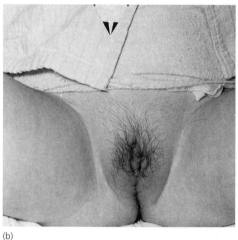

(a) (b)

Fig. 21.2 (a) 9-month-old girl with virilizing adrenal carcinoma with Cushing's syndrome; and (b) pubic hair with enlargement of clitoris.

The tumours are as follows:

Exocrine

(1) Adenoma

(2) Carcinoma

Endocrine

(1) Adenoma of β cells (insulinoma)

(2) Adenoma of non-β cells

(3) Carcinoma of non-β cells

Adenoma

Adenomas of the exocrine pancreas are occasionally found without any symptoms. The mode of presentation in large adenomas is with distension of the upper part of the abdomen with few or no symptoms. A post-traumatic pseudocyst of the pancreas is much more common than a cystic adenoma. The radiological findings in the two conditions are similar. Congenital cysts of the pancreas are often related to von Hippel-Lindau disease. Excision is the treatment of choice.

Carcinoma

Carcinoma of the exocrine pancreas is very rare. Reported tumours arise in the head of the pancreas, and the clinical signs are distension of the gall bladder and jaundice, but more often these symptoms are related to lymphoma infiltrating the pancreas.

Adenoma of the β cell (insulinoma).

Hypersecretion producing hyperinsulinaemia and hypoglycaemia occur as a result of hyperplasia, an adenoma, or sometimes an adenocarcinoma of the β cells. The symptoms are due to this hyperinsulinism. Children may present with 'epileptiform' attacks due to hypoglycaemia. Treatment is surgical; often a total pancreatectomy is needed.

Adenoma and carcinoma of non-β cells

Nesidioblastosis presents with a Zollinger-Ellison syndrome. Hypersecretion of gastric juices produces diarrhoea. Surgery is the treatment of choice.

Pancreaticoblastoma

This is a very rare tumour affecting children in the first decade of life, and usually arising from the head of the pancreas. It is associated with elevated αFP levels and has a characteristic histological appearance with undifferentiated areas, acinar differentiation, gland-like structures, nodules of squamous epithelium (squamoid corpuscles) and occasionally neuro-endocrine differentiation. Complete surgical excision offers the best chance of cure, but treatment with cisplatin and doxorubicin (as for hepatoblastoma) may be effective. Prognosis is better than for other types of pancreatic tumours.

Nasopharyngeal carcinoma

Nasopharyngeal carcinoma has a large variation in incidence around the world. For example, it is very frequent in children in the Mediterranean region: North Africa, Turkey, and the Middle East, but rare in Northern Europe. The aetiology is not clear but there is evidence of association with viral and environmental factors. There is an established association between nasopharyngeal carcinoma and infection with the Epstein-Barr virus. The most frequent clinical presentation is cervical lymphadenopathy in a teenager, with problems of hearing loss, nasal obstruction, otitis media, epistaxis, and pain. Patients with disseminated disease often have severe bone pain due to bone metastasis, but a paraneoplastic syndrome of osteoarthropathy also occurs (Pao *et al.* 1989; Martin and Shah 1994).

The high incidence of metastatic tumours and of metastatic relapse favours primary treatment with systemic chemotherapy. A number of combination chemotherapy regimens have been used with good response. These include platinum derivatives, alkylating agents, etoposide, bleomycin, and methotrexate. Chemotherapy can be followed by surgery but the curative role of surgical treatment is limited due to the site of the tumour. Irradiation of the tumour region after chemotherapy is an essential part of the treatment (Touglass *et al.* 1996).

Carcinoid tumours

The commonest site of carcinoid tumours is the appendix, but they can also be found in other parts of the intestines and in the bronchus. Most carcinoids are found incidentally, often after appendectomy for appendicitis. Further treatment is not needed in these patients. Larger tumours can present with clinical signs of flushing. In these patients, elevated serum levels of metabolites of tryptophan, such as serotonin, are found. Surgical excision is the treatment of choice (Marshall and Bodnarchuk 1993). Malignant carcinoid tumours in children are very rare. In case of malignancy and when metastases are present, treatment with ^{131}I-MIBG is indicated.

Malignant melanoma

Malignant melanoma is an uncommon tumour in children. In 16–40% there is a preexisting condition, for example congenital naevocytic naevus or xeroderma pigmentosum. The clinical aspects of malignancy are changes in the shape, colour, and size of a preexisting pigmented lesion, either congenital or acquired (Fig. 21.3). A new, pigmented, and rapidly growing lesion without preexisting naevus also requires surgical excision for pathological examination. Malignant melanoma is sometimes difficult to differentiate from Spitz' naevus. Complete excision is the treatment for the primary tumour.

Several chemotherapy regimens have been used. These regimens are based on combinations of platinum derivatives, alkylating agents, and epipodophyllotoxin. Thus far, chemotherapy has not been proven to be of any advantage for the patient (Boddie and McBride 1985).

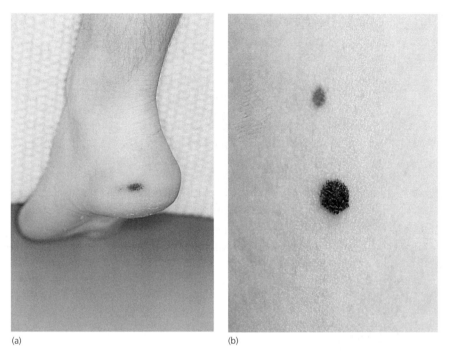

(a)   (b)

Fig. 21.3 (a and b)   Melanoma of the skin (by courtesy of the Department of Dermatology of the Academic Medical Center, Amsterdam).

Xeroderma pigmentosum

Xeroderma pigmentosum is a rare genetic disorder of autosomal recessive inheritance (Fig. 21.4). It is characterized by hypersensitivity to sunlight and the development of cutaneous and ocular tumours. Malignant, cutaneous neoplasms develop after the age of 5 years and include basal-and squamous-cell carcinoma and malignant melanoma.

Diagnosis is usually easy but can be confirmed by *in vitro* studies of DNA repair rates. The severity of the disease increases with decreasing DNA repair rates.

Surgical removal is indicated but other tumours will occur. Topical application of 5- fluorouracil is useful for actinic keratosis. Synthetic retinoids have proved effective in the prevention of cutaneous carcinoma, but high doses are needed.

Kaposi's sarcoma

Kaposi's sarcoma amongst children is very rare, but its incidence is increasing as a result of HIV infection. The tumour, which is often multifocal, presents with slowly growing, raised, pigmented skin lesions. The classical Kaposi's sarcoma with indolent disease occurs initially on the lower limbs. Radiotherapy is the treatment of choice.

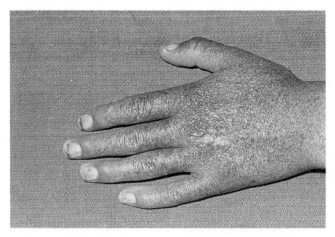

Fig. 21.4   Xeroderma pigmentosum (by courtesy of the Department of Dermatology of the Academic Medical Center, Amsterdam).

The African non-HIV variety has been endemic in Africa for many years and is a more aggressive form of the classical disease, occurring in younger male patients and producing ulcerating lesions. The disease progresses to involve internal organs. This disease does respond to single-agent and combination chemotherapy in which vincristine and alkylating agents are most important.

Kaposi's sarcoma also occurs in immune-suppressed patients, especially when they have been treated with long-term immune suppression to prevent rejection of transplants. The Kaposi's sarcoma of AIDS is also becoming more frequent in children with congenital AIDS. Treatment results are often excellent with radiotherapy, and in widespread Kaposi's syndrome with chemotherapy.

Malignant mesenchymal tumours

Odontogenic and jaw tumours

Admantinomas are tumours of ectodermal origin. They are found in the maxilla but are five times more frequent in the mandible. The tumour generally expands the jaw from within, with a resultant thinning of the buccal or lingual plate. Growth is very slow. Treatment is by adequate surgical removal. Adamantinomas have also been reported as occurring in long bones. The tumour develops in the shaft of the tibia closest to the skin. The aetiology of these tumours is postulated as being the result of trauma.

Malignant schwannoma

This tumour is derived from Schwann cells from the neural crest. It is a tumour most commonly occurring in patients with neurofibromatosis type 1 (NF1). The so-called Triton tumour is a variant of malignant schwannoma with rhabdomyoblastic differentiation. The treatment of choice is surgery with a wide excision if possible. Chemotherapy regimens as used in Ewing's sarcomas or neuroblastomas have not proved to be of much value. The prognosis is generally poor. (Sommelet *et al.* 1991).

Fibrosarcomas

These are composed of fusiform cells with a fasciculated architecture. Varying amounts of collagen are present. Differential diagnosis from certain fusiform-cell forms of rhabdomyosarcoma, monophasic synovial sarcoma, and leiomyosarcoma is sometimes difficult. The most difficult problem remains the differential diagnosis from the aggressive form of fibromatosis. Enzinger and Weiss (1988) proposed that this form of fibromatosis—encountered in children under 1 year of age—be classified among infantile fibrosarcomas. The evolution of fibrosarcoma in infants has a characteristic pattern. Either congenital or occurring during the first year of life, it generally has a favourable outcome, although local recurrence and metastases can occur. Conservative surgery is the treatment of choice, when feasible. If not, initial polychemotherapy as for rhabdomyosarcoma has been shown to be effective in some cases and allows conservative surgery. Clinically, after 1 year of age, these tumours are similar to those found in adult patients, with local recurrences and late pulmonary metastases.

Synovial sarcomas

A translocation X;18 is found in this tumour, which is helpful in diagnosis. The site of predilection is usually, but not always, close to a joint, and the articular origin is not established. Conservative surgery, with radiotherapy in the case of microscopically incomplete excision, can provide local control of the tumour. In children, lymph-node involvement at diagnosis is not seen, thus systematic lymphadenectomy, as is used for adult patients, is not required. In some cases chemotherapy seems effective, allowing conservative surgery. The survival of children with synovial sarcoma is 75% at 5 years. Pulmonary metastasis may occur, which should be surgically removed (Turc-Carel *et al.* 1987).

Neuroepitheliomas

The pathological characteristics of these tumours are similar to those of the adult form. In difficult cases the positivity of enolase helps to differentiate them from rhabdomyosarcoma. Some authors classify this tumour as neuroectodermal.

Askin's tumour, which is described in thoracic sites, should be classified as extraosseous Ewing's sarcoma (round-cell tumour). SIOP has proposed treating these tumours as malignant mesenchymal tumours, although others treat them like Ewing's sarcoma or neuroblastoma.

Esthesioneuroblastoma

This tumour is best classified as a malignant, primitive, neuroectodermal tumour which happens to arise in the olfactory neuroepithelium high in the nasal cavity. The tumour cells contain t(11:22) (q24:q12), identical to that in Askin's/Ewing's tumours (Wang-Peng *et al.* 1978).

These tumours are responsive to chemotherapy and radiotherapy. Treatment regimens as for malignant, primitive, neuroectodermal tumours are used. Delayed surgery to excise residual disease can play a role in the treatment, as does radiotherapy.

Haemangiopericytomas

These occur in the first year of life, and while they can have an appearance of malignant tumour (mitosis, intravascular invasion), the outcome is that of a benign tumour at this age. Differential diagnosis from other malignant mesenchymal tumours can be difficult. Complete surgery is the sole treatment when feasible. Initial chemotherapy in inoperable cases in sometimes effective and allows secondary conservative surgery.

Small round-cell tumours

These tumours are not definitely sarcomas. This question will be clarified by cytogenetic and molecular studies. Extraosseous Ewing's sarcoma is included in this group. Differential diagnosis from other small round-cell tumours, particularly lymphosarcoma, is difficult.

Malignant fibrohistiocytomas (MFH)

In the SIOP mesenchymal malignancy trials (MMT 84 and MMT 89), MFH was the second most common non-rhabdomyosarcoma, soft-tissue sarcoma. In these tumours, chromosomal abnormalities are found, with chromosome bands 19p13, 11p11, 3p12, and 1q11 being most frequently affected. Those with 19p13 show a particularly pronounced tendency to recur.

MFH is one of the commonest types of induced sarcoma. It can be found on the trunk, lower limbs, or on the scalp. Metastases are mostly found in the lung. The treatment of choice is wide surgical excision followed by radiotherapy. Chemotherapy has no clear place in the treatment.

Liposarcomas

Liposarcoma is rarely seen in children. It may originate from previously existing lipoma, but more probably is sarcomatous from the start. It is seen most frequently in the retroperitoneal and perirenal areas, and may grow to a large size causing renal pelvic or urethral distortion. These tumours show an infiltrating growth having a faint resemblance to normal fat. Treatment is surgical, but may be very mutilating because the surgery must be radical.

References

Boddie, A.W. and McBride, C.M. (1985). Melanoma in childhood and adolescence. In: Balch, C. (ed). Cutaneous melanoma. Lippincott, Philadelphia, pp. 63–69.

Enzinger, F.M. and Weiss, S.W. (1988). Malignant soft tissue tumours of uncertain type. Mosby, St. Louis. Chapter 38, 1067–1093.

Exelby, P.E. and Frazell, E.L. (1969). Carcinoma of the thyroid in children. *Surg Clin North Am*, 49: 249–259.

Flack, M.R. and Chrousos, C.P. Cancer of the adrenal cortex. In: Holland, J. (ed). Cancer Medicine, 3rd ed. Philadelphia: Lea and Febiger, 1992.

Hung, W. (1994). Well differentiated thyroid carcinoma in children and adolescents: a review. *Endocrinologist*, 4:117.

Kirk, J.M.W., Mort, C., Grant, D., Touzel, R.J., and Plowman, N. (1992). The usefulness of serum thyroglobulin in the follow-up of differentiated thyroid carcinoma. *Medical and Pediatric Oncology*, 10: 201–8.

Marshall, J.B. and Bodnarchuk, G. (1993). Carcinoid tumours of the gut. An experience over 3 decades and review of the litterature. *J Clin Gastroenterol*, 16: 123.

Martin, W.D. and Shah, J.K. (1994). Carcinoma of the naropharynx in new patients. *Int J Radiat Oncol Biol Phys*, 28: 991.

Pao, W.J., Hustu, A.O., Douglass, E.C., Beckford, N.S., and Kun, L.E. (1989). Pediatric nasopharyngeal syndrome in long term follow-up of 29 patients. *Int J Radiat Oncol Biol Phys*, 17: 299.

Sommelet, D., Flamant, F., and Rodary, C. (1991). A series of 100 soft-tissue sarcoma (STS) in childhood excluding embryonal rhabdomyosarcoma (RMS) and schwannomas. *Med Pediatr Oncol*, 19: 390.

Touglass, J.C., Fontanesi, J., Ribeiro, R.C., and Hawkins, E. (1996). Improved longterm disease free survival in nasopharyngeal carcinoma in childhood and adolescence. *Proc Am Soc Clin Oncol*, 15: 467.

Turc-Carel, C., Dalcin, P., Limon, J., Rao, U., Li, F.P., Corson, J.M., *et al.* (1987). Involvement of chromosome X in primary cytogenetic change in human neoplasia: non random translocation in synovial sarcoma. *Proc Natl Acad Sci USA*, 84: 1981–1985.

Wang-Peng, J., Freter, C.E., Knutsen, T., Nafro, J.J., and Gazdar, A. (1978). Translocation t(11:22) in ethesioneuroblastoma. *Cancer Genet Cytogenet*, 29: 155–157.

Index

Note 1: Page references in **bold** indicate chapter headings.
2: Page references in *italics* indicate a photograph, radiograph or scan.
There may also be textual references on these pages.